T0259466

Cleft Lip and Palate: Current Surgical Management

Editors

THOMAS J. SITZMAN
JEFFREY R. MARCUS

CLINICS IN PLASTIC SURGERY

www.plasticsurgery.theclinics.com

April 2014 • Volume 41 • Number 2

ELSEVIER

1600 John F. Kennedy Boulevard • Suite 1800 • Philadelphia, Pennsylvania, 19103-2899

http://www.theclinics.com

CLINICS IN PLASTIC SURGERY Volume 41, Number 2
April 2014 ISSN 0094-1298, ISBN-13: 978-0-323-29010-4

Editor: Joanne Husovski
Developmental Editor: Donald Mumford

© **2014 Elsevier Inc. All rights reserved.**

This periodical and the individual contributions contained in it are protected under copyright by Elsevier, and the following terms and conditions apply to their use:

Photocopying
Single photocopies of single articles may be made for personal use as allowed by national copyright laws. Permission of the Publisher and payment of a fee is required for all other photocopying, including multiple or systematic copying, copying for advertising or promotional purposes, resale, and all forms of document delivery. Special rates are available for educational institutions that wish to make photocopies for non-profit educational classroom use. For information on how to seek permission visit www.elsevier.com/permissions or call: (+44) 1865 843830 (UK)/(+1) 215 239 3804 (USA).

Derivative Works
Subscribers may reproduce tables of contents or prepare lists of articles including abstracts for internal circulation within their institutions. Permission of the Publisher is required for resale or distribution outside the institution. Permission of the Publisher is required for all other derivative works, including compilations and translations (please consult www.elsevier.com/permissions).

Electronic Storage or Usage
Permission of the Publisher is required to store or use electronically any material contained in this periodical, including any article or part of an article (please consult www.elsevier.com/permissions). Except as outlined above, no part of this publication may be reproduced, stored in a retrieval system or transmitted in any form or by any means, electronic, mechanical, photocopying, recording or otherwise, without prior written permission of the Publisher.

Notice
No responsibility is assumed by the Publisher for any injury and/or damage to persons or property as a matter of products liability, negligence or otherwise, or from any use or operation of any methods, products, instructions or ideas contained in the material herein. Because of rapid advances in the medical sciences, in particular, independent verification of diagnoses and drug dosages should be made.

Although all advertising material is expected to conform to ethical (medical) standards, inclusion in this publication does not constitute a guarantee or endorsement of the quality or value of such product or of the claims made of it by its manufacturer.

Clinics in Plastic Surgery (ISSN 0094-1298) is published quarterly by Elsevier Inc., 360 Park Avenue South, New York, NY 10010-1710. Months of issue are January, April, July, and October. Business and Editorial Offices: 1600 John F. Kennedy Blvd., Suite 1800, Philadelphia, PA 19103-2899. Periodicals postage paid at New York, NY and additional mailing offices. Subscription prices are $490.00 per year for US individuals, $716.00 per year for US institutions, $240.00 per year for US students and residents, $555.00 per year for Canadian individuals, $853.00 per year for Canadian institutions, $630.00 per year for international individuals, $853.00 per year for international institutions, and $305.00 per year for Canadian and foreign students/residents. To receive student/resident rate, orders must be accompanied by name of affiliated institution, date of term, and the *signature* of program/residency coordinator on institution letterhead. Orders will be billed at individual rate until proof of status is received. Foreign air speed delivery is included in all *Clinics* subscription prices. All prices are subject to change without notice. **POSTMASTER:** Send address changes to *Clinics in Plastic Surgery*, Elsevier Health Sciences Division, Subscription Customer Service, 3251 Riverport Lane, Maryland Heights, MO 63043. **Customer Service: 1-800-654-2452 (US and Canada). From outside of the United States and Canada, call 314-447-8871. Fax: 314-447-8029. E-mail:** JournalsCustomerService-usa@elsevier.com **(for print support);** JournalsOnlineSupport-usa@elsevier.com **(for online support).**

Reprints. For copies of 100 or more of articles in this publication, please contact the Commercial Reprints Department, Elsevier Inc., 360 Park Avenue South, New York, New York 10010-1710. Tel.: +1-212-633-3874; Fax: +1-212-633-3820; E-mail: reprints@elsevier.com.

Clinics in Plastic Surgery is covered in *Current Contents, EMBASE/Excerpta Medica, Science Citation Index, MEDLINE/ PubMed (Index Medicus), ASCA, and ISI/BIOMED.*

Printed and bound by CPI Group (UK) Ltd, Croydon, CR0 4YY

Contributors

EDITORS

THOMAS J. SITZMAN, MD
Assistant Professor of Clinical Surgery, Division of Plastic Surgery, Cincinnati Children's Hospital Medical Center, Cincinnati, Ohio

JEFFREY R. MARCUS, MD, FACS, FAAP
Division of Plastic, Maxillofacial and Oral Surgery, Duke Cleft and Craniofacial Center, Duke Children's Hospital, Durham, North Carolina

AUTHORS

FAISAL AL-MUFARREJ, MB BCh
Craniofacial and Pediatric Plastic Surgery Fellow, Division of Plastic Surgery, The Craniofacial Center, Seattle Children's Hospital and Regional Medical Center; Division of Plastic Surgery, Department of Surgery, University of Washington, Seattle, Washington

ALEXANDER C. ALLORI, MD, MPH
Division of Plastic, Maxillofacial, and Oral Surgery, Children's Health Center; Duke Cleft and Craniofacial Center, Duke Children's Hospital, Durham, North Carolina

ARTHUR S. AYLSWORTH, MD
Professor of Pediatrics and Genetics, Departments of Pediatrics and Genetics, University of North Carolina at Chapel Hill, Chapel Hill, North Carolina

ADRIANE L. BAYLIS, PhD, CCC-SLP
Director, Velopharyngeal Dysfunction Program Co-Director, 22q Center Section of Plastic and Reconstructive Surgery, Nationwide Children's Hospital, Clinical Assistant Professor, Department of Plastic Surgery, The Ohio State University College of Medicine, Columbus, Ohio

JAMES P. BRADLEY, MD
Professor and Chief, Section of Plastic and Reconstructive Surgery, Temple University, Philadelphia, Pennsylvania

EDWARD P. BUCHANAN, MD
Division of Plastic Surgery, Michael E. Debakey Department of Surgery, Baylor College of Medicine, Houston, Texas

DAVID M. FISHER, MD, FRCSC, FACS
Division of Plastic and Reconstructive Surgery, Cleft Palate and Lip Program, Hospital for Sick Children, Toronto, Ontario, Canada

MARK D. FISHER, MD
Craniofacial Fellow, Division of Plastic and Reconstructive Surgery, Cleft Palate and Lip Program, Hospital for Sick Children, Toronto, Ontario, Canada; Duke Cleft and Craniofacial Center, Duke Children's Hospital, Durham, North Carolina

MICHAEL S. GART, MD
Division of Plastic and Reconstructive Surgery, Northwestern University Feinberg School of Medicine, Chicago, Illinois

ARUN K. GOSAIN, MD
Division of Plastic and Reconstructive Surgery, Ann and Robert H. Lurie Children's Hospital of Chicago, Chicago, Illinois

LARRY H. HOLLIER Jr, MD, FACS
Division of Plastic Surgery, Michael E. Debakey Department of Surgery, Baylor College of Medicine, Houston, Texas

RICHARD A. HOPPER, MD, MS
Chief, Division of Plastic Surgery, Surgical Director, The Craniofacial Center, Seattle Children's Hospital and Regional Medical Center; Associate Professor, Division of Plastic Surgery, Department of Surgery, University of Washington, Seattle, Washington

DAVID Y. KHECHOYAN, MD
Division of Plastic Surgery, Michael E. Debakey
Department of Surgery, Baylor College of
Medicine, Houston, Texas

RICHARD E. KIRSCHNER, MD, FACS, FAAP
Robert F. and Edgar T. Wolfe Foundation
Endowed Chair in Plastic and Reconstructive
Surgery Chief, Section of Plastic and
Reconstructive Surgery Director, Cleft Lip and
Palate Center and Co-Director, 22q Center
Nationwide Children's Hospital, Professor of
Surgery and Pediatrics, The Ohio State
University College of Medicine, Columbus,
Ohio

**ANN W. KUMMER, PhD, CCC-SLP, ASHA
Fellow**
Senior Director, Division of Speech-Language
Pathology, Professor of Clinical Pediatrics,
Professor of Otolaryngology, Cincinnati
Children's Hospital Medical Center, Cincinnati,
Ohio

JUSTINE C. LEE, MD, PhD
Assistant Professor of Surgery, Division of
Plastic Surgery, University of California,
Los Angeles, California

DANIEL LEVY-BERCOWSKI, DDS, MSD
Associate Professor (Craniofacial
Orthodontics), Department of Orthodontics,
Georgia Regents University, Augusta, Georgia

JOSEPH E. LOSEE, MD
Professor and Executive Vice Chair, Chief,
Pediatric Plastic Surgery, Department of
Plastic Surgery, University of Pittsburgh,
Pittsburgh, Pennsylvania

JEFFREY R. MARCUS, MD, FACS, FAAP
Division of Plastic, Maxillofacial and Oral
Surgery, Duke Cleft and Craniofacial Center,
Duke Children's Hospital, Durham,
North Carolina

ROBERT E. MEYER, PhD, MPH
Director, Birth Defects Monitoring Program,
Division of Public Health, North Carolina
Department of Health and Human Services,

State Center for Health Statistics, Raleigh,
North Carolina

LAURA A. MONSON, MD
Division of Plastic Surgery, Michael E. Debakey
Department of Surgery, Baylor College of
Medicine, Houston, Texas

PEDRO E. SANTIAGO, DMD
Director of Orthodontics, Associate
Consulting Professor of Surgery
(Craniofacial Orthodontics), Division of
Plastic Surgery, Duke University, Durham,
North Carolina

LINDSAY A. SCHUSTER, DMD, MS
Director, Cleft-Craniofacial Orthodontics,
Children's Hospital of Pittsburgh,
Assistant Clinical Professor of Surgery,
University of Pittsburgh, Pittsburgh,
Pennsylvania

THOMAS J. SITZMAN, MD
Assistant Professor of Clinical Surgery,
Division of Plastic Surgery, Cincinnati
Children's Hospital Medical Center,
Cincinnati, Ohio

DARREN M. SMITH, MD
Adminstrative Chief Resident, Department of
Plastic Surgery, University of Pittsburgh,
Pittsburgh, Pennsylvania

RONALD P. STRAUSS, DMD, PhD
Executive Vice Provost and Chief
International Officer, Dental Friends
Distinguished Professor of Dental Ecology,
UNC Center for AIDS Research, UNC School
of Dentistry, Professor of Social Medicine,
UNC School of Medicine, University of North
Carolina at Chapel Hill, Chapel Hill,
North Carolina

**GUY THORBURN, FRCS (Plastic Surgery),
MA**
Department of Plastic Surgery, North Thames
Cleft Centre, Great Ormond Street Hospital for
Children NHS Foundation Trust, London,
United Kingdom

RAJ M. VYAS, MD
Department of Plastic Surgery, NYU School of
Medicine, New York, New York

STEPHEN M. WARREN, MD, FACS
Department of Plastic Surgery, NYU School of
Medicine, New York, New York

**STEPHANIE E. WATKINS, PhD, MSPH,
MSPT**
Post Doctoral Fellow,
Center for Health Promotion and
Disease Prevention, University of North
Carolina at Chapel Hill, Chapel Hill,
North Carolina

Contents

Orofacial clefts (OFCs) include a broad range of facial conditions that differ in cause and disease burden. In the published literature, there is substantial ambiguity in both terminology and classification of OFCs. This article discusses the terminology and classification of OFCs and the epidemiology of OFCs. Demographic, environmental, and genetic risk factors for OFCs are described, including suggestions for family counseling. This article enables clinicians to counsel families regarding the occurrence and recurrence of OFCs. Although much of the information is detailed, it is intended to be accessible to all health professionals for use in their clinical practices.

Modern cleft surgery requires four-dimensional and functional anatomic understanding of the cleft (and noncleft) lip, nose, and alveolus. Some techniques for nasolabial repair rely more on precise anatomic geometry, whereas others afford the surgeon a more flexible design. Consistent anthropometry enables accurate assessment and reporting of long-term outcomes; such reports are needed to guide perioperative care, delineate optimal repair principles, and resolve ongoing controversies.

The understanding of the bilateral cleft lip and associated nasal deformity has evolved over the last 30 years to a point where there now exists general agreement regarding the goals, principles, and strategies for operative repair. This article presents modern tenets for repair of bilateral cleft lip and describes a logical approach to correction of the different possible subtypes.

The authors begin with a discussion of the anatomy relevant to palatoplasty. Perioperative considerations are then addressed. A broad range of surgical options has evolved over time; these are discussed in their historical context. The authors present a detailed description of their preferred surgical approach. Postoperative care is then described. An examination of recent trends and controversies in the field is then offered. Finally, an approach to outcomes assessment is discussed. It is hoped that this monograph will be of use in guiding others as they embark on the highly challenging, but equally rewarding, task of perfecting the palatoplasty.

The neonatal morbidity and mortality associated with Pierre Robin sequence has decreased with improved nonsurgical and surgical methods for airway protection.

With the introduction of distraction osteogenesis and the understanding that improved outcomes occur with a systematic approach to patient management that includes mandibular distraction for appropriate candidates, the proportion of severely micrognathic patients requiring tracheostomies can be decreased. The challenge to institutions is to implement and optimize systematic methods for evaluation and treatment of these neonates to achieve timely, consistent, and cost-effective outcomes.

Orthopedic and orthodontic management of patients born with clefts of the lip, alveolus and palate is based on the application of basic biomechanical principles adapted to the individualized cleft anatomy. This article focuses on orthopedic and orthodontic preparation for 2 stages of interdisciplinary orthodontic/surgical cleft care: presurgical infant orthopedics (nasoalveolar molding) for lip/alveolus/nasal surgical repair and maxillary arch preparation for secondary alveolar bone grafting. These preparatory stages of orthopedic/orthodontic therapy are undertaken with the goal of restoring normal anatomic relationships to assist the surgeon in providing the best possible surgical care.

Cleft surgeons seek to provide the best results in the fewest surgeries. Gingivoperiosteoplasty (GPP) is one option to achieve this goal. Although it may normalize early form and function and obviate secondary alveolar bone grafting, it has been associated with iatrogenic dentofacial restriction requiring more extensive treatment later. GPP technique associated with nasoalveolar molding (NAM) uses passive presurgical molding with strict patient-selection criteria. Data on the benefits of NAM-GPP are favorable but long-term outcome studies are required before its final role in cleft care is determined. This article describes the history, technique, perioperative care, and preliminary outcomes of NAM-GPP.

 Videos of a speech sample, evaluation of nasal emission using a straw, oral examination, nasometry, and nasopharyngoscopy accompany this article

Children with cleft palate are at risk for speech problems, particularly those caused by velopharyngeal insufficiency. There may be an additional risk of speech problems caused by malocclusion. This article describes the speech evaluation for children with cleft palate and how the results of the evaluation are used to make treatment decisions. Instrumental procedures that provide objective data regarding the function of the velopharyngeal valve, and the 2 most common methods of velopharyngeal imaging, are also described. Because many readers are not familiar with phonetic symbols for speech phonemes, Standard English letters are used for clarity.

The primary goal of cleft palate repair is to create an anatomically and functionally intact palate while minimally affecting maxillary growth and development. In order to produce normal speech, a child must have velopharyngeal competence, defined as the ability to completely close the velopharyngeal sphincter that separates the oropharynx and nasopharynx. The absence of this ability, termed velopharyngeal insufficiency (VPI), is seen in a wide range of patients following primary cleft palate repair. This article discusses patient assessment, treatment options, and the surgical management of VPI. Recent trends and future directions in management are also presented.

The 22q11.2 deletion syndrome (22q11DS) may be associated with several palatal abnormalities, including overt cleft palate, submucosal cleft palate, palatopharyngeal disproportion, and velar hypotonia. The syndrome is the genetic disorder most commonly associated with velopharyngeal dysfunction (VPD). The complex causes of VPD in affected patients combine with the complexity of associated medical disorders to render surgical management of the velopharynx particularly challenging. Optimization of surgical outcomes requires precision in diagnosis, surgical management, and multidisciplinary care. This article provides an overview of 22q11DS and provides a review of the assessment and surgical management of VPD in affected individuals.

The cleft nasal deformity remains the most likely stigma of the cleft to remain plainly visible despite vigorous and repeated attempts at correction. This deformity is present at birth, but evolves over time. Certain aspects can be treated early, but some, such as the dorsal and septal deformity continue to develop as facial growth proceeds through adolescence. This article presents a conceptual mechanism and a philosophy of conservative reliable gains starting at the primary operation, with the long-term view of achieving definitive correction at maturity. Cogent planning of longitudinal care of the deformity from infancy leads to solid, predictable results.

To properly treat a patient with a secondary cleft lip or palate deformity, one must make an accurate diagnosis of the underlying problem. Recognition of specific recurring patterns and common deformities will help facilitate the surgical planning process and assist the surgeon during future procedures. Through a combination of accurate analysis, clinical patience, and technical precision, successful correction of secondary cleft lip and palate deformities can be delivered.

Measuring meaningful outcomes in cleft lip and palate surgery is difficult. Many methods of measurement lack validity or reliability, are impractical to implement, or are not consistently used. Yet the power of measuring outcomes is so great, and the potential to improve patients' lives so strong, that these hurdles are worth overcoming. This chapter reviews previous efforts at outcome measurement from cleft centers around the world. It also suggests a framework for adopting outcome measurement within your practice. Challenges of measurement are discussed, along with the role outcome reporting will take in accreditation and quality management.

CLINICS IN PLASTIC SURGERY

RELATED INTEREST

Growth and Development Considerations for Craniomaxillofacial Surgery
Bernard J. Costello, Reynaldo D. Rivera, Jocelyn Shand, Mark Mooney
In Oral and Maxillofacial Surgery Clinics of North America
Volume 26, Issue 1, August 2012
Horswell and Jaskolka, *Editors*

DOWNLOAD
Free App!

Review Articles
THE CLINICS

NOW AVAILABLE FOR YOUR iPhone and iPad

Preface
Cleft Lip and Palate: Current Surgical Management

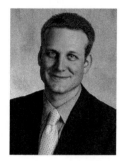 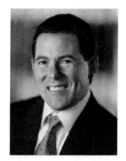

Thomas J. Sitzman, MD   Jeffrey R. Marcus, MD
Editors

We are honored to bring you this issue of *Clinics in Plastic Surgery* focusing on cleft lip and palate. Whether you are the occasional cleft surgeon looking to stay current, or the senior cleft surgeon interested in the approaches of your peers, this issue will reward you with in-depth reviews of modern cleft care using detailed illustrations to highlight each surgeon's technical approach. The authors, all recognized experts in cleft surgery, offer their insights into the complexities of treating patients with cleft lip and palate so that you and the field may grow from their experiences.

Readers may ask if any new information exists in cleft care; the answer is a resounding YES. Our understanding of genetic contributions to cleft lip and palate continues to evolve, giving order to the spectrum of deformities surgeons encounter. There is growing recognition for the importance of anatomic reconstruction of the velar musculature during cleft palate repair. There are new instruments for measuring speech outcomes, and a structured approach to managing velopharyngeal insufficiency is evolving. Controversy

around naso-alveolar molding grows, accompanied by a resurgent interest in gingivoperiosteoplasty. These developments are changing how we care for all children with cleft lip and palate, and each is addressed in this issue of *Clinics in Plastic Surgery*.

Cleft care continues to advance both in how we approach all patients and in our understanding of the nuanced approach necessary for each patient. This issue includes articles detailing approaches to patients with 22q11.2 deletion syndrome and Pierre Robin sequence. These articles highlight the unique features of each condition, including how the treatment approach should be adapted.

Coupled with the evolution in surgical approaches, there is a growing appreciation for the role of outcome measurement in cleft care. The last two decades have witnessed the birth of intercenter outcome comparisons, multinational randomized clinical trials, and the incorporation of outcome reporting into standard care delivery. Each article in this issue includes a

Clin Plastic Surg 41 (2014) xi–xii
http://dx.doi.org/10.1016/j.cps.2014.02.001
0094-1298/14/$ – see front matter © 2014 Elsevier Inc. All rights reserved.

discussion of appropriate outcome measures, including the what, when, and how of applying them. This information is of widespread importance as outcome reporting becomes integrated with clinical care.

We are grateful to Elsevier for the opportunity to be guest editors to this issue of *Clinics in Plastic Surgery*. We are indebted to each of the authors for their valuable contributions, taking time from their professional and personal lives to share their insights. The editorial staff of *The Clinics* is outstanding, in particular, our senior editor, Joanne Husovski. Finally, we would like to thank our wives and families for their understanding and support during this project.

Thomas J. Sitzman, MD
Division of Plastic Surgery
Cincinnati Children's Hospital Medical Center
3333 Burnet Avenue
Cincinnati, OH 45229, USA

Jeffrey R. Marcus, MD
Duke Cleft and Craniofacial Center
Division of Plastic, Maxillofacial & Oral Surgery
Duke Children's Hospital
200 Trent Drive, Erwin Road
Durham, NC 27710, USA

E-mail addresses:
Thomas.Sitzman@cchmc.org (T.J. Sitzman)
jeffrey.marcus@duke.edu (J.R. Marcus)

Classification, Epidemiology, and Genetics of Orofacial Clefts

Stephanie E. Watkins, PhD, MSPH, MSPT[a],*,
Robert E. Meyer, PhD, MPH[b], Ronald P. Strauss, DMD, PhD[c],
Arthur S. Aylsworth, MD[d]

KEYWORDS

- Epidemiology • Orofacial clefts • Classification • Genetics

KEY POINTS

- The following terminology is used when describing orofacial clefts (OFCs): cleft lip alone without cleft palate (CL); cleft lip with or without cleft palate (CL/P), which includes cleft lip only and cleft lip with cleft palate; cleft lip with cleft palate (CLP); posterior cleft palate without cleft lip (CPO); syndromic and nonsyndromic; and familial and nonfamilial (or simplex).
- Prevalence is the suggested measure of disease frequency.
- The source population, the time period of data collection, the clinical case definition, and the method of case ascertainment are important considerations when comparing prevalence estimates of OFCs.
- Both CL/P and CPO may occur in association with other major birth defects. CPO is more commonly syndromic than is CL/P.
- The clinical approach includes a history and physical examination for associated morbidity, a thorough gestational history for possible teratogenic factors, and a detailed family history for possible genetic factors.

HISTORICAL PERSPECTIVE: TERMINOLOGY AND CLASSIFICATION

There is considerable ambiguity in the use of terminology when referring to orofacial clefts (OFCs). Many clinicians incorrectly refer to OFCs as deformities, which are said to be the result of disrupted embryologic development. In 1982, an international working group proposed our currently used concepts and terms to describe errors of morphogenesis, which include OFCs.[1] The term *malformation* should be used for a "morphologic defect of an organ, part of an organ, or larger region of the body resulting from an *intrinsically* abnormal developmental process."[1] On the other hand, a *disruption* is a "morphologic defect of an organ, part of an organ, or a larger region of the body resulting from the *extrinsic* breakdown of or an interference with, an originally normal developmental process."[1] In contrast to a malformation, the developmental potential of the involved organ was originally normal and "an extrinsic factor such as an infection, teratogen, or trauma interfered with the development, which thereafter proceeded abnormally."[1] An example of an OFC caused by a disruption would be one caused by a swallowed amniotic band.

Disclosures: The authors report no conflicts of interest.
a Center for Health Promotion and Disease Prevention, University of North Carolina at Chapel Hill, 1700 Martin Luther King Jr Boulevard, Chapel Hill, NC, USA; b Birth Defects Monitoring Program, Division of Public Health, North Carolina Department of Health and Human Services, State Center for Health Statistics, 222 North Dawson Street, Cotton Building, Raleigh, NC 27603, USA; c UNC Center for AIDS Research, UNC School of Dentistry, UNC School of Medicine, University of North Carolina at Chapel Hill, 104 South Building, CB# 3000, Chapel Hill, NC 27599-3000, USA; d Departments of Pediatrics and Genetics, University of North Carolina at Chapel Hill, CB# 7487, UNC Campus, Chapel Hill, NC 27599-7487, USA
* Corresponding author.
E-mail address: wat@email.unc.edu

plasticsurgery.theclinics.com

The term *deformation* (or deformity) should be reserved for "an abnormal form, shape, or position of a part of the body caused by *mechanical forces*," such as plagiocephaly.[1] Although nasal collapse and skeletal asymmetry may be secondary *deformities* in a child with a repaired cleft lip, the cleft itself is a *malformation* not a *deformity*. Finally, the term *dysplasia* describes "an abnormal *organization of cells into tissues* and its morphologic results."[1] Hence, we have a group of conditions called *ectodermal dysplasias*, which involve derivatives of the embryonic ectoderm and may have associated OFCs, and *skeletal dysplasias*, some of which also have OFCs associated with them.

Most OFCs are considered malformations, unless there is clear evidence that it might be a disruption. Even when a cleft is associated with an underlying bone *dysplasia* or genetic syndrome it is considered a malformation because the process of embryologic tissue growth and fusion was abnormal (because of the underlying syndrome).

The use of the terms *isolated* and *syndromic* is another area of potential confusion when describing OFCs. *Isolated cleft palate* may refer to *cleft palate without cleft lip* or it may be used to describe a patient who does not have any other malformations or anomalies. In addition, nonfamilial clefts are sometimes called *isolated*.

The word *syndrome* means "a pattern of multiple anomalies thought to be pathogenetically related."[1] A malformation is *syndromic* if patients have more than one malformation involving more than one developmental field or region of the body. In clinical practice, this usually means birth defects in more than one organ system. For syndromes, pathogenesis is usually unknown, whereas underlying causal factors may be known or unknown.

Some researchers will use the term *syndromic* in a more restrictive fashion to refer only to patients with syndromes of known or suspected cause (eg, chromosomal syndromes, Mendelian syndromes, eponymic syndromes). The authors suggest calling these syndromes of known cause in order to differentiate them from idiopathic syndromic cases or syndromic cases of unknown cause, which will include OFCs of unknown cause with other major anomalies. A major anomaly is commonly defined as a structural or functional variation from the norm that is of medical, surgical, or cosmetic significance. Both cleft lip with or without cleft palate and posterior cleft palate without cleft lip may occur in association with other major birth defects. Posterior cleft palate without cleft lip is more commonly syndromic than cleft lip with or without cleft palate (**Table 1**).[2–10]

Finally, the difference between sporadic and simplex events should be highlighted. *Sporadic* refers to a chance event, whereas *simplex* refers to a single occurrence of a condition in a family.[11] Simplex, or nonfamilial, cases can result from a variety of genetic and nongenetic causes, whereas truly sporadic cases are pure accidents of development. In most cases of *simplex* OFCs, we simply do not know the cause and, therefore, it is not appropriate to speculate that these are *sporadic*. As Pagon pointed out, we "need to be very clear when we use the term 'sporadic' that it is a chance event with little risk of recurrence and that when we use the term 'simplex,' risk of occurrence in relatives remains a possibility."[11]

Throughout this review, the authors use the terms cleft lip alone without cleft palate (CL), cleft lip with or without cleft palate (CL/P), which includes cleft lip only and cleft lip with cleft palate, cleft lip with cleft palate (CLP), posterior cleft palate without cleft lip (CPO), syndromic and nonsyndromic, and familial and nonfamilial (or simplex) in order to avoid ambiguity.

CLASSIFICATION

Several different classification systems for OFCs have been proposed in the surgical and dental literature. These systems are primarily divided

---

Table 1
Proportion of postnatally diagnosed OFCs that are syndromic or nonsyndromic and proportion of each that are associated with chromosome abnormalities

	Syndromic (%)	Syndromic with Chromosome Abnormality (%)	Nonsyndromic with Chromosome Abnormality (%)
CL	12.1	11.3	1.8
CL/P[a] and CLP	34.6	25.0	0.6
CPO	45.9	18.1	1.6

[a] Some studies did not separate CL from CLP cases. Therefore, this combined category includes some CL cases.

Data from Maarse W, Rozendaal AM, Pajkrt E, et al. A systematic review of associated structural and chromosomal defects in oral clefts: when is prenatal genetic analysis indicated? J Med Genet 2012;49:490–8.

into anatomic systems useful for surgeons and embryology-based systems useful for genetic counseling and research. The disciplines of surgery, genetic counseling, and research require and use different types of OFC data, which has hindered the development of a universally acceptable and useable classification system.[12]

Modern concepts of classification date from the proposal by Kernahan and Stark,[13] which included alveolar ridge clefts with those involving the lip. Based on these concepts a more detailed classification was published.[14,15] A comprehensive history of OFC classification systems is beyond the scope of this article but has been covered in numerous reviews and classification system proposals.[12–14,16–25]

Animal model data, as well as analysis of recurrence in humans, indicate that, in most cases, CL/P is causally and pathogenetically distinct from CPO.[26–28] The normal process of secondary palate closure in the human occurs during gestational weeks 6 through 9.[29,30] Because the lip normally closes by the end of the sixth week and then palate fusion proceeds in a posterior direction over the next several weeks, CPO usually arises from different morphogenetic events than CL/P. Such a view is supported by observations that in families with more than one affected individual, the clefts are usually of the same type. Therefore, traditional empiric recurrence risks given in counseling are risks for CL/P or CPO.[31] There are exceptions to this rule, however, such as the van der Woude and popliteal pterygium syndromes, which are characterized by lower lip pits and either CL/P or CPO.[32] Another example is a Dutch family with 12 affected relatives segregating a causative MSX1 mutation having various combinations of CLP, CPO, and tooth agenesis.[33]

In addition, atypical OFCs[34] include both midline clefts and Tessier oblique clefts,[14] which are relatively rare and are assumed to be both causally heterogeneous and distinct from the more common OFCs.

Midline clefts of the lip deserve a special mention. It is extremely important for clinicians to differentiate between the true median cleft lip with a midline, inverted V-shaped notch similar to that normally seen in rabbits, hares, and numerous other animals (apparently the origin of the colloquial term *harelip*),[35] and a wide cleft with a flat nose and absent columella caused by premaxillary agenesis. The former, true median or midline cleft, is rare and usually involves only the vermilion border but may extend into the alveolar ridge.[36] This type of true midline notch or cleft is frequently associated with syndromes, such as the oral-facial-digital spectrum and Ellis-van Creveld syndrome. On the other hand, the wide midline cleft of the lip and midline alveolar ridge caused by premaxillary agenesis is a hallmark of the holoprosencephaly spectrum of brain malformations. Holoprosencephaly may be caused by numerous chromosomal abnormalities and single gene mutations.[37–40] These holoprosencephaly syndromes are usually associated with significant developmental delay and frequently early lethality. Newborns with any of these midline clefts require early consultation by a pediatric geneticist and diagnostic testing to help direct future care and counseling.

Finally, classification needs to take into account milder microform, or *forme fruste*, examples of OFCs such as small paramedian notches in the upper lip and/or alveolar ridge. A scar on the lip at birth indicates that closure occurred later than usual (ie, a cleft lip healed itself in utero after tissues switched from nonscarring fusion to a scarring type of healing process).[41]

Submucous cleft palate (SMCP) is generally considered to be a microform of CPO, and velopharyngeal insufficiency (VPI) seems to represent the mildest end of the CPO spectrum. This point is illustrated by patients with deletions of chromosome 22q11.2 (DiGeorge syndrome, velocardiofacial syndrome [DGS/VCF]); 69% have a palatal abnormality, more than half of which is VPI, SMCP, or bifid uvula.[42]

Although bifid uvula occurs in the general population as a benign trait, it may also suggest the presence of a submucous cleft. In a study of general pediatric patients with either bifid uvula or an even more subtle small notch in the uvula, most had at least some of the associated anatomic or physiologic pharyngeal abnormalities associated with SMCP.[43] On the other hand, one can have an SMCP without a bifid uvula. The subtlety of these milder microforms ensures that ascertainment for epidemiologic studies will be incomplete and, therefore, these OFCs are usually excluded from epidemiologic research. These microforms do, however, maintain their importance in studies of genetic causation as well as in patient care.

In many epidemiologic studies, CL/P, including both CL and CLP, are studied as a group distinct from CPO because embryology suggests that CLP differs from CL only in severity. Evidence has been presented, however, to suggest that CL may be considered distinct from CLP. In an epidemiologic study of 1.8 million live births in Norway, recurrence risk estimates showed a qualitative difference between the 2 categories of cleft lip (CL and CLP), suggesting that disease severity is not the sole distinguishing factor between the 2 phenotypes.[44] Another study shows a clear separation of risk and transmission patterns between cases with CL and those with CLP.[45]

MEASURES OF OCCURRENCE OF OROFACIAL CLEFTS
Incidence Versus Prevalence

Incidence and prevalence are traditional epidemiologic measures used to quantify the occurrence of disease in a population. Incidence reflects the transition from health to disease where prevalence reflects both the presence of disease as well as how long a person lives with the disease.[46] *Incidence* is defined as the *number of new cases* of disease in a population of individuals at risk for developing the disease in a given time period. This measure can be expressed as either a proportion, with the size of the population at risk in the denominator (**Box 1**), or as a rate whereby the denominator reflects the time at risk in the population. *Prevalence* is a static measure, which describes the proportion of *cases of disease in the population* at a given time point (**Box 2**).[47,48] In published studies of birth defects, both incidence and prevalence have been used to describe the frequency of OFCs. Measuring the true incidence of OFCs and other birth defects, however, is virtually impossible because of the difficulties in ascertaining incident cases, which occur early in the first trimester and are often spontaneously aborted, as well as with defining *the population at risk* (number of conceptions).

Typical OFCs are caused by factors operating during the first 9 weeks of gestation.[29] To measure incidence, one would need to include all embryos during the gestational period when the embryos are at risk for developing an OFC. During this early stage of pregnancy, however, many women are unaware that they are pregnant, and many pregnancy losses go undetected. Thus, it is impossible to quantify the number of conceptions that reach the gestational age when an OFC occurs.[49]

Suggested Measure of Disease Occurrence

Birth prevalence, which in birth defects research is often simply referred to as *prevalence*, is the suggested measure to quantify the frequency of OFCs at the time of delivery. The authors follow that convention here and use the term *prevalence* through the remainder of this article. Prevalence is a function of the number of new cases of OFCs as well as survival of the fetus.[47] Prevalence of birth defects, including OFCs, is estimated using the following formula (see **Box 2**). In birth defects research, prevalence is an estimate usually expressed as a ratio measure of the number of cases of OFCs among live births, spontaneous fetal deaths (usually limited to 20 weeks' gestation or greater), and induced terminations (regardless of gestational age) over the total number of live births in a given time period.[49] The estimate is often expressed per 10,000 live births. For example, a prevalence estimate of 0.001 is typically expressed as 10 cases per 10,000 live births. Because the number of fetal deaths is very small relative to the number of live births, exclusion of fetal deaths from the denominator has little practical influence on the prevalence estimate.[49]

Including both fetal deaths and terminations in the numerator more closely reflects the true prevalence of OFCs at the time of delivery. If one includes only the number of cases among live births, then the true prevalence of OFCs will be underestimated.

Prevalence of Orofacial Clefts

The prevalence of OFCs is often reported as the proportion of children who have CL/P and the proportion of children who have CPO. In a population-based study of approximately 8 million births, the prevalence of CL/P was 9.9 per 10,000 births. These data were collected from 54 birth defect registries across 30 countries between 2000 and 2005. This estimate was consistent with the prevalence of 10.2 per 10,000 births as reported in the United States.[50] The prevalence in Western Europe (12.1 per 10,000 births) was similar to that of the United States, yet the prevalence of CL/P in Japan (20.0 per 10,000 births) was twice that of the United States (**Table 2**).[50]

Thirty-one percent of the cases of CL/P in the United States were CL. Moreover, in the United States, 75% of children with CL/P during this time period were nonsyndromic (no other malformation or only a minor defect), with 8% of cases being associated with a known syndrome and

---

Box 1
Incidence proportion

Number of new cases of disease/population at risk for disease.

From Koepsell TD, Weiss NS. Epidemiologic methods: studying the occurrence of illness. New York: Oxford University Press; 2003.

| Box 2 |
| Prevalence |
| Number of cases of disease/size of the population at a given time point. |
| *From* Koepsell TD, Weiss NS. Epidemiologic methods: studying the occurrence of illness. New York: Oxford University Press; 2003. |

17% of cases having multiple malformations. Both of these trends were similar across Canada, Western Europe, Australia, and Japan.[50]

The prevalence of CPO (in the United States between 2004 and 2006) was 6.5 cases per 10,000 live births.[51] The birth prevalence of CPO, excluding chromosomal disorders, differs considerably by geographic region ranging from 1.2 cases per 10,000 births in areas of sub-Saharan Africa to 11.3 cases per 10,000 births in the Oceania region. In Europe and Central Asia, the average birth prevalence of CPO is 6.0 per 10,000 births.[52]

Surveillance Systems

Measures of the prevalence of birth defects are usually estimated from data reported by population-based surveillance systems. Surveillance systems collect, analyze, and report measures of disease occurrence for given populations over time. The method of case ascertainment and the data source for cases may vary by geographic region and depends on the structure of the health care system.

Case finding in surveillance systems may be described as either active or passive. Active surveillance requires intensive effort on the part of the surveillance staff to find cases and confirm diagnoses. Passive surveillance typically involves submission of case reports from given reporting sources directly to the surveillance system and may or may not involve subsequent case

confirmation to verify diagnoses. Some surveillance systems use a combination of active and passive surveillance. Common data sources for birth defect case ascertainment include hospitals, physician offices, laboratories, prenatal diagnostic clinics, and administrative data.[53]

Given the potential for variability across surveillance systems, one must consider differences in surveillance methodology when comparing published estimates of the prevalence of OFCs. First one must consider the source population of births that are in the catchment area of the surveillance system. Moreover, the time period in which the data were collected, the clinical case definition, and the method of case ascertainment may influence prevalence estimates and should be considered when interpreting such data.[50]

A source of differential case ascertainment is the underreporting of OFCs that occurs with pregnancy terminations.[54] This underreporting seems to be more common among syndromic OFCs, such as trisomy 13, than nonsyndromic cases. In the United States, the frequency of pregnancy terminations is estimated to be approximately 10%, which limits the impact of these missing cases on the estimate of birth prevalence. In regions where the prevalence of pregnancy terminations is higher, the magnitude of this effect may be greater. Additional factors that influence case ascertainment include errors or lack of specificity in diagnostic coding and failure to report births outside of the catchment area.[50]

RISK FACTORS FOR OROFACIAL CLEFTS
Sex, Race, and Ethnicity

Prevalence of OFCs differs by sex, race, and maternal age. The prevalence of CL/P among males is approximately twice that of females, whereas the prevalence for CPO is about two-thirds that of females.[55,56]

The prevalence of all OFCs is less for non-Hispanic blacks compared with non-Hispanic whites.[57] African Americans are 44% less likely to have CL/P compared with non-Hispanic whites. Moreover, the prevalence of CPO was approximately 30% less for African American and Hispanic children when compared with whites.[2,19,58] Maternal age younger than 25 years and older

| Table 2 |
| Prevalence of CL/P between 2000 and 2005 |

Geographic Region	Cases per 10,000 Births	95% Confidence Interval
United States	10.2	9.8, 10.6
Western Europe	12.1	11.1, 13.2
Japan	20.0	18.6, 21.6
Canada	11.5	10.2, 12.9
Australia	9.7	8.5, 11.0

Data from The International Perinatal Database of Typical Oral Clefts (IPDTOC). Cleft Palate Craniofac J 2011;48:66–81.

than 29 years is associated with an increased risk of OFCs compared with mothers aged 25 to 29 years (**Table 3**).[55,59,60]

Environmental Factors

Most nonsyndromic OFCs are thought to be multifactorial in origin, whereby a combination of genetic and environmental factors is involved. An extensive body of research exists regarding possible causes of OFCs. With the exception of family history, relatively few strong associations are clearly established. The risk factors and the magnitude of their effects are different for CL/P and CPO, supporting the idea that these phenotypes are both causally and pathogenetically distinct entities.

Maternal smoking, particularly at high levels, is consistently associated with an increased risk for OFCs in numerous studies.[61–69] The risk seems to be stronger for CL/P than for CPO. Furthermore, the association between maternal smoking and OFCs is substantially modified by the presence of specific genetic variants in the mother and fetus, most notably involving transforming growth factor-alpha polymorphisms.[70–72] Maternal nutritional factors also seem to play a role in the development of OFCs in offspring.[73]

Maternal first-trimester consumption of large amounts of alcohol has been associated with an increased risk for OFCs in several studies, although the results have been somewhat inconsistent.[66,74–80] Questions persist about the risks associated with moderate drinking as well as the type of alcohol consumed. In mouse studies, alcohol causes CL/P when administered as early as 8.25 days' gestation, timing equivalent to early in the fourth week after conception in the human.[81]

Several studies have demonstrated a link between periconceptional intake of multivitamins or folic acid and a reduced risk for both CL/P and for CPO.[82–85] The evidence for a protective effect of folic acid on OFCs is not as strong as that for neural tube defects. Further research is needed to clarify the optimal dosage, timing, and the potential effect on reducing cleft recurrence.[86] The extent of the protective effect of folic acid on OFCs also seems to be mediated by genetic variants, particularly the methylenetetrahydrofolate reductase (MTHFR) 677T and A1298C polymorphisms.[87]

Several prescription medications have been linked to OFCs when taken during the first trimester. Not surprisingly, folate antagonists and certain other drugs that exhibit antifolate properties are associated with an increased risk for OFCs, both CL/P and CPO. These drugs include anticonvulsants, such as carbamazepine, valproic acid, phenytoin, phenobarbital, and trimethadione.[88–90] Retinoic acid and certain corticosteroids are also associated with increased OFC risk.[91,92]

Some maternal diseases and obstetric conditions have been linked to OFCs in the babies of affected women. Prepregnancy diabetes mellitus, but not gestational diabetes, confers an increased risk for several congenital malformations, including CL/P and CPO.[93,94] Maternal obesity (body mass index $\geq$30) is associated with an increased risk for both CL/P and CPO in some studies; but the magnitude of the risk is relatively small, with odds ratios around 1.3.[95,96] The pathogenesis of OFCs associated with diabetes and obesity may be similar because obese patients develop glucose intolerance and increased insulin resistance. Rarely, atypical OFCs may be caused by amniotic bands that deform and disrupt the fetal structures (see **Table 3**).[97]

Several other environmental risk factors have been investigated in relation to OFCs, including chlorinated disinfection byproducts in drinking water; environmental contaminants, such as pesticides, air pollution, and environmental estrogens; and occupational exposures, such as organic solvents. No consistent evidence has been established, however, to indicate these are causally related.

Genetic Factors

OFCs are causally complex phenotypes resulting from the interactions of many different potential factors during development. These factors include programmed and stochastic combinations of genetic and environmental influences, whereby the

Table 3 Risk factors associated with CL/P	
Sex[a]	Prescription medication; folate antagonists, anticonvulsants, retinoic acid[a]
White non-Hispanic race[a]	Maternal first-trimester heavy alcohol consumption
Maternal age	Prepregnancy diabetes mellitus[a]
Maternal smoking	Maternal obesity (BMI $\geq$30)[a]

Abbreviation: BMI, body mass index.
[a] Risk factors associated with CPO.
Data from Refs.[2,55,56,61–63,65–69,74–80,88–96]

genetic contribution may be determined by one or more genes. OFCs can occur along with other structural and/or functional birth defects as *syndromic clefts* or without other major structural or functional developmental anomalies as *nonsyndromic clefts*. A detailed survey of the genetics of OFCs is beyond the scope of this article but is well covered in several recent reviews.[36,98–105]

OFCs, like most other birth defects and common diseases of both childhood and adult life, fit the description of *complex* disorders. These disorders are conditions whereby a single, causative, completely penetrant gene does not always produce the phenotype. Instead, a combination of effects from more than one gene with or without additional environmental (nongenetic) factors may produce the phenotype. Complex phenotypes are causally heterogeneous, which means that over an extended population, the genetic causes of OFCs include *both* low frequency (ie, rare), high penetrance, causative alleles and more common, low penetrance, susceptibility alleles interacting with environmental factors. Most of the common disorders of children and adults seem to be complex phenotypes, including most birth defects, intellectual disability, autism, short stature, cancer, diabetes, cardiovascular disease, hypertension, stroke, psychoses, and so forth.[106,107]

In thinking about malformations, it is helpful to subdivide phenotypes into syndromic and nonsyndromic and then by those of known cause and those of unknown cause (idiopathic). Such an overview of OFCs is shown in **Fig. 1**.

OFC syndromes of known cause
The causes of human malformation syndromes generally fall into 3 categories: (1) chromosome abnormalities and genomic rearrangements; (2) Mendelian or single gene disorders; and (3) complex interactions of genetic, environmental, and stochastic factors, referred to as *multifactorial* earlier. Because teratogens disrupt normal embryonic and fetal morphogenesis, and may interact with predisposing genetic factors, environmental factors must always be considered in a discussion of causes of OFC syndromes. Known genetic factors are usually rare and causal. Variability of expression and incomplete penetrance are also features of these phenotypes.

Chromosomal syndromes In an analysis of 20 studies of associated anomalies and chromosomal defects in OFCs, chromosomal abnormalities were most frequently seen in syndromic OFCs (see **Table 1**).[10] Almost all prenatally diagnosed OFCs with chromosomal defects were in syndromic cases or associated with other ultrasound markers, such as intrauterine growth retardation. This review concluded that "the presence of additional anomalies on ultrasound is the most important predictor of underlying chromosomal defects in fetuses with oral clefts."[10]

Numerous cytogenetic and submicroscopic genomic rearrangements, both deletions and duplications, are known to be causally associated with OFCs.[36] The most frequent interstitial deletion in humans is del(22)(q11.2), with an estimated prevalence of 1 per 4000 live births. This deletion is associated with a wide phenotypic spectrum including the DGS/VCF phenotypes with numerous clinical manifestations described and palatal anomalies in approximately half of the cases. Commonly associated extrapalatal anomalies are cardiovascular malformations (CVMs), immune defects, and neurodevelopmental disabilities. The most common palatal abnormality is VPI, affecting 29% to 50% of cases.[42,108]

The most common clefts associated with DGS/VCF are posterior, including SMCP and CPO; but CLP and even CL may rarely occur. Controversy exists over whether patients with nonsyndromic VPI or CPO should be screened for the VCF deletion. Some have found very low yields and concluded that screening nonsyndromic cases of CPOs is not indicated.[109–111] It is very clear, however, that any patient with a palatal defect *and any other* associated feature of the DGS/VCF spectrum should be screened because the yield is significant, as high as 30% to 40% or even higher in some studies.[108,112–114]

Associated findings that should trigger testing for the DGS/VCF deletion include any CVM, short stature, microcephaly, developmental delay, immune deficiency, history of (or family history of) psychiatric disease, and facial dysmorphism. Many clinicians will screen even apparently nonsyndromic

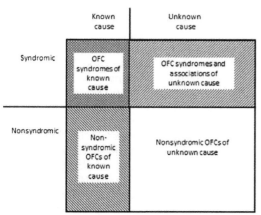

Fig. 1. Classification of OFCs by causation and type.

patients with CPO, SMCP, or VPI that present in infancy when growth and developmental data are still unknown. Patients with typical suggestive findings (palatal abnormalities, CVMs, growth and/or neurodevelopmental disorders) who are negative on fluorescence in situ hybridization (FISH) testing can have further analysis using microarray technology to identify other related but atypical rearrangements, including both neighboring (distal) 22q11.2 deletions as well as duplications that may be missed by FISH.[115] Another advantage of the single nucleotide polymorphism (SNP) arrays is that they will detect rearrangements (both deletions and duplications) elsewhere in the genome in patients with syndromic OFC who do not have typical DGS/VCF phenotypes.

Mendelian syndromes Numerous syndromes caused by the effects of single gene mutations have been reported and are listed in the Online Mendelian Inheritance in Man catalog as well as other general references.[36,116] Notable among these is the van der Woude syndrome and its related phenotype, the popliteal pterygium syndrome, caused by mutations in *IRF6*.[32] These phenotypes are associated with lower lip pits and demonstrate the unusual feature of expressing both CL/P and CPO as a manifestation of the mutation.

Teratogenic syndromes Teratogens, such as alcohol and valproic acid, cause OFCs and other features of VCF, such as CVMs, short stature, brain anomalies, and developmental delay.[76,117–119] Some newer antiepileptic drugs may show less teratogenic potential but have not been well studied.[120] The interaction of these environmental agents with underlying genetic/genomic variation in both mothers and patients with an OFC constitutes an area of intense research interest at present.

Nonsyndromic OFCs of known cause
In this category, one usually thinks of changes in single genes that predispose to clefting rather than cause OFCs a high percentage of the time. Such changes in the coding sequences of single genes produce alleles with relatively low penetrance rather than high penetrance. Numerous Mendelian syndromes have OFCs as major findings; some of the genes responsible for these syndromes, such as IRF6, have also been implicated as causative factors in nonsyndromic OFCs.[99,121] In addition, data now suggests that mutations in BMP4 are causally associated with both CL/P and CL microforms.[122] MSX1 mutations have been implicated as causative in patients with CL/P with and without other features of tooth agenesis.[123,124]

Teratogens, such as smoking, alcohol, and antiepileptic drugs, have also been implicated in causing nonsyndromic and syndromic OFCs (see earlier section on environmental factors).[61–69,88–90]

OFC syndromes and associations of unknown cause
These are multiple malformation associations that are seen often enough to suggest they share common causes and/or pathogenetic pathways. The oral-facial-digital (OFD) group of syndromes includes a spectrum of patients with OFCs (usually midline) and associated anomalies of the tongue and extremities.[125,126] Nosology is complicated, and the causes of most phenotypes in this spectrum are unknown.[125] It has been proposed that some of these may be ciliopathies.[126] The recent identification of *TCTN3* mutations in a patient with an OFD-overlap syndrome seems to support this suggestion.[127]

The oromandibular-limb hypogenesis spectrum includes patients with birth defects that include micrognathia, microstomia, hypoglossia, glossopalatine ankylosis, intraoral bands, cleft palate, sixth and seventh cranial nerve palsy (Moebius sequence), hypodactylia, adactylia, and peromelia. Patients have been reported with combinations of these features, and classification schemes subdivide this spectrum into specific groups of associated anomalies.[128,129] Diagnostic labels given to affected patients include aglossia-adactylia, hypoglossia-hypodactylia, glossopalatine ankylosis, Hanhart, Moebius, and Charlie M syndromes. Reasonably good circumstantial evidence suggests that many of these phenotypes are caused by maternal illness, placental disruption, or hypotension causing fetal hypoperfusion, hypoxemia, and tissue destruction during the first trimester of gestation.[130,131] Several cases have been associated with early chorionic villus sampling.[131]

Nonsyndromic OFCs of unknown cause
In addition to SNP array and whole exome/genome sequencing technologies, genome-wide association studies are also being used to identify loci that are involved in predisposing to clefting. Two of the most significant are *IRF6*[45,121,132–134] and a locus that maps to 8q24.[134–136] Other recent examples include studies of *NAT1* & *NAT2* genes,[137] *DMD* SNPs,[138] maternal or fetal *MTHFR* C677T genotypes,[139] *SOX9* enhancer deletions,[140,141] *MSX1*,[142] neighboring genes of *MSX1*,[143] variants near *MAFB* and *ABCA4*,[144] *ADH1C*,[121] and the influence of maternal genotypes.[103] The Hedgehog pathway has also been implicated.[81] Recent studies of environmental teratogens also show

some low level predisposition of unclear significance, such as with venlafaxine,[145] tobacco, and alcohol.[139,146] There have been several recent general reviews of genetic and environmental predisposing factors.[10,34,98–100,102]

PIERRE ROBIN SEQUENCE

The Robin sequence (commonly referred to as the Pierre Robin Syndrome [PRS]) deserves special mention. Current concepts classify this as a malformation complex or a sequence, in recognition of the embryologic sequence of events involved.[1] PRS is usually defined by the triad of micrognathia/retrognathia,[147] cleft palate (usually U shaped but may be V shaped), and glossoptosis (abnormal posterior placement of the tongue); but there is a significant precedent for using this term to refer to only severe microretrognathia with glossoptosis as originally described by Robin and others.[36,148,149] PRS is present in approximately 1 per 14,000 to 1 per 8500 births.[150] Approximately 40% of PRS is nonsyndromic and 60% syndromic. There are dozens of syndromes of known cause (chromosomal, Mendelian, and teratogenic) that are associated with PRS. Stickler and velocardiofacial syndromes are always important diagnostic considerations in the newborn with PRS.

A sequence constitutes a pattern of "multiple anomalies derived from a single known or presumed prior anomaly or mechanical factor."[1] In other words, a series of events occurs in a *sequence*, which then results in a specific malformation phenotype. After fusion of the primary palate, the tongue is positioned between the secondary palatal shelves, which have grown down on either side of the tongue. Then during the eighth week after conception, the mandible undergoes a growth spurt forward, the tongue drops down, and the palatal shelves rotate up, subsequently growing together and joining as the cells at their epithelial borders break down and fuse.[151,152] Anything that interferes with early aspects of this normal sequence of events, such as external compression on the mandible or failure of the mandible to undergo a growth spurt forward, can result in PRS.[153] Therefore, PRS can be caused by any chromosomal abnormality, single gene mutation, environmental teratogen, or multifactorial combination of genes, environment, and chance that affect this early requirement for mandibular growth. If these early events occur normally, then failure of shelf rotation or of cell division and palatal growth or events related to final joining of the shelves and fusion can lead to CPO without other features of PRS.

PATIENT EVALUATION AND FAMILY COUNSELING

Most parents who have a child with an OFC wonder why this happened to their child and whether they caused it by doing something they should not have done or by not doing something that they should have done. Parents may also be worried about their chance of having the same or more severe malformations affect future pregnancies. Patients with OFCs may have similar concerns about the health of their offspring. Health professionals who care for patients with OFCs should be alert to their patients' needs for genetic counseling.

In 1975, a committee of The American Society of Human Genetics defined genetic counseling as "a communication process which deals with the human problems associated with the occurrence, or the risk of occurrence, of a genetic disorder in a family."[154] Appropriate genetic counseling depends on a correct diagnosis and on the correct application of the principles of human genetics.

Although great advances in knowledge about OFC causes and new testing technologies have evolved since 1985, the clinical approach to patients with an OFC remains largely unchanged.[155,156] The usual modalities of clinical diagnosis are used, namely, history and physical examination. In addition to obtaining a patient's complete medical history and doing a physical examination, one should also take a thorough gestational history to look for possible teratogenic factors as well as a detailed family history to identify possible genetic factors. In this way, one determines if patients have a syndromic or nonsyndromic OFC, a familial or nonfamilial OFC, and whether there are potential teratogenic factors present.

Our understanding of how best to counsel families and how to reduce both recurrences and primary occurrences has proceeded slowly. For example, there is some evidence that folic acid and perhaps other micronutrients may play a role in preventing OFCs; but data have been inconsistent regarding the types of OFCs affected and the magnitude of effects associated with different levels of supplementation.[86] The significance of specific susceptibility gene-environment interactions has yet to be clarified in most cases; currently, testing for susceptibility polymorphisms is only done on a research basis. Nonetheless, the current recommendation is that all women of childbearing age should take 400 μg of folic acid each day, mainly for the preventive effect for neural tube defects but also keeping in mind the potential effect on OFCs and CVMs.[157]

A recent large study in Denmark seems to confirm the traditionally held multifactorial threshold model of inheritance for nonsyndromic CL/P. In families of CL/P probands, these researchers reported recurrence rates of 3.5% (95% confidence interval [CI]: 3.1%–4.0%), 0.8% (95% CI: 0.6%–1.0%), and 0.6% (95% CI: 0.4%–0.8%) for first-, second-, and third-degree relatives, respectively. The recurrence risk also seemed to be related to cleft severity; 4.6% (95% CI: 3.2–6.1) of sibs with bilateral CLP had recurrences as opposed to 2.5% (95% CI: 1.8–3.2) of sibs of probands born with unilateral defects.[31]

Over the past few years, subepithelial defects or discontinuities of the superior orbicularis oris (OO) muscle have been identified in relatives of patients with an OFC as a subphenotype (subclinical trait) for CL/P[158–162]; but it is not clear how widely applicable or practical OO imaging will be for the average craniofacial clinic population. Genome-wide analyses to identify genetic loci associated with the OO muscle defect phenotype have identified BMP4 as one likely candidate.[122]

In family studies, OO defects do seem to segregate through families as microforms of CL/P. In one OFC cohort of 835 families, the occurrence of CL/P was significantly increased in families with OO defects versus those without.[158] These OO defects were seen in 16.4% of first-degree relatives and 17.2% of sibs of individuals with OO defects. On the other hand, although 7.3% of first-degree relatives of individuals with OO defects had CL/P, only 3.3% of siblings had CL/P, a figure similar to the rate found in the large Danish study discussed earlier and similar to figures traditionally quoted in the literature for sib recurrence.

Genetic counseling services are important for families of children with OFCs. Surgeons and craniofacial center professionals are essential contacts that can help families obtain and understand counseling information. These professionals can also help the parents of an unborn child with an OFC understand their baby's birth defect and anticipate the range of issues that might arise during the child's life. Medical advice must be neutral, nonjudgmental, and as accurate as possible. If surgeons and other craniofacial team personnel can be successful in managing this genetic information along with other treatment and management issues, it will make a powerful impact on the ability of these vulnerable families to adapt to caring for their children and to manage their future expectations.

REFERENCES

1. Spranger J, Benirschke K, Hall JG, et al. Errors of morphogenesis: concepts and terms. Recommendations of an international working group. J Pediatr 1982;100:160–5.
2. Croen LA, Shaw GM, Wasserman CR, et al. Racial and ethnic variations in the prevalence of orofacial clefts in California, 1983-1992. Am J Med Genet 1998;79:42–7.
3. Emanuel I, Culver BH, Erickson JD, et al. The further epidemiological differentiation of cleft lip and palate: a population study of clefts in King Country, Washington, 1856-1965. Teratology 1973; 7:271–81.
4. Shprintzen RJ, Siegel-Sadewitz VL, Amato J, et al. Anomalies associated with cleft lip, cleft palate, or both. Am J Med Genet 1985;20:585–95.
5. Rollnick BR, Pruzansky S. Genetic services at a center for craniofacial anomalies. Cleft Palate J 1981;18:304–13.
6. Jones MC. Etiology of facial clefts: prospective evaluation of 428 patients. Cleft Palate J 1988;25: 16–20.
7. Stoll C, Alembik Y, Dott B, et al. Associated malformations in cases with oral clefts. Cleft Palate Craniofac J 2000;37:41–7.
8. Calzolari E, Bianchi F, Rubini M, et al. Epidemiology of cleft palate in Europe: implications for genetic research. Cleft Palate Craniofac J 2004;41:244–9.
9. Calzolari E, Pierini A, Astolfi G, et al. Associated anomalies in multi-malformed infants with cleft lip and palate: an epidemiologic study of nearly 6 million births in 23 EUROCAT registries. Am J Med Genet A 2007;143:528–37.
10. Maarse W, Rozendaal AM, Pajkrt E, et al. A systematic review of associated structural and chromosomal defects in oral clefts: when is prenatal genetic analysis indicated? J Med Genet 2012; 49:490–8.
11. Pagon RA. 2006 ASHG Award for Excellence in Human Genetics Education. GeneTests: integrating genetic services into patient care. Am J Hum Genet 2007;81:658–9.
12. Mooney MP. Classification of orofacial clefting. In: Losee J, Kirschner RE, editors. Comprehensive cleft care. New York: McGraw-Hill Medical; 2009. p. 21–33.
13. Kernahan DA, Stark RB. A new classification for cleft lip and cleft palate. Plast Reconstr Surg Transplant Bull 1958;22:435–41.
14. Tessier P. Anatomical classification facial, craniofacial and latero-facial clefts. J Maxillofac Surg 1976;4:69–92.
15. Harkins CS, Berlin A, Harding RL, et al. A classification of cleft lip and cleft palate. Plast Reconstr Surg Transplant Bull 1962;29:31–9.

16. Kernahan DA. On cleft lip and palate classification. Plast Reconstr Surg 1973;51:578.

17. Kriens O. Lahshal. A concise documentation system for cleft lip, alveolus, and palate diagnoses. In: Kriens O, editor. What is a Cleft Lip and Palate? A Multidisciplinary Update. Stuttgart; New York Thieme 1989:30.

18. Spina V. A proposed modification for the classification of cleft lip and cleft palate. Cleft Palate J 1973; 10:251–2.

19. Tolarova MM, Cervenka J. Classification and birth prevalence of orofacial clefts. Am J Med Genet 1998;75:126–37.

20. Zhou YQ, Ji J, Mu XZ, et al. Diagnosis and classification of congenital craniofacial cleft deformities. J Craniofac Surg 2006;17:198–201.

21. Delestan C, Montoya P, Doucet JC, et al. New neonatal classification of unilateral cleft lip and palate-part 1: to predict primary lateral incisor agenesis and inherent tissue hypoplasia. Cleft Palate Craniofac J 2013. [Epub ahead of print].

22. Doucet JC, Delestan C, Montoya P, et al. New neonatal classification of unilateral cleft lip and palate part 2: to predict permanent lateral incisor agenesis and maxillary growth. Cleft Palate Craniofac J 2013. [Epub ahead of print].

23. Luijsterburg AJ, Rozendaal AM, Vermeij-Keers C. Classifying common oral clefts: a new approach after descriptive registration. Cleft Palate Craniofac J 2013. [Epub ahead of print].

24. Wang BC, Hakimi M, Martin MC. Use of two cleft lip and palate classification systems by nonsubspecialized health care providers. Cleft Palate Craniofac J 2013. [Epub ahead of print].

25. Koch H, Grzonka M, Koch J. Cleft malformation of lip, alveolus, hard and soft palate, and nose (LAHSN)–a critical view of the terminology, the diagnosis and gradation as a basis for documentation and therapy. Br J Oral Maxillofac Surg 1995;33: 51–8.

26. Juriloff DM, Harris MJ. Mouse genetic models of cleft lip with or without cleft palate. Birth Defects Res A Clin Mol Teratol 2008;82:63–77.

27. Murray JC. Gene/environment causes of cleft lip and/or palate. Clin Genet 2002;61:248–56.

28. Mossey PA, Little J, Munger RG, et al. Cleft lip and palate. Lancet 2009;374:1773–85.

29. Sadler T. Langman's medical embryology. 12th edition. Philadelphia: Wolters Kluwer Health/Lippincott Williams & Wilkins; 2012.

30. Sulik K. Orofacial embryogenesis: a framework for understanding clefting sites. In: Fonseca R, Marciani R, Turvey T, editors. Oral and maxillofacial surgery. 2nd edition. St Louis (MO): Saunders/Elsevier; 2009. p. 697–712.

31. Grosen D, Chevrier C, Skytthe A, et al. A cohort study of recurrence patterns among more than 54,000 relatives of oral cleft cases in Denmark: support for the multifactorial threshold model of inheritance. J Med Genet 2010;47:162–8.

32. Kondo S, Schutte BC, Richardson RJ, et al. Mutations in IRF6 cause Van der Woude and popliteal pterygium syndromes. Nat Genet 2002;32:285–9.

33. van den Boogaard MJ, Dorland M, Beemer FA, et al. MSX1 mutation is associated with orofacial clefting and tooth agenesis in humans. Nat Genet 2000;24:342–3.

34. Mangold E, Ludwig KU, Nothen MM. Breakthroughs in the genetics of orofacial clefting. Trends Mol Med 2011;17:725–33.

35. Noll JD. The origin of the term "harelip". Cleft Palate J 1983;20:169–71.

36. Hennekam RC. Gorlin's syndromes of the head and neck. Oxford (United Kingdom), New York: Oxford University Press; 2010.

37. Chen CP. Prenatal sonographic diagnosis of median facial cleft should alert holoprosencephaly with premaxillary agenesis and prompt genetic investigations. Ultrasound Obstet Gynecol 2002;19:421–2.

38. Cohen MM Jr, Sulik KK. Perspectives on holoprosencephaly: part II. Central nervous system, craniofacial anatomy, syndrome commentary, diagnostic approach, and experimental studies. J Craniofac Genet Dev Biol 1992;12:196–244.

39. Yamada S, Uwabe C, Fujii S, et al. Phenotypic variability in human embryonic holoprosencephaly in the Kyoto Collection. Birth Defects Res A Clin Mol Teratol 2004;70:495–508.

40. Solomon BD, Bear KA, Wyllie A, et al. Genotypic and phenotypic analysis of 396 individuals with mutations in Sonic Hedgehog. J Med Genet 2012;49:473–9.

41. Castilla EE, Martinez-Frias ML. Congenital healed cleft lip. Am J Med Genet 1995;58:106–12.

42. McDonald-McGinn D, Emanuel B, Zackai E. 22q11.2 Deletion syndrome. In: Pagon R, Adam M, Bird T, et al, editors. Gene reviews. Seattle (WA): University of Washington Seattle; 1999.

43. Shprintzen RJ, Schwartz RH, Daniller A, et al. Morphologic significance of bifid uvula. Pediatrics 1985;75:553–61.

44. Harville EW, Wilcox AJ, Lie RT, et al. Cleft lip and palate versus cleft lip only: are they distinct defects? Am J Epidemiol 2005;162:448–53.

45. Rahimov F, Marazita ML, Visel A, et al. Disruption of an AP-2alpha binding site in an IRF6 enhancer is associated with cleft lip. Nat Genet 2008;40: 1341–7.

46. Aschengrau A, Seage GR. Essentials of epidemiology in public health. Sudbury (MA): Jones and Barlett Publishers, LLC; 2008.

47. Rothman KJ, Greenland S. Modern epidemiology. 2nd Edition. Philadelphia, PA: Lippincott Raven; 1998.

48. Koepsell TD, Weiss NS. Epidemiologic methods. New York: Oxford University Press; 2003.

49. Mason CA, Kirby RS, Sever LE, et al. Prevalence is the preferred measure of frequency of birth defects. Birth Defects Res A Clin Mol Teratol 2005; 73:690–2.

50. Prevalence at birth of cleft lip with or without cleft palate: data from the International Perinatal Database of Typical Oral Clefts (IPDTOC). Cleft Palate Craniofac J 2011;48:66–81.

51. Parker SE, Mai CT, Canfield MA, et al. Updated national birth prevalence estimates for selected birth defects in the United States, 2004–2006. Birth Defects Res A Clin Mol Teratol 2010.

52. Mossey PA, Modell B. Epidemiology of oral clefts 2012: an international perspective. Front Oral Biol 2012;16:1–18.

53. Buehler JW. Surveillance. In: Rothman K, Greenland S, Lash T, editors. Modern epidemiology. Philadelphia: Lippincott William and Wilkins; 2008.

54. Amini H, Axelsson O, Ollars B, et al. The Swedish Birth Defects Registry: ascertainment and incidence of spina bifida and cleft lip/palate. Acta Obstet Gynecol Scand 2009;88:654–9.

55. Shaw GM, Croen LA, Curry CJ. Isolated oral cleft malformations: associations with maternal and infant characteristics in a California population. Teratology 1991;43:225–8.

56. Hashmi SS, Waller DK, Langlois P, et al. Prevalence of nonsyndromic oral clefts in Texas: 1995-1999. Am J Med Genet A 2005;134:368–72.

57. Genisca AE, Frias JL, Broussard CS, et al. Orofacial clefts in the National Birth Defects Prevention Study, 1997-2004. Am J Med Genet A 2009;149A: 1149–58.

58. Canfield MA, Honein MA, Yuskiv N, et al. National estimates and race/ethnic-specific variation of selected birth defects in the United States, 1999-2001. Birth Defects Res A Clin Mol Teratol 2006;76:747–56.

59. DeRoo LA, Gaudino JA, Edmonds LD. Orofacial cleft malformations: associations with maternal and infant characteristics in Washington State. Birth Defects Res A Clin Mol Teratol 2003;67:637–42.

60. Reefhuis J, Honein MA. Maternal age and nonchromosomal birth defects, Atlanta–1968-2000: teenager or thirty-something, who is at risk? Birth Defects Res A Clin Mol Teratol 2004;70:572–9.

61. Khoury MJ, Weinstein A, Panny S, et al. Maternal cigarette smoking and oral clefts: a population-based study. Am J Public Health 1987;77:623–5.

62. Khoury MJ, Gomez-Farias M, Mulinare J. Does maternal cigarette smoking during pregnancy cause cleft lip and palate in offspring? Am J Dis Child 1989;143:333–7.

63. Van den Eeden SK, Karagas MR, Daling JR, et al. A case-control study of maternal smoking and congenital malformations. Paediatr Perinat Epidemiol 1990;4:147–55.

64. Werler MM. Teratogen update: smoking and reproductive outcomes. Teratology 1997;55:382–8.

65. Lieff S, Olshan AF, Werler M, et al. Maternal cigarette smoking during pregnancy and risk of oral clefts in newborns. Am J Epidemiol 1999;150: 683–94.

66. Lorente C, Cordier S, Goujard J, et al. Tobacco and alcohol use during pregnancy and risk of oral clefts. Occupational Exposure and Congenital Malformation Working Group. Am J Public Health 2000;90:415–9.

67. Little J, Cardy A, Munger RG. Tobacco smoking and oral clefts: a meta-analysis. Bull World Health Organ 2004;82:213–8.

68. Little J, Cardy A, Arslan MT, et al. Smoking and orofacial clefts: a United Kingdom-based case-control study. Cleft Palate Craniofac J 2004;41:381–6.

69. Honein MA, Rasmussen SA, Reefhuis J, et al. Maternal smoking and environmental tobacco smoke exposure and the risk of orofacial clefts. Epidemiology 2007;18:226–33.

70. Hwang SJ, Beaty TH, Panny SR, et al. Association study of transforming growth factor alpha (TGF alpha) TaqI polymorphism and oral clefts: indication of gene-environment interaction in a population-based sample of infants with birth defects. Am J Epidemiol 1995;141:629–36.

71. Shaw GM, Wasserman CR, Lammer EJ, et al. Orofacial clefts, parental cigarette smoking, and transforming growth factor-alpha gene variants. Am J Hum Genet 1996;58:551–61.

72. Zeiger JS, Beaty TH, Liang KY. Oral clefts, maternal smoking, and TGFA: a meta-analysis of gene-environment interaction. Cleft Palate Craniofac J 2005;42:58–63.

73. Shaw GM, Carmichael SL, Laurent C, et al. Maternal nutrient intakes and risk of orofacial clefts. Epidemiology 2006;17:285–91.

74. Hassler JA, Moran DJ. Effects of ethanol on the cytoskeleton of migrating and differentiating neural crest cells: possible role in teratogenesis. J Craniofac Genet Dev Biol Suppl 1986;2:129–36.

75. Werler MM, Lammer EJ, Rosenberg L, et al. Maternal alcohol use in relation to selected birth defects. Am J Epidemiol 1991;134:691–8.

76. Munger RG, Romitti PA, Daack-Hirsch S, et al. Maternal alcohol use and risk of orofacial cleft birth defects. Teratology 1996;54:27–33.

77. Shaw GM, Lammer EJ. Maternal periconceptional alcohol consumption and risk for orofacial clefts. J Pediatr 1999;134:298–303.

78. Meyer KA, Werler MM, Hayes C, et al. Low maternal alcohol consumption during pregnancy

and oral clefts in offspring: the Slone Birth Defects Study. Birth Defects Res A Clin Mol Teratol 2003; 67:509–14.

79. Martinez-Frias ML, Bermejo E, Rodriguez-Pinilla E, et al. Risk for congenital anomalies associated with different sporadic and daily doses of alcohol consumption during pregnancy: a case-control study. Birth Defects Res A Clin Mol Teratol 2004;70: 194–200.

80. Romitti PA, Sun L, Honein MA, et al. Maternal periconceptional alcohol consumption and risk of orofacial clefts. Am J Epidemiol 2007;166: 775–85.

81. Lipinski RJ, Song C, Sulik KK, et al. Cleft lip and palate results from Hedgehog signaling antagonism in the mouse: phenotypic characterization and clinical implications. Birth Defects Res A Clin Mol Teratol 2010;88:232–40.

82. Shaw GM, Lammer EJ, Wasserman CR, et al. Risks of orofacial clefts in children born to women using multivitamins containing folic acid periconceptionally. Lancet 1995;346:393–6.

83. Munger R, Romitti P, West N, et al. Maternal intake of folate, vitamin B-12, and zinc and risk of orofacial cleft birth defects. Am J Epidemiol 1997;145.

84. Kelly D, O'Dowd T, Reulbach U. Use of folic acid supplements and risk of cleft lip and palate in infants: a population-based cohort study. Br J Gen Pract 2012;62:e466–72.

85. Li S, Chao A, Li Z, et al. Folic acid use and nonsyndromic orofacial clefts in China: a prospective cohort study. Epidemiology 2012;23:423–32.

86. Wehby GL, Murray JC. Folic acid and orofacial clefts: a review of the evidence. Oral Dis 2010;16: 11–9.

87. van Rooij IA, Vermeij-Keers C, Kluijtmans LA, et al. Does the interaction between maternal folate intake and the methylenetetrahydrofolate reductase polymorphisms affect the risk of cleft lip with or without cleft palate? Am J Epidemiol 2003;157:583–91.

88. Matalon S, Schechtman S, Goldzweig G, et al. The teratogenic effect of carbamazepine: a meta-analysis of 1255 exposures. Reprod Toxicol 2002; 16:9–17.

89. Hernandez-Diaz S, Werler MM, Walker AM, et al. Folic acid antagonists during pregnancy and the risk of birth defects. N Engl J Med 2000;343: 1608–14.

90. Holmes LB, Wyszynski DF, Lieberman E. The AED (antiepileptic drug) pregnancy registry: a 6-year experience. Arch Neurol 2004;61:673–8.

91. Lammer EJ, Chen DT, Hoar RM, et al. Retinoic acid embryopathy. N Engl J Med 1985;313:837–41.

92. Carmichael SL, Shaw GM. Maternal corticosteroid use and risk of selected congenital anomalies. Am J Med Genet 1999;86:242–4.

93. Aberg A, Westbom L, Kallen B. Congenital malformations among infants whose mothers had gestational diabetes or preexisting diabetes. Early Hum Dev 2001;61:85–95.

94. Correa A, Gilboa SM, Besser LM, et al. Diabetes mellitus and birth defects. Am J Obstet Gynecol 2008;199:237.e1–9.

95. Cedergren M, Kallen B. Maternal obesity and the risk for orofacial clefts in the offspring. Cleft Palate Craniofac J 2005;42:367–71.

96. Stott-Miller M, Heike CL, Kratz M, et al. Increased risk of orofacial clefts associated with maternal obesity: case-control study and Monte Carlo-based bias analysis. Paediatr Perinat Epidemiol 2010;24:502–12.

97. Muraskas JK, McDonnell JF, Chudik RJ, et al. Amniotic band syndrome with significant orofacial clefts and disruptions and distortions of craniofacial structures. J Pediatr Surg 2003;38:635–8.

98. Vieira AR. Genetic and environmental factors in human cleft lip and palate. Front Oral Biol 2012;16: 19–31.

99. Kohli SS, Kohli VS. A comprehensive review of the genetic basis of cleft lip and palate. J Oral Maxillofac Pathol 2012;16:64–72.

100. Stuppia L, Capogreco M, Marzo G, et al. Genetics of syndromic and nonsyndromic cleft lip and palate. J Craniofac Surg 2011;22:1722–6.

101. Bae HT, Sebastiani P, Sun JX, et al. Genome-wide association study of personality traits in the long life family study. Front Genet 2013;4:65.

102. Dixon MJ, Marazita ML, Beaty TH, et al. Cleft lip and palate: understanding genetic and environmental influences. Nat Rev Genet 2011;12: 167–78.

103. Jugessur A, Shi M, Gjessing HK, et al. Maternal genes and facial clefts in offspring: a comprehensive search for genetic associations in two population-based cleft studies from Scandinavia. PLoS One 2010;5:e11493.

104. Shi M, Mostowska A, Jugessur A, et al. Identification of microdeletions in candidate genes for cleft lip and/or palate. Birth Defects Res A Clin Mol Teratol 2009;85:42–51.

105. Jugessur A, Farlie PG, Kilpatrick N. The genetics of isolated orofacial clefts: from genotypes to subphenotypes. Oral Dis 2009;15:437–53.

106. Sebastiani P, Timofeev N, Dworkis DA, et al. Genome-wide association studies and the genetic dissection of complex traits. Am J Hematol 2009; 84:504–15.

107. Manolio TA, Collins FS, Cox NJ, et al. Finding the missing heritability of complex diseases. Nature 2009;461:747–53.

108. Monteiro FP, Vieira TP, Sgardioli IC, et al. Defining new guidelines for screening the 22q11.2 deletion based on a clinical and dysmorphologic evaluation

of 194 individuals and review of the literature. Eur J Pediatr 2013;172(7):927–45.

109. Reish O, Finkelstein Y, Mesterman R, et al. Is isolated palatal anomaly an indication to screen for 22q11 region deletion? Cleft Palate Craniofac J 2003;40:176–9.

110. Mingarelli R, Digilio MC, Mari A, et al. The search for hemizygosity at 22qll in patients with isolated cleft palate. J Craniofac Genet Dev Biol 1996;16:118–21.

111. Ruiter EM, Bongers EM, Smeets D, et al. No justification of routine screening for 22q11 deletions in patients with overt cleft palate. Clin Genet 2003;64:216–9.

112. Oh AK, Workman LA, Wong GB. Clinical correlation of chromosome 22q11.2 fluorescent in situ hybridization analysis and velocardiofacial syndrome. Cleft Palate Craniofac J 2007;44:62–6.

113. Sivertsen A, Lie RT, Wilcox AJ, et al. Prevalence of duplications and deletions of the 22q11 DiGeorge syndrome region in a population-based sample of infants with cleft palate. Am J Med Genet A 2007;143:129–34.

114. Sandrin-Garcia P, Richieri-Costa A, Tajara EH, et al. Fluorescence in situ hybridization (FISH) screening for the 22q11.2 deletion in patients with clinical features of velocardiofacial syndrome but without cardiac anomalies. Genet Mol Biol 2007;30:21–4.

115. Fagerberg CR, Graakjaer J, Heinl UD, et al. Heart defects and other features of the 22q11 distal deletion syndrome. Eur J Med Genet 2013;56:98–107.

116. Online Mendelian Inheritance in Man, OMIM®. McKusick-Nathans Institute of Genetic Medicine, Johns Hopkins University (Baltimore, MD), {2013}. Available at: http://www.omim.org/.

117. Kini U. Fetal valproate syndrome: a review. Paediatr Perinat Drug Ther 2006;7:123–30.

118. Kini U, Adab N, Vinten J, et al, Liverpool and Manchester Neurodevelopmental Study Group. Dysmorphic features: an important clue to the diagnosis and severity of fetal anticonvulsant syndromes. Arch Dis Child Fetal Neonatal Ed 2006;91:F90–5.

119. Boyles AL, DeRoo LA, Lie RT, et al. Maternal alcohol consumption, alcohol metabolism genes, and the risk of oral clefts: a population-based case-control study in Norway, 1996-2001. Am J Epidemiol 2010;172:924–31.

120. Koo J, Zavras A. Antiepileptic drugs (AEDs) during pregnancy and risk of congenital jaw and oral malformation. Oral Dis 2013;19(7):712–20.

121. Jugessur A, Shi M, Gjessing HK, et al. Genetic determinants of facial clefting: analysis of 357 candidate genes using two national cleft studies from Scandinavia. PLoS One 2009;4:e5385.

122. Suzuki S, Marazita ML, Cooper ME, et al. Mutations in BMP4 are associated with subepithelial, microform, and overt cleft lip. Am J Hum Genet 2009;84:406–11.

123. Suzuki Y, Jezewski PA, Machida J, et al. In a Vietnamese population, MSX1 variants contribute to cleft lip and palate. Genet Med 2004;6:117–25.

124. Jezewski PA, Vieira AR, Nishimura C, et al. Complete sequencing shows a role for MSX1 in nonsyndromic cleft lip and palate. J Med Genet 2003;40:399–407.

125. Gurrieri F, Franco B, Toriello H, et al. Oral-facial-digital syndromes: review and diagnostic guidelines. Am J Med Genet A 2007;143A:3314–23.

126. Toriello HV. Are the oral-facial-digital syndromes ciliopathies? Am J Med Genet A 2009;5:32799.

127. Thomas S, Legendre M, Saunier S, et al. TCTN3 mutations cause Mohr-Majewski syndrome. Am J Hum Genet 2012;91:372–8.

128. Hall BD. Aglossia-adactylia. Birth Defects Orig Artic Ser 1971;7:233–6.

129. Chicarilli ZN, Polayes IM. Oromandibular limb hypogenesis syndromes. Plast Reconstr Surg 1985;76:13–24.

130. Allanson E, Dickinson JE, Charles AK, et al. Fetal oromandibular limb hypogenesis syndrome following uterine curettage in early pregnancy. Birth Defects Res A Clin Mol Teratol 2011;91:226–9.

131. Firth H, Boyd PA, Chamberlain P, et al. Limb defects and chorionic villus sampling. Lancet 1996;347:1406 [author reply: 7–8].

132. Zucchero TM, Cooper ME, Maher BS, et al. Interferon regulatory factor 6 (IRF6) gene variants and the risk of isolated cleft lip or palate. N Engl J Med 2004;351:769–80.

133. Jugessur A, Rahimov F, Lie RT, et al. Genetic variants in IRF6 and the risk of facial clefts: single-marker and haplotype-based analyses in a population-based case-control study of facial clefts in Norway. Genet Epidemiol 2008;32:413–24.

134. Rojas-Martinez A, Reutter H, Chacon-Camacho O, et al. Genetic risk factors for nonsyndromic cleft lip with or without cleft palate in a Mesoamerican population: evidence for IRF6 and variants at 8q24 and 10q25. Birth Defects Res A Clin Mol Teratol 2010;88:535–7.

135. Blanton SH, Burt A, Stal S, et al. Family-based study shows heterogeneity of a susceptibility locus on chromosome 8q24 for nonsyndromic cleft lip and palate. Birth Defects Res A Clin Mol Teratol 2010;88:256–9.

136. Nikopensius T, Ambrozaityte L, Ludwig KU, et al. Replication of novel susceptibility locus for nonsyndromic cleft lip with or without cleft palate on chromosome 8q24 in Estonian and Lithuanian patients. Am J Med Genet A 2009;149A:2551–3.

137. Song T, Wu D, Wang Y, et al. Association of NAT1 and NAT2 genes with nonsyndromic cleft lip and palate. Mol Med Rep 2013;8:211–6.

138. Patel PJ, Beaty TH, Ruczinski I, et al. X-linked markers in the Duchenne muscular dystrophy gene associated with oral clefts. Eur J Oral Sci 2013;121:63–8.

139. Butali A, Little J, Chevrier C, et al. Folic acid supplementation use and the MTHFR C677T polymorphism in orofacial clefts etiology: an individual participant data pooled-analysis. Birth Defects Res A Clin Mol Teratol 2013;97(8):509–14.

140. Amarillo IE, Dipple KM, Quintero-Rivera F. Familial microdeletion of 17q24.3 upstream of SOX9 is associated with isolated Pierre Robin sequence due to position effect. Am J Med Genet A 2013; 161A:1167–72.

141. Fukami M, Tsuchiya T, Takada S, et al. Complex genomic rearrangement in the SOX9 5′ region in a patient with Pierre Robin sequence and hypoplastic left scapula. Am J Med Genet A 2012; 158A:1529–34.

142. Jagomagi T, Nikopensius T, Krjutskov K, et al. MTHFR and MSX1 contribute to the risk of nonsyndromic cleft lip/palate. Eur J Oral Sci 2010;118:213–20.

143. Ingersoll RG, Hetmanski J, Park JW, et al. Association between genes on chromosome 4p16 and non-syndromic oral clefts in four populations. Eur J Hum Genet 2010;18:726–32.

144. Beaty TH, Murray JC, Marazita ML, et al. A genome-wide association study of cleft lip with and without cleft palate identifies risk variants near MAFB and ABCA4. Nat Genet 2010;42:525–9.

145. Polen KN, Rasmussen SA, Riehle-Colarusso T, et al, National Birth Defects Prevention Study. Association between reported venlafaxine use in early pregnancy and birth defects, national birth defects prevention study, 1997-2007. Birth Defects Res A Clin Mol Teratol 2013;97:28–35.

146. Molina-Solana R, Yanez-Vico RM, Iglesias-Linares A, et al. Current concepts on the effect of environmental factors on cleft lip and palate. Int J Oral Maxillofac Surg 2013;42:177–84.

147. Allanson JE, Cunniff C, Hoyme HE, et al. Elements of morphology: standard terminology for the head and face. Am J Med Genet A 2009;149A:6–28.

148. Randall P, Krogman WM, Jahins S. Pierre Robin and the syndrome that bears his names. Cleft Palate J 1965;36:237–46.

149. Gangopadhyay N, Mendonca DA, Woo AS. Pierre robin sequence. Semin Plast Surg 2012;26:76–82.

150. Izumi K, Konczal LL, Mitchell AL, et al. Underlying genetic diagnosis of Pierre Robin sequence: retrospective chart review at two children's hospitals and a systematic literature review. J Pediatr 2012; 160:645–50.e2.

151. Sulik K, Bream P Jr. Palate development. In: Embryo images: normal and abnormal mammalian development. Chapel Hill (NC): University of North Carolina at Chapel Hill; 1994. Available at:

https://syllabus.med.unc.edu/courseware/embryo_images/unit-hednk/hednk_htms/hednk037.htm; 1994.

152. Hill M. Palate development. 2013. Available at: http://php.med.unsw.edu.au/embryology/index.php?title=Palate_Development. Accessed August 6, 2013.

153. Hanson JW, Smith DW. U-shaped palatal defect in the Robin anomalad: developmental and clinical relevance. J Pediatr 1975;87:30–3.

154. Genetic counseling. Am J Hum Genet 1975;27: 240–2.

155. Aylsworth AS. Genetic considerations in clefts of the lip and palate. Clin Plast Surg 1985;12:533–42.

156. Aylsworth AS. The prediction of risk and genetic counseling for craniofacial abnormalities. In: Bader JD, editor. Risk assessment in dentistry. Chapel Hill (NC): University of North Carolina Dental Ecology; 1990. p. 261–6.

157. Centers for Disease Control and Prevention. Folic acid recommendations. Atlanta, GA: Centers for Disease Control and Prevention; 2013. Available at: http://www.cdc.gov/ncbddd/folicacid/recommendations.html.

158. Klotz CM, Wang X, DeSensi RS, et al. Revisiting the recurrence risk of nonsyndromic cleft lip with or without cleft palate. Am J Med Genet A 2010; 152A(11):2697–702.

159. Weinberg SM, Brandon CA, McHenry TH, et al. Rethinking isolated cleft palate: evidence of occult lip defects in a subset of cases. Am J Med Genet A 2008;146A:1670–5.

160. Marazita ML. Subclinical features in nonsyndromic cleft lip with or without cleft palate (CL/P): review of the evidence that subepithelial orbicularis oris muscle defects are part of an expanded phenotype for CL/P. Orthod Craniofac Res 2007;10:82–7.

161. Neiswanger K, Weinberg SM, Rogers CR, et al. Orbicularis oris muscle defects as an expanded phenotypic feature in nonsyndromic cleft lip with or without cleft palate. Am J Med Genet A 2007; 143A:1143–9.

162. Rogers CR, Weinberg SM, Smith TD, et al. Anatomical basis for apparent subepithelial cleft lip: a histological and ultrasonographic survey of the orbicularis oris muscle. Cleft Palate Craniofac J 2008;45:518–24.

FURTHER READING

Readers interested in a more detailed discussion of current concepts regarding terminology and classification of malformations are directed to Hennekam RC, Biesecker LG, Allanson JE, et al. Elements of morphology: general terms for congenital anomalies. Am J Med Genet A 2013;161(11):2726–33. http://dx.doi.org/10.1002/ajmg.a.36249.

Unilateral Cleft Lip Repair

Raj M. Vyas, MD, Stephen M. Warren, MD*

KEYWORDS

- Cleft lip • Cleft alveolus • Cleft nasal deformity • Nasoalveolar molding
- Presurgical infant orthopedics • Cheiloplasty • Gingivoperiosteoplasty • Primary cleft nasal surgery

KEY POINTS

- Modern cleft surgery requires four-dimensional and functional anatomic understanding of the cleft (and noncleft) lip, nose, and alveolus.
- Some techniques for nasolabial repair rely more on precise anatomic geometry, whereas others afford the surgeon a more flexible design.
- Consistent anthropometry enables accurate assessment and reporting of long-term outcomes; such reports are needed to guide perioperative care, delineate optimal repair principles, and resolve ongoing controversies.

INTRODUCTION

Since 390 BCE, the treatment of upper lip clefts has challenged generations of surgeons.[1] Cleft care is now concentrated in specialized, high-volume centers where multidisciplinary teams can best serve patients and their families. The American Cleft Palate–Craniofacial Association (ACPA) has established a framework for such centers that guides multidisciplinary team composition, interdisciplinary communication, cultural competence, psychosocial services, and outcomes assessment (www.acpa-cpf.org). Modern cleft reconstruction requires three-dimensional (3D) and functional anatomic understanding of the cleft (and noncleft) lip, nose, and alveolus. Accurate nomenclature defines shared challenges, improves classification schema, and builds consensus (where possible). Multiple repair techniques and modifications reflect the rich variety and continuous evolution of operative principles in cleft reconstruction. Diligent anthropometry enables accurate assessment of outcomes over time, the so-called fourth dimension.[2]

EMBRYOLOGY AND EPIDEMIOLOGY

Lip development occurs from the fourth to the seventh weeks of gestation.[3,4] The frontonasal prominence is formed from mesenchymal tissue ventral to the forebrain and leads to development of the medial and lateral nasal prominences.[5] The paired maxillary and mandibular prominences are formed from neural crest cells migrating from the first pharyngeal arch.[6] The primary palate, or premaxilla, similarly forms from the fusion of the medial palatine processes. A unilateral cleft lip occurs when there is failure of complete fusion between the advancing maxillary prominence and the fused medial nasal prominences on one side (Fig. 1). The cleft of the lip extends through the maxillary dentoalveolus to the incisive foramen when the medial palatine processes fail to fuse. The secondary palate, posterior to the incisive foramen, develops from the 6th to the 12th weeks of gestation as the lateral palatine processes fuse. A cleft palate occurs when there is incomplete fusion of the lateral palatine processes with the medial palatine process and/or nasal septum (Fig. 2). Various anomalous combinations in lip and palate development occur; it is more common to have cleft lip and palate (46%) than isolated cleft palate (33%) or isolated cleft lip (21%).[7] Additional failures of mesenchymal penetration result in an array of facial clefts.

Cleft lip (with or without cleft palate) occurs most commonly in boys and has a 6:3:1 ratio of

Department of Plastic Surgery, NYU School of Medicine, 33rd Street, New York, NY 10016, USA
* Corresponding author. 875 Park Avenue, New York, NY 10075
E-mail address: stephen.warren.md@gmail.com

0094-1298/14/$ – see front matter © 2014 Elsevier Inc. All rights reserved.

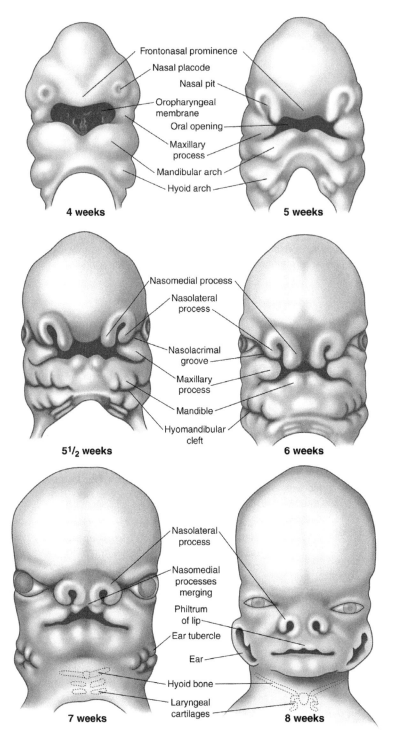

Fig. 1. Embryology of the normal lip. The face is initially made up of 5 prominences: a central frontonasal prominence, paired maxillary prominences, and paired mandibular prominences. These primordial structures appear during the fourth week of development and surround the primitive mouth. The maxillary prominence gives rise to the upper jaw, lip (lateral to the philtral column), orbital floor, and inferior portion of the lateral nasal wall. Rapid growth of the maxillary prominences, along with the medial nasal processes, during weeks 4 to 8 leads to a shift of the frontonasal process away from the stomodeum. The medial nasal processes fuse and give rise to the intermaxillary segment, which ultimately becomes the philtrum of the lip, the premaxilla, and the primary palate. (*From* Carlson BM. Head and neck. In: Carlson BM, editor. Human Embryology and Developmental Biology, Fifth Edition. Philadelphia: Elsevier Saunders, 2014; with permission.)

left/right/bilateral involvement.[7] If a child is born with a cleft lip, the risk of having another child with cleft lip is 4% and 9% after 2 affected children.[7] If a mother and child are affected, the risk to the second child is 15.3%.[7] The condition occurs in approximately 2 of 1000 Asians, 1 of 1000 white people, and 0.5 of 1000 African Americans.[8] Unlike isolated cleft palate, cleft lip is usually sporadic and associated with only a few syndromes: van der Woude (autosomal dominant, lip pits), 22q deletion

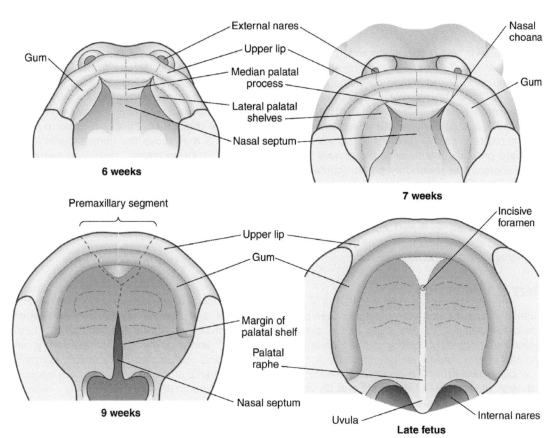

Fig. 2. Embryology of the normal palate. Palate formation occurs from gestational weeks 6 to 10 and involves 4 primary structures: the median palatine process, a pair of lateral palatine processes (palatal shelves), and the nasal septum. The median palatine process forms the primary palate, which is often referred to as the premaxillary component of the maxilla. This structure ultimately houses the 4 maxillary incisors. The secondary palate is formed by the lateral palatine processes, which begin to fuse during the seventh week. The nasal septum then joins the fused palatal shelves to complete the formation of the secondary palate. (*From* Carlson BM. Head and neck. In: Carlson BM, editor. Human Embryology and Developmental Biology, Fifth Edition. Philadelphia: Elsevier Saunders, 2014; with permission.)

(DiGeorge anomaly, conotruncal malformation, velocardiofacial syndrome), and Stickler (type 2 collagen mutation, retinal detachment).

APPLIED ANATOMY

Restoration of normal surface, muscle, and mucosal anatomy is paramount in patients with cleft lip. The upper lip is lined posteriorly with non-keratinized oral mucosa and anteriorly by keratinized vermillion and hair-bearing skin. The red line divides labial mucosa from vermillion, whereas the vermillion border separates vermillion from white roll. The white roll is a shiny, hairless convexity lying just above the vermillion border. The normal philtrum is composed of a central depression between 2 ridges that emanate upward from the peaks of Cupid's bow toward the medial footplates of the lower lateral nasal cartilages. Philtral ridges are normally formed by decussating fibers

of orbicularis oris muscle that insert superficially into overlying dermis.[9] The orbicularis oris has 2 functional components: lip retraction (fibers originating superficially from facial mimetic muscles) and oral sphincter closure (fibers originating deeper from modiolus).[10] Within vermillion, orbicularis oris becomes superficial and concave. Known here as the pars marginalis, its shape contributes to the lip's natural pout.

In a unilateral cleft, the medial lip is short with a flat philtral ridge and narrow vermillion. The lateral lip also has deficient mucosa, vermillion, and white roll medial to the Noordhoff point (of maximum vermillion height).[11] The orbicularis oris is deficient, with aberrant muscle insertions into the alar base, nasal sill, columella, and dermal cleft margins.[12,13] The cleft nasal deformity is variable and corresponds with severity of the cleft lip.[14,15] The columella is short and the anterior nasal spine/caudal septum deviates away from the cleft.[16,17] In complete unilateral clefts, the nasal sill, nasal floor, alveolus, and primary palate are also disrupted, allowing unrestricted growth of the greater (medial) maxillary segment, which splays the maxillary arch. The cleft-side ala and associated lower lateral cartilage are widened and distorted by the ala's attachments to the collapsed lesser (lateral) maxillary segment. The primary palate (containing premaxilla, central alveolus, and philtrum) is anterior to the incisive foramen, whereas the secondary palate (containing maxilla, palatine bones, palatal musculature, uvula, and pterygoid plates) is posterior. The incisive foramen is important because it distinguishes the complete cleft lip defect from a cleft palate defect, and also because it contains the nasopalatine nerves and sphenopalatine artery.

CLEFT CLASSIFICATION

Numerous classification schemas have been proposed for cleft lip[18–22]; we think that a simple system with objective, clearly defined anatomic features is most useful for practitioners. A cleft lip is distinguished by 2 main characteristics: (1) unilateral versus bilateral deformity and (2) complete versus incomplete deformity. A complete cleft lip is characterized by through-and-through involvement of the lip, nasal sill, nasal floor, and alveolus, whereas incomplete clefts show partial penetrance through these structures. Thirty percent of patients with complete cleft lip still show a Simonart band.[23,24]

Veau[25] described the spectrum of incomplete unilateral clefts. Various colloquialisms such as minimal and occult have since been used to describe the array of incomplete labial, muscular, and dental cleft phenotypes.[26–29] Yuzuriha and Mulliken[30] describe lesser form labial clefts (those at the far end of the unilateral incomplete spectrum) as minor form (notched vermillion-cutaneous junction extending 3 mm or more above the normal Cupid's bow peak), microform (notch less than 3 mm above the normal Cupid's bow peak), or mini-microform (disrupted vermilion-cutaneous junction without elevation of Cupid's bow peak) (**Fig. 3**).[30] For each, nasal severity reflects that of the lip. Yuzuriha and Mulliken's[30] classification is practical because it guides optimal operative technique by cleft severity.

ANTHROPOMETRIC ANALYSIS AND PLANNING

Anthropometry is the measurement of the human individual and permits comparison of anatomy under normal and abnormal conditions. Dr Leslie Farkas,[31] father of medical anthropometry, and Farkas and colleagues,[32] provided normative measurements of the lip and nose. Cleft surgeons use anthropometry to objectively measure aesthetic outcomes over time. With an applied understanding of the fourth dimension (growth), these data are retrospectively applied to improve the initial 3D design at primary nasolabial repair.[33]

There are fundamental nasolabial anthropometric landmarks essential to cleft surgery (**Fig. 4**): alare (ala) is the most lateral point of each ala, subalare (sbal) is the most inferior point of each alar base, the highest point of columella

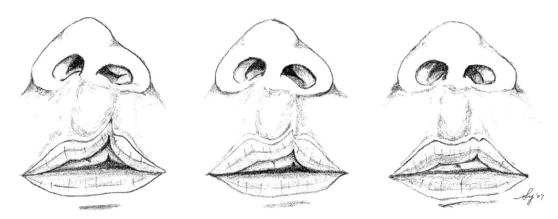

Fig. 3. Incomplete unilateral clefts. Mulliken described unilateral incomplete spectrum as minor form (notched vermillion-cutaneous junction extending 3 mm or more above the normal Cupid's bow peak), microform (notch less than 3 mm above the normal Cupid's bow peak), or mini-microform (disrupted vermilion-cutaneous junction without elevation of Cupid's bow peak). For each condition, the severity of the nasal difference correlates with the severity of the lip cleft. (*From* Yuzuriha S, Mulliken JB. Minor-form, microform, and mini-microform cleft lip: anatomical features, operative techniques, and revisions. Plast Reconstr Surg 2008;122(5):1485–93; with permission.)

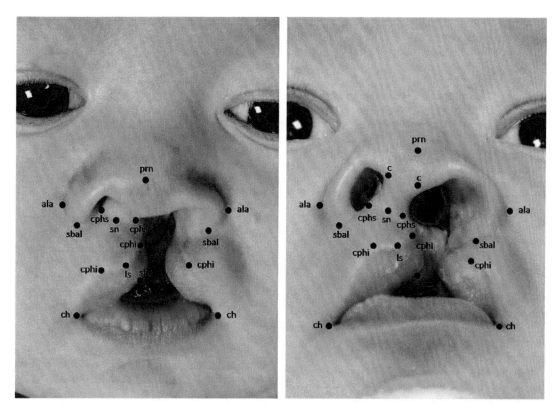

Fig. 4. Anthropometry. Anthropometric landmarks for unilateral nasolabial repair; anterior (*left*) and subnasal (*right*) views. Alare (al) is the most lateral point of each ala, subalare (sbal) is the most inferior point of each alar base, the highest point of columella (c) lies atop each hemicolumella and is level with each nostril peak, subnasale (sn) defines the angle between columellar base and upper lip, crista philtri superior (cphs) is atop each philtral column at the same horizontal line drawn through sn, crista philtri inferior (cphi) lies at the base of each philtral column (each Cupid's bow peak), labiale superius (ls) lies at the midpoint of the upper vermilion (Cupid's bow trough), stomion (sto) is the point along the vertical facial midline that bisects the free margin of the upper lip, and cheilion (ch) is located at each labial commissure. Relevant lip and nose measurements for unilateral cleft deformities include heminasal width (sn-al), nasal width (al-al), nasal tip projection (sn-prn), columellar length on each side (sn-c), columellar width (c-c), labial height (sn-cphi, sbal-cphi), and lip length (cphi-ch).

(c) lies atop each hemicolumella and is level with each nostril peak, subnasale (sn) defines the angle between columellar base and upper lip, crista philtri superior (cphs) is atop each philtral column at the same horizontal line drawn through sn, crista philtri inferior (cphi) lies at the base of each philtral column (each Cupid's bow peak), labiale superius (Ls) lies at the midpoint of the upper vermilion (Cupid's bow trough), stomion (sto) is the point along the vertical facial midline that bisects the free margin of the upper lip, and cheilion (ch) is located at each labial commissure.[33]

Anthropometric measurements can be obtained by direct or indirect methods. Direct anthropometry is the gold standard, but requires experience and a cooperative patient. For young patients, this is most accurately obtained in the operating room under general anesthesia. Indirect anthropometry can be obtained by two-dimensional

(2D) photography but requires image standardization and calibration for linear measurements; 2D photography is best for discerning proportions and angles. As an alternative, 3D photography allows photographs to be analyzed with software accompanying 3D camera systems. This technique has gained favor as an alternative to direct anthropometry in children because images are captured in as little as 3.5 milliseconds. Wong and colleagues[34] evaluated the validity and reliability of nasolabial anthropometry using 3D photography compared with direct anthropometry and found that linear measurements were highly correlated and overall precision of 3D measurements were within 1 mm of direct measurements.

Relevant lip and nose measurements for unilateral cleft deformities include heminasal width (sn-al), nasal width (al-al), nasal tip projection (sn-prn), columellar length on each side (sn-c), columellar width (c-c), labial height (sn-cphi, sbal-cphi), and lip length (cphi-ch). Understanding future growth is crucial when performing primary cleft lip repair. The surgeon must normalize nasolabial measurements not at the time of repair but when the child reaches 5 to 10 years of age. Mulliken and LaBrie[2] studied anthropometric changes over time after unilateral nasolabial repair and found that heminasal width (sn-al) increases more on the cleft side than noncleft side during the first 6 years of life. Lateral drift of the alar base was also described by Millard,[35] who secured the alar base to the caudal septum to reduce alar creep. Byrd preserves a muscular roll below the alar base that he sutures to soft tissue adjacent to the anterior nasal spine and contralateral medial crural footplate.[36] Slow-growing structures such as nasal tip projection (sn-prn) and columellar length (sn-c) should be made longer than those of age-matched, gender-matched, and ethnicity-matched subjects at the time of primary repair. Fast-growing features such as nasal width (al-al) and prolabial width (cphs-cphs and cphi-cphi in bilateral deformities) are intentionally made narrower than those of normative subjects.[33] Vermilion-mucosal height is a fast-growing features that is intentionally made longer because of concern for deficiency of tissue in the median tubercle.[33]

GOALS OF SURGERY

Nasolabial repair of the unilateral cleft deformity should restore normal midfacial anatomic relationships and obtain long-term symmetry. Regardless of the technique used, a primary goal is to achieve lip height (sn-cphi and sbal-cphi) on the cleft side that matches the noncleft side. An ideal technique allows for more adjustments and produces a favorable scar pattern. Blair[16] delineated the stigmata of the unilateral cleft nasal deformity: deviation of the tip and caudal septum to the noncleft side, dislocated lower lateral cartilage, obtuse angle between middle and lateral crura, posterolaterally displaced alar base, and short columella on the cleft side. Primary correction of these deformities is variously undertaken in repair of unilateral cleft nose, with anthropometric studies indicating improvements in nasal symmetry following certain repair strategies.[37–40]

CURRENT PRACTICE
Presurgical Molding

Most cleft centers currently use presurgical molding to align skeletal and soft tissues in preparation for definitive repair. Both passive molding, such as

lip taping and (naso)alveolar molding, and active molding, such as the pin-retained (Latham) device, take advantage of the malleable tissues and rapid facial growth of infancy. Presurgical molding is an important, well-studied topic and detail is provided in the article "Management of the Alveolar Cleft" elsewhere in this issue by Pedro E. Santiago, Lindsay A. Schuster, and Daniel Levy-Bercowski.

Lip Adhesion

Lip adhesion is sometimes done for operative molding before definitive nasolabial repair. It restrains the alveolar segments and reduces cleft gaps by up to 60%.[41,42] Adhesion is accomplished by ligating tissue along each cleft margin that is normally discarded during labial repair; various descriptions exist. Lip adhesion requires that the infant undergoes an additional operation and might compromise the outcome by restrictive scarring.[43–45] Supporters argue it improves definitive repair by approximating the alveolar cleft, thereby facilitating gingivoperiosteoplasty and decreasing tension along the labial closure.[46–48] Ridgway and colleagues[49] used ultrasonography to show that the lateral orbicularis oris is thickened after lip adhesion, potentially aiding philtral construction. In addition, lip adhesion begins early nasal molding and provides 2 opportunities to correct cleft nasal asymmetry.[49] As with presurgical molding, preference for lip adhesion is based on cleft severity, available expertise, and family/surgeon preference.[8]

Triangular Repair

Tennison[50] designed his repair after learning of Le-Mesurier's use of (unilimb[51]) Z-plasty to lengthen the cleft lip. Unlike LeMesurier, whose backcut along the lateral lip element translated to a transverse philtral scar, Tennison[50] made the backcut for his unilimb Z-plasty from cphi of the medial lip toward the philtral dimple (**Fig. 5**). This incision opens to achieve the desired height of the medial lip; the deficit is satisfied with a laterally based triangular flap. Randall[52] built on Tennison's[50] design by adding key anatomic landmarks and geometric techniques to seek mathematic symmetry at closure.

In the Tennison-Randall repair, a point is chosen along the medial and lateral cleft nasal floor so that closure at these landmarks optimizes nasal symmetry (sn-al, sn-c, and sn-prn). An incision is marked from the medial point of closure to cphi; the predicted medial lip deficiency is then recorded. From the lateral nasal point of closure, an incision of equivalent length is marked toward the chosen lateral cphi point. The gap between the inferior end of this line and cphi defines the

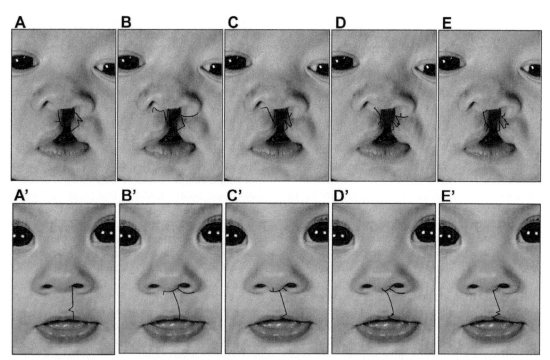

Fig. 5. Unilateral lip markings. Preoperative markings (*top row*) and postoperative pattern of closure (*bottom row*) for unilateral cleft nasolabial repair. *A* and *A'*, Tennison-Randall repair; *B* and *B'*, Millard repair; *C* and *C'*, Mohler repair; *D* and *D'*, Mulliken repair; *E* and *E'*, Fisher repair.

base of the lateral triangular flap that fills the medial lip backcut. The exact pattern of closure along the lateral lip margin (including triangle) is designed while being mindful of (1) the equivalent length of the lines drawn from each point of nasal closure, and (2) the deficiency in medial lip height. Swinging calipers help finalize this pattern by tracing intersecting arches from both the lateral nasal point of closure and cphi (see **Fig. 5**).

The Tennison-Randall approach is most useful for wide clefts or clefts with severe vertical deficiency. Cronin[53] suggested designing the triangular flap 1 mm above the vermillion border to avoid disruption of the white roll. Critics argue that the technique produces excess lip height (sn-cphi, sbal-cphi); Brauer and Cronin[54] suggested a 1-mm initial undercorrection and possible full-thickness excision below the ala (particularly for incomplete clefts).[55] A major limitation of this technique is the triangular philtral scar.

Rotation-Advancement: Millard and Modifications

Millard[56] introduced the rotation-advancement repair in 1955 to move the line of closure away from the philtral dimple and into the anatomically camouflaged cleft philtral column. Rotation-advancement advocates that all available tissue

be rearranged for nasolabial construction with minimal tissue discard. Millard proposed a medial curvilinear incision from cleft cphi up along the cleft margin to cleft cphs at the columella, continuing along the lip-columella junction just short of noncleft cphs (see **Fig. 5**). The resulting flap rotates inferiorly, providing height but leaving a defect in the central upper lip. Millard[47,57] embodied a cut-as-you-go mindset; when he needed more lip height, he added a backcut made from the end of his rotation incision down toward the noncleft philtral column. He filled the resulting gap with a portion of his superiorly-based C-flap, otherwise used to close the nasal sill.[47,57]

At the side, cphi is carefully chosen to ensure both sufficient lip height (sbal-cphi) and advancement flap dimensions that fill the upper medial lip rotation deficit. A more medially selected cphi results in a more deficient white roll, vermillion, and mucosa; collectively limiting the fullness of the median tubercle. A more laterally selected cphi gives better quality tissues and more vertical (but less horizontal) lip length. Using the Noordhoff point maximizes the quality of incorporated labial tissues, but does not guarantee adequate vertical height.[58] Cleft surgeons generally tolerate less horizontal lip (cphi-ch) with potential vermillion thinning to avoid the more noticeable asymmetry of vertical lip deficiency (sbal-cphi).[2,59] Millard[57] emphasized aggressive lateral dissection to ensure adequate lateral lip advancement. He even modified his original design by extending the transverse incision around the cleft ala.

No technique has been more widely adopted and modified than Millard's rotation-advancement. In a 2005 worldwide survey of leading cleft centers, 84% of surgeons used some variation of rotation-advancement to repair unilateral clefts.[60] Several noteworthy modifications now provide cleft surgeons a variety of tools to customize desired elements of nasolabial repair. In 1987, Mohler[61] introduced the concept of using columella to lengthen the medial lip (cleft cphi-cphs). Instead of the traditional backcut through the upper philtrum, Mohler's[61] rotation incision extends onto the columella and a backcut is made to the lip-columellar junction (see **Fig. 5**). Cutting popularized a similar technique; his incision is less bowed toward the cleft margin and extends up onto the columella 1.5 to 2.0 mm above the nasolabial junction and just past midline.[59] Cutting's lip repair allows a wider C-flap to fill the medial defect and results in a near–straight-line anatomic closure. Detailed, step-by-step videos and simulations demonstrating this technique are publically available (https://smile-train.biodigitalhuman.com/home). Stal uses an S-shaped rotation incision to gain medial lip height; he extends onto the columella and uses a backcut when needed.[62] Like Mohler, Mulliken's rotation incision is curved toward the cleft margin and extends into the columella.[51] However, instead of a backcut toward noncleft cphs, Mulliken uses a perpendicular releasing incision further up the columella into which the C-flap is inset (lengthening cleft-side sn-c). Because there is a smaller upper lip rotation defect, Mulliken's advancement flap neither crosses nor effaces the philtral column (see **Fig. 5**).[51,62]

Millard[56,63] introduced the concept of using a flap of lateral lip medial to cphi to augment the deficient median tubercle. Noordhoff[11] further defined this flap as a unilimb Z-plasty of available lateral lip vermillion that is inset as a taper into a releasing incision at the cleft mucovermillion junction. Mulliken and Cutting both use a variation of this Noordhoff flap.[51,59] Millard[57,64] stressed interdigitation of flaps at the vermillion-cutaneous junction to avoid the more conspicuous effects of linear scar contracture. Mulliken uses a unilimb Z-plasty to introduce a small triangle carrying skin and white roll medial to cphi of the lateral lip into a 2.0-mm to 2.5-mm vertical defect created by a releasing incision along the vermillion-cutaneous junction of the medial lip (see **Fig. 5**).[51]

Millard pioneered many aspects of primary nasal repair during rotation-advancement. He designed his C-flap to assist in closure of the nasal floor/sill, emphasized maneuvers to correct the deviated septum and asymmetric columella, and divided the lateral cleft element into a labial advancement flap (to narrow sn-al) and a separate alar base flap (for nasal floor closure and 3D flexibility).[56,57,63,64] Millard[56,63,64] dissected the nasal soft tissue envelope off the lower lateral cartilages and elevated the cleft nasal mucosa off the piriform to allow anterior movement. Byrd maintains a muscular roll under the cleft alar base that he sutures to periseptal tissues to augment the deficient maxilla and build a platform that projects the cleft ala.[36] McComb, Salyer, and Cutting reposition and suspend the lower lateral cartilage with internal sutures,[45,59,62] and Stal uses a transdermal alar suspension technique.[65] Mulliken straightens and fixates the deviated anterocaudal septum during primary repair and includes the medial crural footplate with his C-flap to correct columellar asymmetry.[51] By placing a suture from the medial alar base to underlying periosteum of the lateral incisor fossa, Mulliken prevents alar creep and restores the native (z-axis) depression of the nasal sill. Mulliken uses a semiopen technique with bilateral marginal rim incisions to dissect soft tissue off both lower lateral cartilages and the ipsilateral upper lateral cartilage; interdomal and intercartilaginous resorbable sutures internally suspend the cleft ala into an overcorrected position.[51]

Anatomic Subunit Repair

Fisher[66] recently introduced a geometric repair that places the line of closure between anatomic subunits, eliminating scars on or below the columella (see **Fig. 5**). The design requires identification of 25 anatomic landmarks and relies heavily on direct anthropometry.[8] Central and noncleft landmarks supply normal anthropometrics from which corresponding cleft-side landmarks are derived. Although it requires extensive attention to detail, this technique emphasizes anatomic geometry rather than surgeon experience to produce reliable results.

Identification of sn and noncleft cphs determines cleft cphs. While manually correcting the nose, 2 noncleft alar landmarks are identified: sbal and the alar insertion point (junction of ala and nasal sill). An arbitrary point within the normal nasal sill is chosen that is collinear with these two points as well as with sn/noncleft cphs (Tse). Mirroring the distance between this point and the noncleft alar insertion point determines the superiormost aspect of the lateral lip incision; mirroring the distance between this point and noncleft cphs determines the superiormost aspect of the medial lip incision. Uniting these superior points corrects the cleft nasal sill.

The incision runs medially from this established superiormost point of closure within the cleft nasal sill down the base of the cleft-side medial crural footplate to cleft cphs and then straight down to the white roll atop cphi. The incision continues perpendicular to the white roll and red line and then toward the gingivobuccal sulcus. The incision is designed laterally between 2 fixed landmarks: the previously established superiormost point of closure within the cleft nasal sill and the Noordhoff point (cphi). Between these two points, 3 elements are designed to match the medial lip's line of closure. First, a limb is drawn matching the length and curvature of the medial lip's incision along the medial crural footplate; the end of this limb establishes cphs laterally. Second, the lateral philtral column is traced, matching the medial lip's cphs-cphi length. Third, a small triangular flap is designed for inset into a backcut above the medial lip white roll; its base measures the deficiency between cleft and noncleft philtral heights (minus 1 mm to account for the Rose-Thompson effect). In contrast with preset medial lip markings, the 3 components of the lateral lip incision are tailored to each patient depending on lateral lip height and cleft severity.[66] For lesser form clefts, the small lateral triangle can be omitted. Fisher[66] also uses a unilimb Z-plasty to incorporate lateral lip vermillion medial to Noordhoff point into the deficient median tubercle (see **Fig. 5**).

POSTOPERATIVE CARE

Most cleft surgeons admit infants overnight for observation following nasolabial repair. However, a 2009 review of 23 US children's hospitals showed that 28% of patients are discharged on the day of surgery; on average such children are older, without comorbidities, and treated in higher-volume cleft centers.[67] To protect the lip and nose from traumatic dehiscence, most surgeons use a variety of tools from elbow restraints to the Logan bow.[68–72] Video surveillance shows that, without arm restraints, young infants touch their lips, but do so innocuously.[73] Large retrospective series show no complications and some cost savings by forgoing restraints.[74,75] Postoperative nutrition is essential but care must be taken to protect the repair while feeding. Special cleft nipples (eg, Haberman feeder) can be helpful, and surgeon preference decides return to breast-feeding. In Asian centers, nasal stenting for 3 to 6 months is shown to improve long-term nasal symmetry but requires motivated, compliant caregivers.[38,76] Long-term nasal stenting is less

popular in the United States and is currently being studied at our institution and others.

TRENDS AND CONTROVERSIES

Presurgical molding of the unilateral cleft defect is either active or passive and can include or preclude the nose. There is debate regarding potential growth disturbance from these devices,[77–80] which is discussed elsewhere in this issue. Nevertheless, nasal and/or alveolar molding effectively aligns the maxillary elements, facilitating nasolabial repair and permitting gingivoperiosteoplasty (GPP). The GPP, as described by Skoog[81] and modified by Latham and Millard,[82,83] creates a gingivoperiosteal tunnel that bridges the cleft alveolar segments; this environment supports bridging bone and critical bone generation around the tooth roots mesial and distal to the cleft.[82,83] When accomplished, primary GPP reduces the need for,[84] and improves results from,[85] secondary alveolar bone grafting. Furthermore, it stabilizes the alveolar segments, eliminates fistulas, and enables eruption of the primary dentition.[85] Some argue that primary GPP restricts maxillary growth[77–80]; our long-term analysis shows no significant midfacial growth restriction up to the age of puberty.[86,87]

Repair of the unilateral cleft nasal deformity is a four-dimensional challenge.[2] Some surgeons think that operative scarring compromises the final result and, therefore, advocate minimum nasal intervention until after skeletal maturity and orthognathic correction. Others advocate early correction of nasal asymmetries and take advantage of all available opportunities to restore nasal anatomy. For example, Mulliken straightens and fixates the caudal septum, closes the nasal floor, recreates the multidimensional nasal sill, (over)corrects sn-al distance, (over)suspends the dislocated lower lateral cartilage, and discards excess vestibular tissue.[51] These maneuvers during primary nasolabial repair help maximize long-term outcome and minimize later rhinoplasty revisions.[51]

Many surgical outreach organizations participate in cleft lip repair; each has a unique governing philosophy, organizational structure, and method of assessing quality and safety. Little has been reported on the frequency of emergency scenarios, near-miss events, or adverse outcomes encountered by the multitude of surgical humanitarian outreach providers. In 1999, Operation Smile reported 18 deaths while treating 50,000 patients (0.04% mortality).[88] In 2002, the International task Force collectively evaluated 10 large overseas cleft surgery organizations having treated

3500 total patients and reported that 7 groups experienced notable morbidities (unspecified) whereas 2 reported a combined 4 mortalities (0.11% mortality).[89] Quality assurance guidelines and emergency response protocols have recently been established to promote the highest level of care in overseas cleft outreach.[90–92] In addition to optimizing patient care and safety, enforcing quality standards and ensuring emergency preparedness deliver a strong message of compassion to host nations that builds trust, provides additional credibility to surgical outreach teams, and bolsters existing partnerships.[92]

ASSESSING OUTCOMES OF NASOLABIAL REPAIR

Dentoalveolar and nasolabial impressions are taken in our office before nasoalveolar molding, in the operating room at the time of nasolabial repair, and again in the operating room at the time of palate repair. From these impressions, stone casts are constructed to allow direct anthropometry and assessment of nasolabial shape and symmetry. More recently, we have begun using 3D photography to document nasolabial morphology. Using validated software, indirect anthropometric measurements are made with high fidelity and new metrics are possible (nostril diameter, nostril surface area). At a minimum, 3D photographs are taken before nasoalveolar molding, 6 months after nasolabial repair, and as the child approaches school age. In addition to adding to the medical record, routine photogrammetric assessment enables review (and modification, if necessary) of the surgical technique and provides the potential for improved outcomes.

SUMMARY

Modern cleft surgery requires four-dimensional and functional anatomic understanding of the cleft (and noncleft) lip, nose, and alveolus. Some techniques for nasolabial repair rely more on precise anatomic geometry, whereas others afford the surgeon a more flexible design. Consistent anthropometry enables accurate assessment and reporting of long-term outcomes; such reports are needed to guide perioperative care, delineate optimal repair principles, and resolve ongoing controversies.

REFERENCES

1. Perko M. The history of treatment of cleft lip and palate. Prog Pediatr Surg 1986;20:238–51.
2. Mulliken JB, LaBrie RA. Fourth-dimensional changes in nasolabial dimensions following rotation-advancement repair of unilateral cleft lip. Plast Reconstr Surg 2012;129(2):491–8.
3. Mossey PA, Little J, Munger RG, et al. Cleft lip and palate. Lancet 2009;374(9703):1773–85.
4. Diewert VM. Development of human craniofacial morphology during the late embryonic and early fetal periods. Am J Orthod 1985;88(1):64–76.
5. Kirschner RE, LaRossa D. Cleft lip and palate. Otolaryngol Clin North Am 2000;33(6):1191–215.
6. Tapadia MD, Cordero DR, Helms JA. It's all in your head: new insights into craniofacial development and deformation. J Anat 2005;207(5):461–77.
7. Grabb WC. Grabb and Smith's plastic surgery. 6th edition. New York: Lippincott Williams & Wilkins; 2006. p. 201–24.
8. Tse R. Unilateral cleft lip: principles and practice of surgical management. Semin Plast Surg 2012;26: 145–55.
9. Latham RA, Deaton TG. The structural basis of the philtrum and the contour of the vermilion border: a study of the musculature of the upper lip. J Anat 1976;121(Pt 1):151–60.
10. Nicolau PJ. The orbicularis oris muscle: a functional approach to its repair in the cleft lip. Br J Plast Surg 1983;36(2):141–53.
11. Noordhoff MS. Reconstruction of vermilion in unilateral and bilateral cleft lips. Plast Reconstr Surg 1984;73(1):52–61.
12. Dado DV, Kernahan DA. Anatomy of the orbicularis oris muscle in incomplete unilateral cleft lip based on histological examination. Ann Plast Surg 1985; 15(2):90–8.
13. De Mey A, Van Hoof I, De Roy G, et al. Anatomy of the orbicularis oris muscle in cleft lip. Br J Plast Surg 1989;42(6):710–4.
14. Stenstrom SJ, Oberg TR. The nasal deformity in unilateral cleft lip: some notes on its anatomic bases and secondary operative treatment. Plast Reconstr Surg 1961;28(3):295–305.
15. McComb H. Primary correction of unilateral cleft lip nasal deformity: a 10-year review. Plast Reconstr Surg 1995;75(6):791–7.
16. Blair VP. Nasal deformities associated with congenital cleft of the lip. JAMA 1925;84:185–7.
17. Li AQ, Sun YG, Wang GH, et al. Anatomy of the nasal cartilages of the unilateral complete cleft lip nose. Plast Reconstr Surg 2002;109(6):1835–8.
18. Kernahan DA, Stark RB. A new classification for cleft lip and cleft palate. Plast Reconstr Surg Transplant Bull 1958;22(5):435–41.
19. Kernahan DA. The striped Y – a symbolic classification for cleft lip and palate. Plast Reconstr Surg 1971;47(5):469–70.
20. Sandham A. Classification of clefting deformity. Early Hum Dev 1985;12(1):81–5.
21. Smith AW, Khoo AK, Jackson IT. A modification of the Kernahan "Y" classification in cleft lip and

palate deformities. Plast Reconstr Surg 1998; 102(6):1842–7.

22. Kriens O. LAHSHAL: an easy system of cleft lip alveolus and palate documentation. In: Kriens O, editor. Proceedings of the advanced workshop "what is a cleft?". Stuttgart (Germany): G Thieme; 1989. p. 30–4.

23. Gibson T. Gustav Simon (1824–1876): Simonart(s)(z) of the band? Br J Plast Surg 1977; 30(4):255–60.

24. Da Silva Filho OG, Santamaria M Jr, da Silva Dalben G, et al. Prevalence of a Simonart's band in patients with complete cleft lip and alveolus and complete cleft lip and palate. Cleft Palate Craniofac J 2006;43(4):442–5.

25. Veau V. Bec-de lievre: formes cliniques-chirurgie (avec la collaboration de J. Recamier). Paris: Masson et Cie; 1938.

26. Cosman B, Crickelair GF. The minimal cleft lip. Plast Reconstr Surg 1966;37(4):334–40.

27. Lehman JA, Artz JS. The minimal cleft lip. Plast Reconstr Surg 1976;58(3):306–9.

28. Heckler FR, Oesterle LG, Jabalay ME. The minimal cleft lip revisited: clinical and anatomic corrections. Cleft Palate J 1979;16(3):240–7.

29. Chen PK, Yeow VK, Noordhoff MS, et al. Augmentation of the nasal floor with surgical in primary lip repair: a prospective study showing no efficacy. Ann Plast Surg 1999;42(2):149–53.

30. Yuzuriha S, Mulliken JB. Minor-form, microform, and mini-microform cleft lip: anatomical features, operative techniques, and revisions. Plast Reconstr Surg 2008;122(5):1485–93.

31. Farkas LG. Anthropometry of the head and face. New York: Raven Press; 1994.

32. Farkas LG, Posnick JC, Hreczko TM, et al. Growth patterns of the nasolabial region: a morphometric study. Cleft Palate Craniofac J 1992;29:318–24.

33. Mulliken JB, Burvin R, Farkas LG. Repair of bilateral complete cleft lip: intraoperative nasolabial anthropometry. Plast Reconstr Surg 2001;107: 307–14.

34. Wong JY, Oh AK, Ohta E, et al. Validity and reliability of craniofacial anthropometric measurement of 3D digital photogrammetric images. Cleft Palate Craniofac J 2008;45:232–9.

35. Millard DR Jr. Earlier correction of the unilateral cleft lip nose. Plast Reconstr Surg 1982;70:64–73.

36. Byrd HS, Salomon J. Primary correction of the unilateral cleft nasal deformity. Plast Reconstr Surg 2000;106:1276–86.

37. Farkas LG, Hajnis K, Posnick JC. Anthropometric and anthroposcopic findings of the nasal and facial region in cleft patients before and after primary lip and palate repair. Cleft Palate Craniofac J 1993;30: 1–12.

38. Chang CS, Por YC, Liou EJ, et al. Long-term comparison of four techniques for obtaining nasal symmetry in unilateral complete cleft lip patients: a single surgeon's experience. Plast Reconstr Surg 2010;125:1276–84.

39. Wong GB, Burvin R, Mulliken JB. Resorbable internal splint: an adjunct to primary correction of unilateral cleft lip-nasal deformity. Plast Reconstr Surg 2002;110:385–91.

40. Barillas I, Dec W, Warren SM, et al. Nasoalveolar molding improves long-term nasal symmetry in complete unilateral cleft lip-cleft palate patients. Plast Reconstr Surg 2009;123:1002–6.

41. Gatti GL, Lazzeri D, Romeo G, et al. Effect of lip adhesion on maxillary arch alignment and reduction of a cleft's width before definitive cheilognathoplasty in unilateral and bilateral complete cleft lip. Scand J Plast Reconstr Surg Hand Surg 2010; 44(2):88–95.

42. Rintala A, Haataja J. The effect of the lip adhesion procedure on the alveolar arch. With special reference to the type and width of the cleft and the age at operation. Scand J Plast Reconstr Surg Hand Surg 1979;13(2):301–4.

43. Scrimshaw GC. Lip adhesion – a passing fad? Ann Plast Surg 1979;2(3):183–8.

44. Anderl H, Hussl H, Ninkovic M. Primary simultaneous lip and nose repair in the unilateral cleft lip and palate. Plast Reconstr Surg 2008;121(3): 959–70.

45. Salyer KE, Xu H, Genecov ER. Unilateral cleft lip and nose repair; closed approach Dallas protocol completed patients. J Craniofac Surg 2009; 20(Suppl 2):1939–55.

46. Hamilton R, Graham WP III, Randall P. The role of the lip adhesion procedure in cleft lip repair. Cleft Palate J 1971;8:1–9.

47. Millard DR. Cleft craft. the evolution of its surgery, volume 1: the unilateral deformity. Philadelphia: Lippincott Williams & Wilkins; 1976.

48. Randall P. In defense of lip adhesion. Ann Plast Surg 1979;3(3):290–1.

49. Ridgway EB, Estroff JA, Mulliken JB. Thickness of orbicularis oris muscle in unilateral cleft lip: before and after labial adhesion. J Craniofac Surg 2011; 22(5):1822–6.

50. Tennison CW. The repair of the unilateral cleft lip by the stencil method. Plast Reconstr Surg 1952;9(2): 115–20.

51. Mulliken JB, Martinez-Perez D. The principle of rotation advancement for repair of unilateral complete cleft lip and nasal deformity: technical variations and analysis of results. Plast Reconstr Surg 1999;104(5):1247–60.

52. Randall P. A triangular flap operation for the primary repair of unilateral clefts of the lip. Plast Reconstr Surg Transplant Bull 1959;23(4):331–47.

53. Cronin TD. A modification of the Tennison-type lip repair. Cleft Palate J 1966;3:376–82.

54. Brauer RO, Cronin TD. The Tennison lip repair revisited. Plast Reconstr Surg 1983;71(5):633–42.

55. Brauer RO, Wolf LE. Design for unilateral cleft lip repair to prevent a long lip. Plast Reconstr Surg 1978;61(2):190–7.

56. Millard DR Jr. A radical rotation in single harelip. Am J Surg 1958;95(2):318–22.

57. Millard DR Jr. Extensions of the rotation-advancement principle for wide unilateral cleft lips. Plast Reconstr Surg 1968;42(6):535–44.

58. Boorer CJ, Cho DC, Vijayasekaran VS, et al. Presurgical unilateral cleft lip anthropometrics: implications for the choice of repair technique. Plast Reconstr Surg 2011;127(2):774–80.

59. Cutting CB, Dayan JH. Lip height and lip width after extended Mohler unilateral cleft lip repair. Plast Reconstr Surg 2003;111(1):17–23 [discussion: 24–6].

60. Weinfeld AB, Hollier LH, Spira M, et al. International trends in the treatment of cleft lip and palate. Clin Plast Surg 2005;32:19–23.

61. Mohler LR. Unilateral cleft lip repair. Plast Reconstr Surg 1987;80(4):511–7.

62. Stal S, Brown RH, Higuera S, et al. Fifty years of the Millard rotation-advancement: looking back and moving forward. Plast Reconstr Surg 2009;123(4):1364–7.

63. Millard DR Jr. Complete unilateral clefts of the lip. Plast Reconstr Surg 1960;25:595–605.

64. Millard DR Jr. Refinements in rotation-advancement cleft lip technique. Plast Reconstr Surg 1964;33:26–38.

65. Stal S, Hollier LH. Correction of secondary deformities of the cleft lip nose. Plast Reconstr Surg 2002;109:1386–92.

66. Fisher DM. Unilateral cleft lip repair: an anatomical subunit approximation technique. Plast Reconstr Surg 2005;116(1):61–71.

67. Hopper RA, Lewis C, Umbdenstock R, et al. Discharge practices, readmission, and serious medical complications following primary cleft lip repair in 23 U.S. children's hospitals. Plast Reconstr Surg 2009;123(5):1553–9.

68. Nagy K, Mommaerts MY. Postoperative wound management after cleft lip surgery. Cleft Palate Craniofac J 2011;48(5):584–6.

69. Muraoka M, Taniguchi T, Harada T. A restraining device of elbow flexion made from flowerpot bottle net. Plast Reconstr Surg 2002;110(1):368.

70. Serel S, Can Z, Yormuk E. Arm restraint in children with cleft lip and palate. Plast Reconstr Surg 2003;112(2):712 [author reply: 712].

71. Sommerlad BC, Kangesu T. Arm restraint in children with cleft lip/palate. Plast Reconstr Surg 2003;112(1):331–2 [author reply: 332].

72. Skoll PJ, Lazarus DA. Arm restraint in children with cleft lip and palate. Plast Reconstr Surg 2004;113(5):1523.

73. Tokioka K, Park S, Sugawara Y, et al. Video recording study of infants undergoing primary cheiloplasty: are arm restraints really needed? Cleft Palate Craniofac J 2009;46(5):494–7.

74. Michelotti B, Long RE, Leber D, et al. Should surgeons use arm restraints after cleft surgery? Ann Plast Surg 2012;69(4):387–8.

75. O'rlain S. Cleft lip surgery without postoperative restraints. Br J Plast Surg 1977;30(2):140–1.

76. Yeow VK, Chen PK, Chen YR, et al. The use of nasal splints in the primary management of unilateral cleft nasal deformity. Plast Reconstr Surg 1999;103(5):1347–54.

77. Berkowitz SA. Comparison of treatment results in complete bilateral cleft lip and palate using a conservative approach versus Millard-Latham PSOT procedure. Semin Orthod 1996;2:169–84.

78. Berkowitz SA. Apoplectic or apocalyptic? [Letter]. J Oral Maxillofac Surg 2001;59:1252–4.

79. Berkowitz SA. Primary repair of cleft lip and nasal deformity [Letter]. Plast Reconstr Surg 2002;109:2158–61.

80. Henkel KO, Gundlach KK. Analysis of primary gingivoperiosteoplasty in alveolar cleft repair. Part I: facial growth. J Craniomaxillofac Surg 1997;25(5):266–9.

81. Skoog T. The use of periosteal flaps in the repair of clefts of the primary palate. Cleft Palate J 1965;2:332–9.

82. Millard DR Jr, Latham RA. Improved primary surgical and dental treatment of clefts. Plast Reconstr Surg 1990;86(5):856–71.

83. Millard DR Jr, Latham RA, Huifen X, et al. Cleft lip and palate treated by presurgical orthopedics, gingivoperiosteoplasty, and lip adhesion (POPLA) compared with previous lip adhesion method: a preliminary study of serial dental casts. Plast Reconstr Surg 1999;103(6):1630–44.

84. Santiago PE, Grayson BH, Cutting CB, et al. Reduced need for alveolar bone grafting by presurgical orthopedics and primary gingivoperiosteoplasty. Cleft Palate Craniofac J 1998;35(1):77–80.

85. Sato Y, Grayson BH, Garfinkle JS, et al. Success rate of gingivoperiosteoplasty with and without secondary bone grafts compared with secondary alveolar bone grafts alone. Plast Reconstr Surg 2008;121(4):1356–67.

86. Wood RJ, Grayson BH, Cutting CB. Gingivoperiosteoplasty and midfacial growth. Cleft Palate Craniofac J 1997;34(1):17–20.

87. Lee CT, Grayson BH, Cutting CB, et al. Prepubertal midface growth in unilateral cleft lip and palate following alveolar molding and gingivoperiosteoplasty. Cleft Palate Craniofac J 2004;41(4):375–80.

88. Magee B. Operation smile. In: Mars M, Habel A, Sell D, editors. Management of cleft lip and palate

in the developing world. 1st edition. West Sussex (United Kingdom): John Wiley; 2008. p. 59–69.

89. Yeow VK, Lee ST, Lambrecht TJ, et al, International Task Force on Volunteer Cleft Missions. International Task Force on Volunteer Cleft Missions. J Craniofac Surg 2002;13(1):18–25.

90. Eberlin KR, Zaleski KL, Snyder D, et al. Quality assurance guidelines for surgical outreach programs: a 20-year experience. Cleft Palate Craniofac J 2008;45(3):246–55.

91. Vyas RM, Eberlin KR, Hamdan US. Implementation of an emergency response protocol for overseas surgical outreach initiatives. Plast Reconstr Surg 2013;131(4):631e–6e.

92. Vyas RM, Eberlin KR, Patel KB, et al. International surgical outreach initiatives: planning, execution, and safety. In: Rogers D, Hartnick CJ, Hamdan US, editors. Video atlas of cleft lip and palate surgery. San Diego (CA): Plural Publishing; 2013. p. 17–38 Print.

Modern Tenets for Repair of Bilateral Cleft Lip

Alexander C. Allori, MD, MPH, Jeffrey R. Marcus, MD*

KEYWORDS

- Bilateral cleft lip • Cleft lip nasal deformity

KEY POINTS

- The functional and aesthetic outcome of bilateral cleft lip should be comparable with (or even surpass) that of repaired unilateral cleft lip.
- Modern tenets of repair include maintaining symmetry; recessing the projecting premaxilla; making accommodations for "fourth-dimensional" changes that occur with growth; constructing a full median tubercle using lateral labial elements; deepening the gingivolabial sulcus using premaxillary mucosa; establishing muscular continuity primarily; and addressing the nasal deformity synchronously.
- Different forms of bilateral cleft lip (eg, symmetric complete, incomplete, and lesser-form; and asymmetric) require different approaches to maintain symmetry.
- Although revisions of the labial repair per se should rarely be needed, small nasolabial adjustments are frequently warranted because of the secondary/tertiary stigmata that develop with growth.

Too many infants born with bilateral cleft lip undergo old-fashioned, often multi-staged, procedures, and later have to endure sundry revisions throughout childhood and adolescence. Despite the surgeon's efforts, the stigmata of the repaired cleft lip and nose remain painfully obvious – even at a distance. To the contrary, ... the appearance of a child with repaired bilateral cleft lip should be comparable to, and in many instances surpass, that of a repaired unilateral cleft lip.

—John B. Mulliken[1]

INTRODUCTION

Bilateral cleft lip (bCL) has been described as the greatest of surgical challenges, and the undertaking of its correction as the most onerous of responsibilities.[2] The rich and varied surgical history[1,3] related to its repair not only illustrates the considerable difficulty of the clinical problem but also stands as a testament to plastic surgery's ingenuity, perseverance, and indomitable spirit in its pursuit for excellence. Early, radical procedures, such as excision of the premaxilla, gave way to premaxillary setback by vomerine ostectomy and ultimately to preoperative repositioning by dentofacial orthopedics. With better understanding of blood supply and tension-reducing maneuvers, staged labial repair yielded to synchronous bilateral repair. Intricate geometric rearrangements (eg, triangular and quadrangular flaps) gave way to simpler straight line (Veau III-type) techniques, and Millard applied rotation-advancement principles. Staged procedures were accomplished safely in single stages. With deeper appreciation for growth characteristics, intentional lengthening of the prolabium (eg, König, Barsky, and others) was discontinued in favor of carefully designed, narrow philtral flaps. The relative inattention initially given to the cleft nasal deformity, other than columellar lengthening, has gradually given way to primary nasal correction and even to preoperative manipulation (ie, by nasoalveolar molding). It is by reading these stories that many important insights can

Division of Plastic, Maxillofacial & Oral Surgery, Duke Cleft and Craniofacial Center, Duke Children's Hospital, 200 Trent Drive, Erwin Road, Durham, NC 27710, USA
* Corresponding author.
E-mail address: jeffrey.marcus@duke.edu

be gleaned. For the so-inclined, excellent histories have been recounted by Millard[3] and Mulliken.[1]

Over time, there emerged a relative consensus regarding the goals, design principles, and operative strategies concerning bCL and nasal deformity. This article summarizes the contemporary approach. The article focuses on primary repair and related revisions. Palatal repair, alveolar bone grafting, and other aspects that complete the spectrum of care for these patients are presented elsewhere in this issue.

CONTEMPORARY PRINCIPLES

As operative strategies and techniques for repair of bCL have evolved over the last 30 years, various precepts have been clarified.[4–8] These can be distilled into the following tenets for repair of the bCL:

1. Maintain (or establish) symmetry
2. Prepare the projecting premaxilla
3. Anticipate fourth-dimensional changes that occur with growth
4. Construct a full central lip using lateral labial elements and discard prolabial vermilion
5. Deepen the gingivolabial sulcus using premaxillary mucosa
6. Establish muscular continuity primarily
7. Address the nasal deformity synchronously

Maintain (or Establish) Symmetry

Mulliken has famously written that symmetry is the one advantage that bCL has over its unilateral counterpart.[9] Accordingly, symmetry takes pride of place as the quintessential guiding principle.

Staged repair of each side was once advocated to reduce tension on the lip, but it necessarily destroys the symmetry. Consequently, this practice should be abandoned in favor of synchronous bilateral repair.[10] The exception to this rule is the asymmetric bCL, for which various strategies exist to improve symmetry first before undertaking labial repair.[11–13] For example, in the case of a complete with incomplete CL, a nasolabial adhesion should first be performed on the greater (complete) side (in essence converting it to a symmetric bilateral incomplete CL) before attempting definitive cheiloplasty in a secondary stage.

Symmetry must be maintained throughout all stages of operative treatment; even small imperfections may become more noticeable with later growth, requiring further revisions.

Prepare the Projecting Premaxilla

The projecting premaxilla makes tension-free lip closure difficult and makes establishment of muscular continuity impossible. Recession of the premaxilla was advocated by Cronin[14] and Monroe,[15] among others. History credits Desault in the late eighteenth century with preoperative preparation of the premaxilla by way of linen bandages that applied external pressure over time.[1] This might be considered the precedent for the modern process of dentofacial orthopedics, of which there are two principal methods: passive processes, such as nasoalveolar molding[16–18]; and use of active devices, such as pin-retained (Georgiade-Latham) appliances.[19,20] The merits and demerits of passive and active dentofacial orthopedics are controversial and lie beyond the scope of this article, but they are considered elsewhere in this issue (see the article on nasoalveolar molding in this issue). Regardless of the method used, preoperative repositioning of the premaxilla is critical to establishing symmetry, narrowing the alveolar gap, and aligning the alveolar arches, and thus is quintessential to permitting tension-free closure of the lip, completion of the gingivoperiosteoplasty, and closure of the primary palate.

Anticipate Fourth-Dimensional Changes that Occur with Growth

Straight-line labial repairs (eg, Veau III, Manchester[2]) preserved all or most of the prolabial skin, resulting in an excessively wide central segment. Millard later reduced the width to better simulate a "natural" philtral column, preserving the remainder of the prolabial skin as forked flaps.[21,22] However, with growth over time, the result was still a wide, shield-shaped philtrum that is one of the major secondary nasolabial stigmata.

Recent advances in the study of facial growth have not only explained this occurrence but also helped develop strategies to compensate for these changes. Using direct anthropometry, Farkas and coworkers[23] studied craniofacial growth in developmentally normal white children aged 1 to 18 years (albeit in cross-sectional, not longitudinal, fashion). His findings reveal that some facial features are fast-growing, attaining near-adult size by age 5 years, whereas others are slow-growing. Nearly all nasolabial landmarks are fast-growing, with the notable exception of two slow-growing features: columellar length and nasal tip projection. However, philtral width (and lip in general) is a fast-growing structure. If the philtral flap is designed with normal dimensions, by age 5 years it will have widened 2.5-fold superiorly (crista philtri superioris–crista philtri superioris) and two-fold inferiorly (crista philtri inferioris–crista philtri inferioris).[4]

Consequently, the surgeon should make accommodations for these relative growth characteristics by undercorrecting fast-growing structures and overcorrecting slow-growing structures. Mulliken[5] discusses this at length and says that CL and nasal deformity should be corrected "in three-dimensions based on knowledge of anticipated changes in the fourth-dimension." Also, see the article on nasoalveolar molding and the article on cleft nasal deformity and its treatment elsewhere in this issue.

Construct a Full Central Lip Using Lateral Labial Elements and Discard Prolabial Vermilion

One notable exception to the preceding rule is the median tubercle. Although it is a fast-growing structure in the normal child, it becomes slow-growing in the operated lip. Therefore, the vermilion and median tubercle specifically should be treated as a slow-growing structure and overcorrected.[24]

Because the prolabial vermilion is thin and insufficient, it should be discarded; techniques that preserve it (eg, Manchester) should not be used because they create a "whistle deformity," one of the more striking secondary stigmata of bCL. Rather, the central lip should be constructed from lateral labial elements and made to be as full as possible. To facilitate tension-free closure of the lateral labial elements in the midline, the soft tissue overlying the maxilla should be undermined widely in the supraperiosteal plane.

Deepen the Gingivolabial Sulcus Using Premaxillary Mucosa

Early attempts at bCL repair adapted the techniques of unilateral repair. As such, the lateral labial elements were brought toward the midline to join a prolabium/premaxilla that was largely undisturbed. A consequence of this was that the shallow central gingivolabial sulcus was left uncorrected.

Millard[3] concluded that "methods that accept the prolabium's attachment to premaxilla, of course, never achieve a sulcus." As later operative strategies focused on joining the lateral labial elements in the midline behind an elevated prolabial/philtral flap, the labial mucosa creates a new anterior wall for a deepened central sulcus. To create the posterior wall, premaxillary mucosa is re-draped over the premaxilla and sutured high to the periosteum. The original description of this technique is credited by Millard to DeHaan,[25] although similar methods are also described by

Mulliken and Noordhoff. An excellent history and explanation of the preferred technique was written by Marcus and coworkers.[26]

Establish Muscular Continuity Primarily

Early attempts at establishing continuity of the orbicularis oris muscle were hampered by the projecting premaxilla and could only be accomplished in secondary stages.[1] Modern presurgical premaxillary repositioning simplifies this challenge tremendously. Muscular continuity is essential to function (eg, puckering, whistling) and has significant aesthetic implications.

Address the Nasal Deformity Synchronously

The nasal deformity in bCL is obvious and consists of a broad, flattened nose with widened nostrils, splayed alae, recurvatum of the lower lateral cartilages (LLC), and a short columella.[27] Early efforts either deferred nasal correction entirely or only focused on lengthening the columella by recruiting prolabial tissue (eg, forked flaps),[21,22,28] often in delayed or staged fashion. Eventually, the old perception that "prolabial skin belongs to the columella" was replaced by a new mantra, "the columella is in the nose"[5]; that is, by directly addressing aspects of the nasal deformity per se, the columella can be lengthened. Early proponents of primary correction of the CL nasal deformity include Broadbent and Woolf,[29] McComb,[30,31] Mulliken,[27] Trott and Mohan,[32] and Cutting and coworkers.[33] Both open and semiopen ("closed") approaches have been described, and the use of preoperative nasoalveolar molding. Pigott assessed nasolabial aesthetic outcome of primary nasal correction versus no nasal correction (in unilateral CL) using a panel-based evaluation method, showing significantly improved symmetry and aesthetic outcome with primary repair.[34]

REPAIR OF BILATERAL COMPLETE CLEFT LIP

Contemporary technique for repair of bilateral complete CL in the style of Mulliken[1,4,5,35,36] is presented next. A superb and expertly illustrated explanation of all steps is available.[1] Alternative approaches to bCL repair have also been described by Chen and Noordhoff,[8] Byrd and coworkers,[6] and Monson and coworkers.[37]

Markings

A double-ball retractor placed in the nostrils to gently elevate the nasal tip is useful to preserve symmetry while facilitating visualization. Marking begins with identification of standard anthropometric reference points, including nasion (n), pronasale (prn), columella nasi (c), subnasale (sn), ala nasi (al), subalaris (sbal), labiale superius (ls), crista philtri superioris (cphs), crista philtri inferioris (cphi), stomion (sto), chelion (ch), and endocanthion (en). When taking measurements for symmetry, point sn serves as the main reference for the prolabial markings, and point sbal serves as the main reference for the lateral lip markings. The junction between vermilion and labial mucosa ("red line") should also be indicated with a dotted line (**Fig. 1**).

On the prolabium, the philtral flap is drawn. For a child younger than 1 year of age, the philtral flap should measure 6 to 7 mm in vertical height (sn-ls), which is often the total available height of the cutaneous prolabium. The philtral flap should be made 2-mm wide at its superior aspect (cphs-cphs) and 4-mm wide at its inferior aspect (cphi-cphi), and its sides should bow slightly inward. Extracutaneous prolabium on each side of the philtral flap may be de-epithelialized to create "flanking flaps" measuring approximately 2 to 3 mm in width. These flanking flaps provide the extra bulk needed to simulate a philtral ridge when buried under the advanced lateral labial flaps (for clarity in the markings, the flanking flaps are usually denoted with a striped pattern). The remainder of the prolabial skin and vermilion are discarded. Premaxillary mucosa is used to construct the posterior lining of the gingivolabial sulcus.

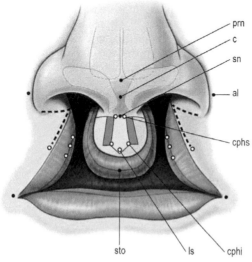

Fig. 1. Markings for the Mulliken repair of bilateral cleft lip. Black dots represent anthropometric points pronasale (prn), subnasale (sn), ala nasi (al), crista philtri superior (cphs), crista philtri inferior (cphi), labiale superius (ls), stomion (sto). Point c marks the highest point on the columella. Open circles mark tattooed dots.

On each lateral lip element, the peak of Cupid's bow (cphi') is placed as far medial as possible where there is still adequate vermilion for the median tubercle and where at least 3 mm of well-defined white roll still exists medially. It is important not to choose a point too medially, where the white roll has already become indistinct or where the vermilion has begun to taper; doing so has been shown to correlate with retained cleft tissue within the repair and poorer aesthetic and functional outcomes.[38] The lateral labial advancement flap on each side is drawn as large as possible, noting that it is trimmed later during inset and closure. It is marked medially following the mucosal-cutaneous junction and inferiorly along the vermilion-cutaneous border, just above the white roll, extending to the marked cphi' point. Superiorly, it curves around the alar base and extends up to, or just beyond, point sbal. It is important that this mark stay just above the crease of the normal alar base-labial junction.

A dilute solution of lidocaine and bupivacaine with epinephrine is infiltrated. Key landmarks (eg, chpi') are tattooed, and a scalpel may be used to score the markings.

Labial Dissection

A mini-blade or #15c scalpel is used to incise the markings of the philtral flap, and the flanking flaps are de-epithelialized. The remaining prolabial skin is discarded. Using a fine double hook and sharp scissors, the philtral flap is elevated (en bloc with the paired flanking flaps) in the subcutaneous plane to the level of the anterior nasal spine.

The lateral labial flaps are incised. Sharp scissors are used to separate the vermilion-mucosal flaps from the musculocutaneous portion. After this is accomplished, sharp dissection is continued beneath the muscle down to the maxilla, and a Tessier elevator is used to widely mobilize the soft tissue in the supraperiosteal plane as far as the malar eminences. Wide mobilization is a critical maneuver to reduce tension on the midline mucosal, muscle, and vermilion closure. Next, the scalpel or sharp scissors are used to dissect free the orbicularis oris muscle from overlying skin and underlying mucosa for a distance of approximately 1 cm.

Closure of the Nasal Floor

Medial and lateral nasal mucosal flaps are elevated from the premaxilla and inferior turbinates, respectively, and closure of the nasal floor is begun. Later in the procedure, the alar base flaps are transposed medially and sutured to the C-flaps, completing the closure of the nasal floor.

Gingivoperiosteoplasty and Mucosal Flap for Deepening of the Gingivolabial Sulcus

Previously, the philtral flap and paired flanking flaps were elevated in the subcutaneous plane, and excess prolabial skin was excised. At this point, the thin strip of prolabial vermilion is removed, and the premaxillary mucosa is cleaned of any residual subcutaneous fat. The gingiva and periosteum of the lateral alveolar segments are then incised vertically, and gingivoperiosteoplasty is performed using chromic suture, beginning posteriorly and proceeding anteriorly. Gentle pressure on the premaxilla may be applied to facilitate closure. Subsequently, the remaining inferiorly based mucosal flap[24] is pulled upward and secured to the premaxillary periosteum using polydioxanone (PDS) suture. This forms the new posterior wall of a deepened gingivolabial sulcus (**Fig. 2**).

Labial Closure

Gentle traction is applied to advance the lateral labial elements toward the midline, and the mucosa is closed using chromic suture, creating the anterior wall of the central sulcus. A small back-cut in the mucosa may be necessary for adequate advancement and tension-free closure.

Orbicularis oris muscle is approximated using PDS suture in simple or horizontal mattress fashion, proceeding from pars marginalis inferiorly toward pars alaris superiorly (**Fig. 3**). The superiormost aspect is sutured using Prolene to the periosteum of the anterior nasal spine.

The vermilion flaps are then approximated using chromic suture beginning at a point 3 mm medial to the tattooed cphi' points on each side. Care must be taken to perfectly align the white roll. Closure proceeds inferiorly down the midline,

trimming excess from the flap to form an adequately sized median tubercle.

Myrtiform Suture

After labial mucosal closure but before approximation of muscle or closure of vermilion, a long PDS suture is placed in the maxillary periosteum on each side medial to the canine fossa and left untied with needle attached (**Fig. 3**). The suture is clamped and placed superolaterally so that muscular repair may be completed. The needle is reloaded, the suture is passed through dermis at the midpoint of the nasal base, and the suture tied. These sutures replicate the function of the myrtiformis or depressor alae nasi mucles, which establish the depressed shape of the nasal floor and oppose alar elevation during smiling.

Nasal Correction

Primary nasal correction is accomplished through a semiopen approach using bilateral rim incisions. Marginal or infracartilaginous incisions used in standard rhinoplasty are also an option but do not allow for excision of redundant skin in the alar domes, a component of the nasal deformity that must be addressed. Rim incisions make this excision easy, but the scars are often visible on close inspection.

Through the rim incisions, scissors are used to dissect between skin and underlying LLC, which are left attached to the underlying nasal mucosa. Dissection continues superiorly to the upper lateral cartilages (ULC) and medially to the contralateral LLC. Fibrofatty tissue is removed, and the cartilages are cleaned for adequate visualization of its parts. The cephalic border of the LLC is disengaged from its pathologic relationship with the ULC.

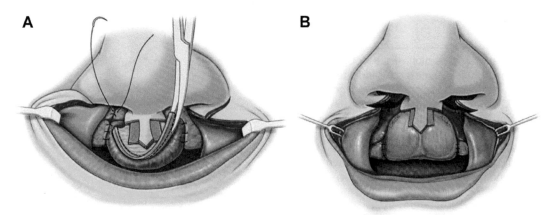

Fig. 2. After completion of the gingivoperiosteoplasty, premaxillary vermilion is trimmed (*A*) and the mucosal flap is sutured to premaxillary periosteum to form the new posterior wall of a deepened gingivolabial sulcus (*B*).

A   B

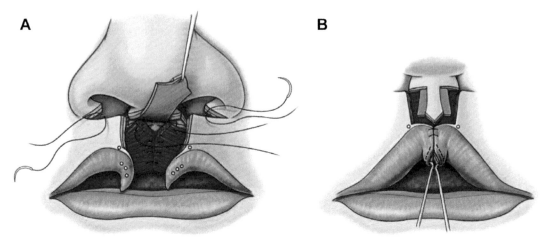

Fig. 3. (A) Orbicularis oris muscle is approximated in the midline, with the superior-most suture placed through the periosteum of the anterior nasal spine. Note the two myrtiform sutures through the nasal floor. (B) Labial closure and trimming of vermilion flaps.

Interdomal reapproximation is accomplished by suturing the genu in horizontal mattress fashion using PDS suture. The LLC is elevated and secured to the ULC with two horizontal mattress stitches to recreate the normal "scroll."

A Prolene cinch suture is used to narrow the interalar distance (al-al) to less than 25 mm. This is slightly smaller than normal for age to compensate for fourth-dimensional widening. The cinch suture is secured to the dermis of the alar base on each side and passed deep to the philtral flap.

Rim incisions are then closed with fine chromic suture. Redundant skin near the soft triangle is removed by crescentic excision. Alar webbing within the nasal vestibule, if present, is addressed through lenticular excision of mucosa.

Note that the principles and techniques used for primary nasal correction are worthy of lengthy discussion and are presented formally elsewhere in this issue in the article on cleft nasal deformity and its treatment.

Skin Closure

To complete the operation, the tip of the philtral flap is inset into Cupid's bow, and the corners joined to the lateral labial flaps at the tattooed cphi' points. Closure is performed in two layers, using 6-0 Vicryl for dermal closure and 7-0 nylon for skin closure. The tip of the lateral labial flaps is trimmed to conform to the shape of the closed nasal sill, and closure is completed in two layers proceeding from lateral to medial (**Fig. 4**).

Postoperative Anthropometry

For documentation and research purposes, the following anthropometric measurements may be recorded[22]: intercanthal distance (en-en), interalar distance (al-al), nasal projection (sn-prn), nasal length (n-sn), columellar length (sn-c), philtral width superiorly (cphs-cphs), philtral width inferiorly (cphi-cphi), philtral height (sn-ls), upper lip height (sn-sto), and median tubercle height (ls-sto).

Postoperative Care

Controversy exists regarding the safety and efficacy of long-term stenting using nasal conformers. It is our practice to place a temporary vented stent (Xeroform gauze wrapped around a 19-gauge

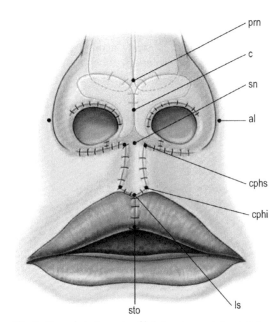

Fig. 4. Completed repair of bilateral complete cleft lip.

angiocatheter tube) in each nostril for 2 days. A Logan bow holds chilled saline-dampened gauze over the wound, changed as needed for 24 hours. This greatly reduces the amount of serosanguinous crusting on the suture line. After 24 hours, the gauze is discontinued, and parents are instructed in gentle wound care. Nylon sutures are removed under anesthesia (mask induction and insufflation) around postoperative Day 5, after which a Steri-Strip is applied across the lip and replaced as need for the next 6 weeks. Elbow immobilizers are used for a total of 4 weeks.

TECHNICAL VARIATIONS

The previous description pertains to bilateral complete CL. Technical modifications may be appropriate for the less-common variants, which include symmetric incomplete, symmetric lesser-form, and asymmetric bCL.

Bilateral Incomplete Cleft Lip

Mulliken and Kim[39] published the results of serial anthropometry in 22 male and 26 female patients with bilateral incomplete CL following repair. Their results confirm that the modern principles described previously hold true in the case of the incomplete bCL, and little variation from the operative technique for complete bCL was necessary. Of note, the prolabium of the incomplete bCL tends to be short, requiring that the philtral flap be designed to use its full height. Despite this effort, the authors note that philtral height (sn-ls) was statistically significantly shorter postoperatively (7.2 mm at 5 months, compared with normal 10.8 ± 1.7 mm) and remained so in the long term (10.4 mm at 9 years, compared with normal 13.3 ± 1.8 mm). Other anthropometric features followed the normal growth curve.

In the bilateral incomplete CL, nasal tip protrusion was found to be near normal[39]; however, other aspects of the cleft nasal deformity were invariably present. Therefore, the authors advocate primary nasal correction in all cases, including elevation of the LLC, interdomal apposition, and narrowing of the interalar distance.

Bilateral Lesser-Form Cleft Lip

The lesser-forms of CL include minor-form, microform, and mini-microform, in decreasing order of severity as defined by the degree of notching and displacement of the vermilion (>3 mm displacement, <3 mm displacement, and discontinuity in vermilion-cutaneous junction without elevation, respectively).[12] The degree of nasal deformity, muscular depression, deficiency of vermilion, and alveolar involvement follow the hierarchy accordingly, with the minor-form being most similar to an incomplete CL.

The operative approach for treatment of lesser-form CL differs from that of a complete or incomplete CL[12]:

1. The most severe of the lesser-forms, minor-form CL, may be treated by an abridged rotation-advancement repair and synchronous correction of the nasal deformity.
2. Microform CL may be treated by double unilimb Z-plasty at the vermilion-cutaneous junction (white roll) and at the vermilion-mucosal junction (red line), and by a dermal graft to augment the philtral ridge. The nasal deformity associated with microform CL is addressed by Y-V-plasty to reduce the alar base width, and semiopen cartilaginous repositioning and tip work, if required.
3. The least severe case, mini-microform CL, is corrected by vertical lenticular excision across the vermilion-cutaneous junction. If there is any degree of nasal deformity, it is amenable to lenticular excision across the nasal sill to narrow the alar base. Cartilaginous repositioning is not required.

In a consecutive case series of lesser-form bCL repair, revisions were required in 8 (73%) of 11 patients with minor-form and 10 (67%) of 15 patients with microform CL; no revisions were required for mini-microform CL.[12] Most commonly, these revisions included augmentation of the philtral ridge using a dermal autograft, trimming of the free mucosal margin, and re-elevation of the LLC.

Asymmetric Bilateral Cleft Lip

Asymmetric bCL occurs when the two clefts differ in severity and thus may be any combination of complete, incomplete, and lesser-form (minor-form, microform, or mini-microform). A retrospective review of 309 patients with bCL found asymmetric bCL in 72 patients (23%).[13] Of these, 32 cases (44%) presented as complete with incomplete CL, 18 cases (25%) as complete with lesser-form CL, and 22 cases (31%) as incomplete with lesser-form CL. Of the 40 patients with a lesser-form CL on one side, seven cases (18%) were minor-form, six cases (15%) were microform, and 27 cases (68%) were mini-microform.[13] For consistency of terminology, the more-severe cleft is referred to as the "greater side," and the less-severe cleft as the "lesser side."

The obvious challenge in asymmetric bCL is the loss of symmetry. Accordingly, the operative decision-making process for asymmetric bCL necessarily entails consideration of how best to re-establish symmetry: synchronously or in a staged fashion. Yuzuriha and colleagues[13] present an elegant decisional tree for planning staged repair based on consideration of the greater and lesser sides:

Greater side:
- All combinations in which the greater side is complete should undergo preliminary dentofacial orthopedics followed by nasolabial adhesion and gingivoperiosteoplasty to convert it to an incomplete form before definitive repair by rotation-advancement.
- All combinations in which the greater side is incomplete do not require dentofacial orthopedics and may proceed straight to definitive repair by rotation-advancement.

Lesser side:
- An incomplete lesser side should undergo synchronous repair by bilateral rotation-advancement following the preliminary nasolabial adhesion on the contralateral complete cleft. In this situation, the nasolabial adhesion[40] converts the greater (complete) side to an incomplete cleft, restoring symmetry and permitting synchronous repair. Preliminary nasolabial adhesion was preferred by the authors over synchronous repair of the complete-with-incomplete bCL.
- A minor-form lesser side should undergo repair synchronously with the greater side. A unilimb Z-plasty may be necessary on the lesser side to compensate for vertical inequality of vermilion. Synchronous repair was preferred by the authors over staged repair (ie, initial definitive repair of the greater side and delayed correction of the minor-form).
- A microform lesser side should undergo delayed double unilimb Z-plasty, after successful repair of the greater side. Because a microform CL lacks a defined Cupid's bow peak, synchronous repair is difficult. It is advisable to repair the microform cleft later by mirroring the neoanatomic landmarks and measurements of the repaired greater side.
- A mini-microform lesser side could be repaired either synchronously or in delayed fashion by vertical lenticular excision.

PREMAXILLARY SETBACK

In some cases, preoperative dentofacial orthopedics is not available or a child may present late when presurgical premaxillary repositioning is no longer an option. If the premaxilla is sufficiently procumbent to preclude tension-free labial closure, the premaxilla must be acutely repositioned by ostectomy and setback.

The need for ostectomy necessarily and significantly changes the treatment plan. Because the ostectomy abrogates one source of blood supply to the premaxilla, the philtral (prolabial) flap should not be elevated. This precludes definitive lip repair. In this circumstance, two options are possible: premaxillary setback with gingivoperiosteoplasty and palatoplasty; or premaxillary setback and intermediary nasolabial adhesion. Definitive labial repair is completed in a secondary stage.

CLEFT LIP REVISIONS

A study of 50 consecutive cases of bCL repair found the overall revision rate to be 33% in bCL and palate and 12% in bCL with or without alveolus (with intact secondary palate).[5] Two revisions were necessary in approximately 25% of the patients who needed revisions (8% of all study subjects). No patients in the study required more than two revisions.

With proper planning and execution of the primary cheiloplasty, revisions of the lip repair itself (ie, cutaneous scars, philtral height/width, columellar length, and so forth) should be extremely rare.

The most common revisions of the lip include the following:

- Central sulcoplasty: The most common revision of all, this entails debulking and resuspension of the mucosa to the premaxillary periosteum.
- Correction of furrowing of the median tubercle: This occurs when the vermilion-mucosal flaps from the lateral labial elements are left too large during closure of the vermilion and creation of the median turbercle.
- Augmentation of the median tubercle: The postoperative median tubercle becomes a slow-growing structure, and may not keep up with the rest of facial growth. This becomes readily apparent in adolescence with eruption of permanent teeth. Dermal graft augmentation of the median tubercle may be performed at the time of alveolar bone grafting.
- Adjustment of the vermilion-cutaneous junction: Asymmetry of Cupid's bow peaks is a relatively rare cause for revision and is corrected by unilimb Z-plasty on the side that needs to be lowered.

Although not technically a revision, excision from a bulky, everted lower lip (the so-called cleft-lip lower-lip deformity) is sometimes warranted to rectify disproportion between the upper and lower lip.[41]

The number of nasal revisions required by adolescence is lower for bilateral CL compared with unilateral CL, where asymmetries are more apparent. Still, nasal tip cartilaginous repositioning by semi-open approach and narrowing of the columella may be necessary. Open, functional septorhinoplasty is commonly required in young adulthood, after completion of midfacial advancement.

SUMMARY

Treatment of bCL has undergone significant evolution during the last 30 years. Its guiding principles are now well-established and accepted, techniques have become refined, and outcomes predictable.

REFERENCES

1. Mulliken JB. Repair of bilateral cleft lip. In: Neligan PC, Rodriguez ED, Losee JE, editors. Plastic surgery, vol. 3. Philadelphia: Saunders-Elsevier Health Sciences; 2012. p. 343–60.
2. Manchester WM. The repair of the bilateral cleft lip and palate. Br J Surg 1965;52:878.
3. Millard DR Jr. Cleft craft: the evolution of its surgery, vol. 2. Boston: Little, Brown & Co; 1977.
4. Mulliken JB. Principles and techniques of bilateral complete cleft lip repair. Plast Reconstr Surg 1985; 75:477–86.
5. Mulliken JB, Wu JK, Padwa BL. Repair of bilateral cleft lip: review, revisions, and reflections. J Craniofac Surg 2003;14:609.
6. Byrd HS, Ha RY, Khosla RK, et al. Bilateral cleft lip and nasal repair. Plast Reconstr Surg 2008;122(4): 1181–90.
7. Noordhoff MS. Bilateral cleft lip reconstruction. Plast Reconstr Surg 1986;78(1):45–54.
8. Chen PK, Noordhoff MS. Bilateral cleft lip and nose repair. In: Losee JE, Kirshner RE, editors. Comprehensive cleft care. New York: McGraw-Hill Professional; 2008. p. 343–60.
9. Mulliken JB. Bilateral cleft lip. Clin Plast Surg 2004; 31(2):209–20.
10. Mulliken JB. Bilateral complete cleft lip and nasal deformity: an anthropometric analysis of staged to synchronous repair. Plast Reconstr Surg 1995;96:9–23.
11. Kim SW, Hyon WS, Kim CW. One stage correction of the severe asymmetric bilateral cleft lip. J Korean Plast Reconstr Surg 1997;24:1283.
12. Yuzuriha S, Mulliken JB. Minor-form, microform, and mini-microform cleft lip: anatomical features, operative techniques, and revisions. Plast Reconstr Surg 2008;122(5):1485–93.
13. Yuzuriha S, Oh AK, Mulliken JB. Asymmetrical bilateral cleft lip: complete or incomplete and contralateral lesser defect (minor-form, microform, or mini-microform). Plast Reconstr Surg 2008; 122(5):1494–504.
14. Cronin TD. Surgery of the double cleft lip and protruding premaxilla. Plast Reconstr Surg 1957;19: 389–400.
15. Monroe CW. Recession of the premaxilla in bilateral cleft lip and palate: a follow-up study. Plast Reconstr Surg 1965;35:512–30.
16. Grayson BH, Cutting CB, Wood R. Preoperative columellar lengthening in bilateral cleft lip and palate. Plast Reconstr Surg 1993;92:1422.
17. Grayson BH, Santiago PE, Brecht LE, et al. Presurgical nasoalveolar molding in infants with cleft lip and palate. Cleft Palate Craniofac J 1999;36(6): 486–98.
18. Grayson BH, Cutting CB. Presurgical nasoalveolar orthopedic molding in primary correction of the lip, and alveolus of infants born with unilateral and bilateral clefts. Cleft Palate Craniofac J 2001;38:193.
19. Georgiade NG, Mason RM, Riefkohl RE, et al. Preoperative positioning of the protruding premaxilla in the bilateral cleft lip patient. Plast Reconstr Surg 1989;83(1):32–8 [discussion: 83(1):39; reply: 84(2): 372–3].
20. Millard DR Jr, Latham RA. Improved primary surgical and dental treatment of clefts. Plast Reconstr Surg 1990;86:856–71.
21. Millard DR Jr. Bilateral cleft lip and a primary forked flap: a preliminary report. Plast Reconstr Surg 1967; 39:59.
22. Millard DR Jr. Closure of bilateral cleft lip and elongation of columella by two operations in infancy. Plast Reconstr Surg 1971;47:324.
23. Farkas LG, Posnick JC, Hreczko TM, et al. Growth patterns of the nasolabial region: a morphometric study. Cleft Palate Craniofac J 1992;29:318.
24. Mulliken JB, Burvin R, Farkas LG. Repair of bilateral complete cleft lip: intraoperative nasolabial anthropometry. Plast Reconstr Surg 2001;107:307–14.
25. DeHaan CR. Initial repair of the cleft lip. In: Stark RB, editor. Cleft palate: a multidiscipline approach. New York: Harper & Row; 1968. p. 128–33.
26. Marcus JR, Fisher DM, Lenz GJ, et al. Inadequate gingivolabial sulcus remains an avoidable problem after bilateral cleft lip repair. Plast Reconstr Surg 2005;115(1):220–5.
27. Mulliken JB. Correction of the bilateral cleft lip nasal deformity: evolution of a surgical concept. Cleft Palate Craniofac J 1992;29:540–5.
28. Cronin TD, Upton J. Lengthening of the short columella associated with bilateral cleft lip. Ann Plast Surg 1978;1:75.
29. Broadbent TR, Woolf RM. Cleft lip nasal deformity. Ann Plast Surg 1984;12:216–34.

30. McComb H. Primary repair of the bilateral cleft lip nose: a 15-year review and a new treatment plan. Plast Reconstr Surg 1990;86:882–93.

31. McComb H. Primary repair of the bilateral cleft lip nose: a 4-year review. Plast Reconstr Surg 1994; 94:37–47.

32. Trott JA, Mohan N. A preliminary report on open tip rhinoplasty at the time of lip repair in bilateral cleft lip and palate: the Alor Setar experience. Br J Plast Surg 1993;46:215–22.

33. Cutting C, Grayson B, Brecht L, et al. Presurgical columellar elongation and primary retrograde nasal reconstruction in one-stage bilateral cleft lip and nose repair. Plast Reconstr Surg 1998;101:630.

34. Cussons PD, Murison MS, Fernandez AE, et al. A panel based assessment of early versus no nasal correction of the cleft lip nose. Br J Plast Surg 1993; 46(1):7–12.

35. Mulliken JB. Mulliken repair of bilateral cleft lip and nasal deformity. In: Losee JE, Kirschner RE, editors. Comprehensive cleft care. New York: McGraw-Hill Medical; 2009. p. 343–60.

36. Mulliken JB. Primary repair of bilateral cleft lip and nasal deformity. Plast Reconstr Surg 2001;108:181–94.

37. Monson LA, Kirschner RE, Losee JE. Primary repair of cleft lip and nasal deformity. Plast Reconstr Surg 2013;132(6):1040e–53e.

38. Losee JE, Selber JC, Arkoulakis N, et al. The cleft lateral lip element: do traditional markings result in secondary deformities? Ann Plast Surg 2003;50(6): 594–600.

39. Mulliken JB, Kim DC. Repair of bilateral incomplete cleft lip: techniques and outcomes. Plast Reconstr Surg 2013;132(4):923–32.

40. Ridgway EB, Estroff JA, Mulliken JB. Thickness of orbicularis oris muscle in unilateral cleft lip: before and after labial adhesion. J Craniofac Surg 2011;22(5): 1822–6.

41. Pensler JM, Mulliken JB. The cleft lip lower-lip deformity. Plast Reconstr Surg 1988;82(4):602–10.

Cleft Palate Repair

Darren M. Smith, MD[a], Joseph E. Losee, MD[b],*

KEYWORDS

- Palatoplasty • Cleft palate repair • Speech surgery

KEY POINTS

- The palate is divided functionally into the hard palate, which provides structural support and is a growth center for the maxilla, and the soft palate, which provides velopharyngeal competence.
- The levator vela palatini muscles are the principal motors of the velar component of velopharyngeal closure.
- In the cleft palate, the levators are positioned *sagittally*, running *posterior to anterior* and inserting onto the posterior edge of the hard palate. This configuration prevents the levator from exerting its upward, backward, and lateral pull.
- Cleft palate repair must include complete release of the levator from its abnormal attachments to the posterior edge of the hard palate medially, the tensor aponeurosis, and the superior constrictor laterally.
- Outcome measures for cleft palate repair include speech quality and palatal integrity.

INTRODUCTION

Human speech is supported by complex anatomic structures and nuanced physiologic processes. A cleft palate is a developmental rent through this system and must be approached in this regard. Palatoplasty is speech surgery. The surgeon addressing a cleft palate must do so with an eye toward repairing the form and function of the dynamic physical structures that work in complex harmony to manipulate air pressure emanating from the respiratory tract into sounds intelligible to others as speech. Herein, the authors begin with a discussion of the anatomy relevant to palatoplasty. Perioperative considerations are then addressed. A broad range of surgical options has evolved over time; these are discussed in their historical context. Next, the authors present a detailed description of their preferred surgical approach. Postoperative care is then described. An examination of recent trends and controversies in the field is then offered. Finally, an approach to outcomes assessment is discussed. It is hoped that this monograph will be of use in guiding others as they embark on the highly challenging, but equally rewarding, task of perfecting the palatoplasty.

PERTINENT ANATOMY

The primary palate includes all structures anterior to the incisive foramen (the premaxilla). The secondary palate comprises the hard palate posterior to the incisive foramen and the soft palate. The muscular soft palate, or velum, is found posterior to the hard palate. Clefts of the secondary palate take the form of a midline bony deficiency resulting in the dissociation of the vomer from the hard palate.[1]

The soft palate may be divided into 3 sections from a functional perspective: the anterior 25%, the middle 50%, and the posterior 25%. In

Disclosures: The authors have nothing to disclose.
[a] Department of Plastic Surgery, University of Pittsburgh, Scaife Hall, Suite 6B, 3550 Terrace Street, Pittsburgh, PA 15261, USA; [b] Pediatric Plastic Surgery, Department of Plastic Surgery, University of Pittsburgh, Scaife Hall, Suite 6B, 3550 Terrace Street, Pittsburgh, PA 15261, USA
* Corresponding author.
E-mail address: joseph.losee@chp.edu

plasticsurgery.theclinics.com

a series of fresh cadaver dissections, Huang and colleagues[2,3] found that fibers of the levator veli palatine occupy the middle 50% of the soft palate. The levators take their origin from the posteromedial aspect of the junction of the cartilaginous and bony segments of the eustachian tube. The left and right levators insert into one another in the palatal midline, forming a sling suspending the soft palate from the cranial base (**Fig. 1**). The levator functions as the motor of the velum.[3] Also in the middle 50% of the soft palate, the palatopharyngeus muscle originates with an inferior head on the oral surface of the levator and a superior head on the nasal surface of the levator and runs inferiorly as the posterior tonsillar pillar.[3,4] Originating from the dorsolateral transverse fibers of the tongue, the palatoglossus travels cephalad as the anterior tonsillar pillar before fanning out to insert in the middle 50% of the soft palate as the most superficial muscle of the velum.[4–7] The anterior 25% of the soft palate is relatively static. Specifically, the tensor veli palatini originates from the greater wing of the sphenoid and the superolateral aspect of the eustachian tube. It then descends nearly vertically to hook around the anterior aspect of the hamulus and inserts into the fibrous tensor aponeurosis in the anterior 25% of the velum (see **Fig. 1**; **Fig. 2**).[2] The palatopharyngeus, palatoglossus, and muscularis

uvulae are found in the posterior 25% of the soft palate. The muscularis uvulae takes its origin at the tensor aponeurosis and courses posteriorly as a paired midline structure to terminate at the base of the uvula.[8]

In the normal palate, the levator forms a muscular sling that suspends the soft palate from the cranial base (see **Fig. 1**A). Running from its origins at the cranial base to its insertion into its partner in the velum, the levator takes a downward, forward, and medial course that facilitates a cranial, posterior, and lateral pull on the soft palate during velopharyngeal closure.[3] In the normal state, the levators take a *transverse course*, running *horizontally* within the middle 50% of the velum, whereas the cleft palate's levators are positioned *sagittally*, running *posterior to anterior* inserting onto the posterior edge of the hard palate. This clefted configuration prevents the levator, the principal motor of the velar component of velopharyngeal closure, from exerting its upward, backward, and lateral pull. Moreover, in the cleft palate, the levator has 3 abnormal associations that must be addressed in repairing the defect: an insertion onto the posterior medial edge of the hard palate, associations with the aponeurosis of the tensor veli palatini, and lateral adhesions to the superior pharyngeal constrictor (see **Fig. 1**B; **Fig. 3**).

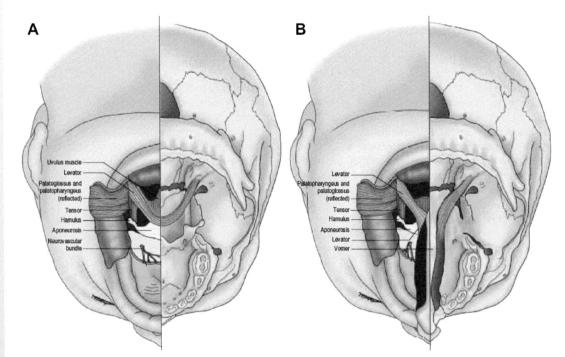

Fig. 1. (*A*) Anatomy of the normal palate. (*B*) Anatomy of the cleft palate. (*From* Losee JE, Smith DM. Cleft palate repair. In: Butler C, editor. Head and neck reconstruction with DVD: a volume in the procedures in reconstructive surgery series. Philadelphia: Saunders Ltd; 2008. p. 271–94; with permission.)

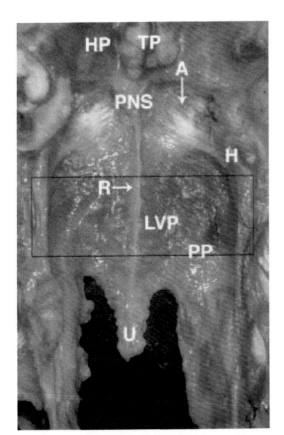

Fig. 2. Dissection of the normal soft palate. Black rectangle denotes middle 50% of velum where levator veli palatini (LVP) resides. A, tensor aponeurosis; H, hamulus; HP, hard palate; LVP, levator veli palatini; PNS, posterior nasal spine; PP, palatopharyngeus; R, midline raphe; TP, torus palatine. (*Data from* Huang MH, Lee ST, Rajendran K. Anatomic basis of cleft palate and velopharyngeal surgery: implications from a fresh cadaveric study. Plast Reconstr Surg 1998;101:613–27; and *From* Losee JE, Smith DM. Cleft palate repair. In: Butler C, editor. Head and neck reconstruction with DVD: a volume in the procedures in reconstructive surgery series. Philadelphia: Saunders Ltd; 2008. p. 271–94; with permission.)

As the levator and tensor take their origins from the eustachian tube, the effects of clefting on this structure must also be considered. Although there is controversy as to whether the tensor or the levator is more significant in tubal dilation, there is likely a synergistic mechanism. In one suggested configuration, the tensor contracts to exert a force on the lateral eustachian tube, dilating the lumen, while the levator rotates the medial lip of the tubal cartilage to optimize the tensor's vector.[4] It stands to reason that the altered morphology of the levator and tensor in the cleft palate may impair their function as tubal dilators.[2]

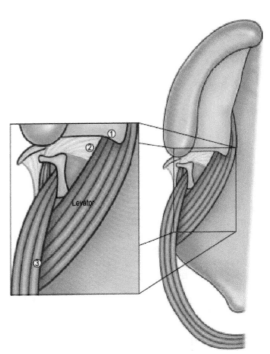

Fig. 3. The cleft levator has 3 abnormal insertions: (1) the hard palate, (2) the tensor aponeurosis, and (3) the superior constrictor. (*From* Losee JE, Smith DM. Cleft palate repair. In: Butler C, editor. Head and neck reconstruction with DVD: a volume in the procedures in reconstructive surgery series. Philadelphia: Saunders Ltd; 2008. p. 271–94; with permission.)

GOALS OF SURGERY

Velopharyngeal competence that supports normal speech production is sine qua non for success in palatoplasty. Velar anatomy must also be restored to maximize eustachian tube function and support hearing, thus minimizing the risk for the development of recurrent otitis media secondary to insufficient tubal dilation and impaired drainage. Nasal air emission and subsequent hypernasality and speech distortion must be obfuscated by a watertight barrier between the oral and nasal cavities. Separating the oral cavity from the nasal cavity will also prevent the nasal regurgitation of fluid and food. A universal requirement essential to all these goals is a tension-free watertight repair of the palate to minimize subsequent scarring and fistula formation (**Fig. 4**).

PATIENT ASSESSMENT AND PERIOPERATIVE CONSIDERATIONS
Timing of the Repair

The palate is divided functionally into the hard palate (serving as structural support and a growth

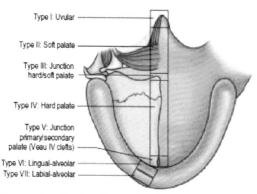

Type I: Uvular
Type II: Soft palate
Type III: Junction hard/soft palate
Type IV: Hard palate
Type V: Junction primary/secondary palate (Veau IV clefts)
Type VI: Lingual-alveolar
Type VII: Labial-alveolar

Fig. 4. The Pittsburgh Fistula Classification System. (*From* Losee JE, Smith DM. Cleft palate repair. In: Butler C, editor. Head and neck reconstruction with DVD: a volume in the procedures in reconstructive surgery series. Philadelphia: Saunders Ltd; 2008. p. 271–94; with permission.)

center for the maxilla) and the soft palate (providing velopharyngeal competence). Because maxillary growth and speech development do not occur in unison, there is disagreement as to the timing of palatoplasty that is most compatible with normal speech development without harming midface growth.[9–14] Some fear that a soft palate cleft persisting past 1 year of age may impair speech development and, therefore, favor early palatoplasty. Those concerned that early palatoplasty may impair midface growth argue for delaying intervention until midface growth is nearing completion.[13] Some address this discrepancy by temporally separating soft palate repair from hard palate repair to uncouple the perceived deleterious effects of a late soft palate repair (impaired speech development) from those of an early hard palate repair (stunted maxillary growth).

The literature on this controversy is difficult to parse because of the variability in surgical timing (3 months to 2 years of age for velum and 6 months to adolescence for hard palate) and technique.[14] Rohrich and colleagues[9,10] detected a statistically significant speech deficiency with delayed (48.6 months) versus early (10.8 months) hard palate closure and no improvements in maxillofacial growth with later repair.[9,10] In a series of 2000 patients, Koberg and Koblin[12] observed that palatoplasty between 8 and 15 years of age caused the greatest degree of maxillary growth disturbance and argued that hard palate repair should be delayed until after 15 years of age. Alternatively, Robertson and Jolleys[14] saw no difference in occlusion or facial profile between patients undergoing palatoplasty from 12 to 15 months of age and those undergoing palatoplasty at 5 years of age. The authors hold that the presently available evidence of impaired midface growth secondary to early

palatoplasty is not sufficiently convincing to justify sacrificing the opportunity to correct soft palate anatomy and facilitate normal speech development with early palatoplasty. These data are also not so robust as to rationalize the additional morbidity and cost associated with a 2-stage repair protocol. It is the authors' standard practice to repair palatal clefts in a single-stage procedure at approximately 1 year of age.

Feeding

Palatal clefts directly affect normal feeding mechanisms: the connection between the oral and nasal cavities permits nasal regurgitation of fluid and food, and swallowing may potentially be affected by velopharyngeal incompetence (VPI). Swallowing difficulties may be addressed by positioning the infant at 45° to 60° from horizontal to exploit gravity during feeding.[15] The clefted velum renders the creation of an intraoral vacuum impossible. A cleft lip in addition to cleft palate yields difficulties in forming a labial seal around the nipple and impairs sucking.

Feedings should be delivered to the posterior portion of the tongue to minimize the infant's dependence on achieving a vacuum.[15] Specialized bottles (Pigeon [Philips Healthcare, Andover, MA] and Haberman feeders [Medela, Inc, McHenry, IL]) are marketed and are designed to allow the caregiver to actively dispense the liquid. Ideally, the infant is weaned entirely from the bottle and drinking from a sippy cup before palatal repair.

Airway Compromise and Pierre Robin Sequence

Patients with cleft palates may preoperatively have airway compromise caused by associated multilevel airway disease. Postoperatively, alterations in airway anatomy secondary to manipulation of the velopharynx or swelling (in the immediate postoperative period) may also result in airway compromise. A thorough evaluation for airway compromise, which may be heralded by episodes of desaturation during feeding or sleep, is mandatory.[16] Should evidence of airway compromise be detected, a complete multilevel examination in conjunction with an otolaryngologist is necessary.[16] The airway in children with Pierre Robin sequence (PRS) is of particular concern. PRS is a constellation of physical findings including posterior displacement of the tongue (glossoptosis), a receding mandible (retrognathia), and resulting compromise of the airway.[17] The U-shaped palatal clefts frequently seen with this condition are thought to result from the retropositioned mandible and posteriorly displaced tongue interfering with the fusion of the palatal shelves (Editor note: PRS is discussed in the article "Surgical Considerations in Pierre Robin Sequence" elsewhere in this issue by Justine Lee and James P. Bradley).[18]

CURRENT PRACTICE AND ITS ORIGINS
Repair of the Hard Palate

Hard palate repair can be divided into techniques that use bipedicled and/or unipedicled flaps. Bipedicled flaps are based on the incisive foramen pedicle anteriorly and the greater palatine pedicle posteriorly. The von Langenbeck repair is a popular technique that incorporates bipedicled flaps. In unipedicled flaps, the anterior pedicle is divided and the palatal flaps are based exclusively on the greater palatine pedicle. The Veau–Wardill–Kilner repair (VWK or VY push-back) and the 2-flap palatoplasty are common examples of a unipedicled repair.[19]

Von Langenbeck described his bipedicled repair in the nineteenth century.[13] Adopting Dieffenbach's[13] earlier introduction of the lateral relaxing incision, this repair raises bilateral bipedicled mucoperiosteal flaps. The lateral border of these flaps is an incision along the attached gingiva that runs posteriorly to a point lateral to the hamulus, approximately 1 cm posterior to the maxillary tuberosity. A mucosal incision along the border of the cleft, between the oral and nasal mucosa, marks the flap's medial extent.[19] Nasal mucosa flaps are sutured to one another in the midline to repair the nasal lining defect (often incorporating a vomer flap). The bipedicled hard palate flaps are advanced to close the oral side of the defect.

The VWK repair and the 2-flap palatoplasty are based on bilateral unipedicled flaps for hard palate reconstruction. The VWK repair took its origins from Veau's VY advancement flap series of 1922.[13] Although conceptually similar to the von Langenbeck repair described earlier, the anterior pedicle is divided to yield unipedicled flaps, and the mucoperiosteal flaps are approximated with the incorporation of an anteriorly based VY advancement flap. Some individuals hold that this repair lengthens the soft palate as the mucoperiosteal flaps are advanced posteriorly and may, therefore, improve velopharyngeal competence. Others express concern that the degree of hard palate periosteal dissection that is necessary may impair midface growth.[19] The authors of this work are unsure of the degree to which hard palate push back contributes to velar length or function. In the 2-flap palatoplasty (also a unipedicled flap technique), flaps similar to those of the VWK repair are raised but extend anteriorly to incorporate the alveolar mucosa when involved.[19]

Repair of the Soft Palate

Although the hard palate is a static structure, the soft palate rapidly changes its configuration to determine the aperture of the velopharynx, thus mediating speech production. Von Graefe and Roux first approached velar repair in the early nineteenth century, focusing their efforts on approximating the 2 sides of the defect.[20] Although these researchers addressed the velum's aberrant morphology, Veau, Wardill, and Kilner endeavored to improve velar dynamics with their push back or straight-line procedures designed to lengthen the soft palate with repair of the hard palate in an effort to better position the velum to participate in velopharyngeal function.[20] The anatomic basis for cleft velar dynamics was first directly addressed in 1969 by Kriens, with his intravelar veloplasty (IVVP).[20] The IVVP reoriented the clefted velar levators from their pathologic sagittal course to their physiologic horizontal course, repairing the levator sling. Furlow[21] described his "double-opposing Z-plasty" in 1986. This imaginative soft palate repair uses paired Z-plasty flaps to simultaneously repair the levator sling and lengthen the soft palate. The effectiveness of the IVVP incorporated into the Furlow repair stems from the fact that the levator is transferred *within* a vascularized mucosal-muscular flap, eliminating the need to completely dissect the levator free from both the nasal and oral mucosae. In transferring the abnormal levators from a sagittal to horizontal configuration, they are overlapped and placed on functional tension to reconstruct the levator sling. Because Z-plasties typically lengthen in one direction at the expense of shortening tissue perpendicularly, by lengthening the velum via a Z-plasty, the Furlow palatoplasty narrows the caliber of the velopharyngeal port. The double-opposing Z-plasty, thus, simultaneously serves as a palatoplasty *and* a pharyngoplasty.

Two-Stage Palatoplasty

Because of the controversy regarding the timing of palatoplasty discussed earlier, certain researchers prefer to separate hard and soft palate repair into 2 phases. This practice is well described by Rohrich and Gosman,[9] who advocate a 2-stage repair whereby both stages are performed fairly early. In brief, Rohrich and Gosman's[9] protocol consists of cleft lip and soft palate repair at 3 to 6 months, with hard palate repair following at 15 to 18 months.[9] It is posited that isolated repair of the lip and velum before hard palate repair molds the anterior and posterior alveolar arch segments, respectively. This molding is thought to yield a narrowed hard palate cleft that allows a tension-free repair with minimized mucoperiosteal elevation (and its attendant adverse growth effects) at the second stage operation.[9]

THE AUTHORS' APPROACH: FURLOW PALATOPLASTY
Soft Palate

Markings
The double-opposing Z-plasties are comprised of 2 oral flaps and 2 nasal flaps. These flaps include 2 anteriorly based mucosal flaps and 2 posteriorly based musculomucosal flaps. The posteriorly based oral musculomucosal flap is designed on the patients' left side by convention. The velar relaxing incisions (**Fig. 5**) are drawn in the crease at the junction of the vertical cheek sidewalls and the horizontal velar shelves. The relaxing incisions extend posteriorly from the maxillary tuberosity to the region of the mandibular retromolar trigone. Anteriorly, they extend onto the hard palate along the attached gingiva. Then, marks are placed on the hamuli, uvular bases, and junctions of the hard and soft palates bilaterally. The medial cleft margin incision is marked. This incision is made slightly on the oral side of the cleft margin in an effort to cheat extra tissue for the nasal lining repair. The medial uvular surfaces are marked to be demucosalized. The lateral limb incision of the left-sided posteriorly based oral musculomucosal flap is designed by joining the marked left hamulus laterally to the junction of the hard and soft palates medially, creating an approximately 60° flap. The lateral limb incision of the right-sided anteriorly based oral mucosal flap is designed by joining the right-sided uvular base medially to the right-sided marked hamulus laterally, creating a flap between 60° and 90°. A mucosal bridge must be preserved between the relaxing incisions and the lateral extent of the lateral limb incisions.

Incisions and flap elevation
The medial uvular halves are demucosalized (**Fig. 6**) and tagged with a suture in each distal tip. The left-sided cleft-margin incision and the lateral limb incision of the left-sided posteriorly based oral musculomucosal flap (**Fig. 7**) are made. Dissection begins near the junction of the hard and soft palates on the left side; the levator is identified medially at its insertion into the posterior edge of the hard palate. This connection is severed, and dissection continues laterally (**Fig. 8**). The tensor aponeurosis is identified at the posterior edge of the hard palate with its abnormal attachment to the levator. The aponeurosis is incised. Lateral dissection releases the levator from its abnormal associations with the superior constrictor (**Fig. 9**). The tip of the left-sided, posteriorly based oral musculomucosal flap is tagged with a traction stitch. Dissection proceeds posteriorly, between the left-sided levator and the nasal mucosa, until the junction of the uvula and velum is reached, leaving submucosa with the nasal lining. The levator is bluntly swept free from any remaining association with the superior constrictor (**Figs. 10** and **11**) and radically retroposed to its anatomic transverse orientation (**Fig. 12**). The levator and the superior constrictor are now at nearly 90° to one another (see **Fig. 11B**). Again, the levator must be completely released from its abnormal attachments to the posterior edge of the hard palate medially, the

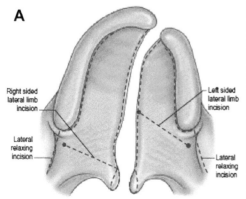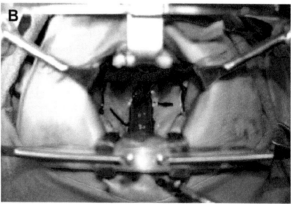

Right sided lateral limb incision

Lateral relaxing incision

Left sided lateral limb incision

Lateral relaxing incision

Fig. 5. (A) The markings for the double-opposing Z-plasty include velar relaxing incisions, the hamuli, the junction of the hard and soft palate medially, the uvular bases, the medial cleft margin, and the medial surfaces of the uvulae. (B) Operative photograph of the markings depicted in (A). (From Losee JE, Smith DM. Cleft palate repair. In: Butler C, editor. Head and neck reconstruction with DVD: a volume in the procedures in reconstructive surgery series. Philadelphia: Saunders Ltd; 2008. p. 271–94; with permission.)

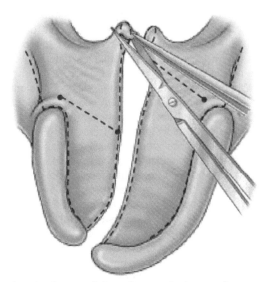

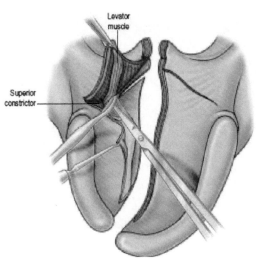

Fig. 6. The medial surfaces of the uvulae are democusalized. (*From* Losee JE, Smith DM. Cleft palate repair. In: Butler C, editor. Head and neck reconstruction with DVD: a volume in the procedures in reconstructive surgery series. Philadelphia: Saunders Ltd; 2008. p. 271–94; with permission.)

Fig. 8. Scissor dissection of the plane between the left levator and nasal mucosa. The levator is released from the posterior edge of the hard palate medially and the tensor aponeurosis and superior constrictor laterally. (*From* Losee JE, Smith DM. Cleft palate repair. In: Butler C, editor. Head and neck reconstruction with DVD: a volume in the procedures in reconstructive surgery series. Philadelphia: Saunders Ltd; 2008. p. 271–94; with permission.)

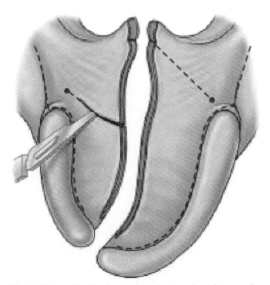

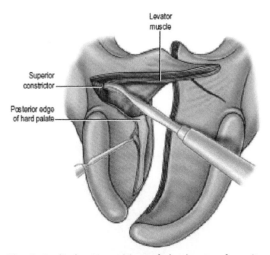

Fig. 7. The left-sided posteriorly based oral musculo-mucosal flap and the right-sided anteriorly based oral mucosal flap are created. (*From* Losee JE, Smith DM. Cleft palate repair. In: Butler C, editor. Head and neck reconstruction with DVD: a volume in the procedures in reconstructive surgery series. Philadelphia: Saunders Ltd; 2008. p. 271–94; with permission.)

Fig. 9. Radical retroposition of the levator from its pathologic sagittal orientation to its normal horizontal orientation after being freed from its abnormal connections to the hard palate, the tensor aponeurosis, and the superior constrictor (see **Fig. 3**). (*From* Losee JE, Smith DM. Cleft palate repair. In: Butler C, editor. Head and neck reconstruction with DVD: a volume in the procedures in reconstructive surgery series. Philadelphia: Saunders Ltd; 2008. p. 271–94; with permission.)

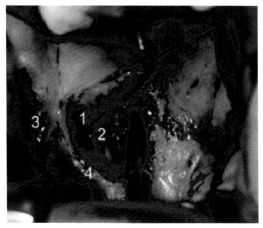

Fig. 10. View of the surgical field highlighting the left-sided, posteriorly based oral musculomucosal flap. Visible are the levator (1), nasal mucosa (2), uncut marking for lateral relaxing incision (3), and posterior edge of hard palate (4). (*From* Losee JE, Smith DM. Cleft palate repair. In: Butler C, editor. Head and neck reconstruction with DVD: a volume in the procedures in reconstructive surgery series. Philadelphia: Saunders Ltd; 2008. p. 271–94; with permission.)

tensor aponeurosis, and the superior constrictor laterally, as achieved in this dissection (see **Figs. 3** and **12**).

The right-sided, cleft-margin incision and right-sided lateral limb incision are then made (**Fig. 13**). The right-sided anteriorly based oral mucosal flap is elevated, bringing the submucosa

with it. The palatopharyngeus and palatoglossus muscles in the posterior velum are left down beneath the elevated anteriorly based mucosal flap (**Fig. 14**). Dissection continues anteriorly to the posterior edge of the hard palate.

When the cleft width is wide, relaxing incisions are liberally made. The mucosal velar relaxing incisions are made from the retromolar trigone posteriorly to the maxillary tuberosity anteriorly (**Fig. 15**). The blade is positioned parallel to the vertical cheek and perpendicular to the horizontal velum to avoid exposing buccal fat laterally. The incision is carried around the maxillary tuberosity and onto the hard palate, within the crease made by the junction of the palatal mucosa and the attached gingiva. The blade is aimed laterally (perpendicular to the mucosa) during this hard palate portion of the incision to protect the underlying pedicle. The hamulus is palpated with the scissor tips through the relaxing incision; with the blades medial to the hamulus and superior constrictor, the scissors are pushed several millimeters posteriorly into the space of Ernst. The tensor tendon is identified rounding the hamulus through the relaxing incision and divided medial to the hamulus (**Fig. 16**). Some individuals think that placing a stitch to pexy (affix) the tensor tendon to the hamulus, before its division, is functionally advantageous to eustachian tube dilation.[22] The hard palate's posterior edge must be dissected free of soft tissue. The hard palate's posterior edge is palpated with a small periosteal elevator through the lateral relaxing

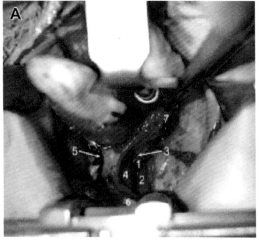

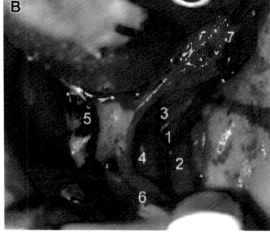

Fig. 11. (*A*) Intraoperative depiction of the left-sided, posteriorly based oral musculomucosal flap demonstrating the levator (1), nasal mucosa (2), cut tensor aponeurosis (3), superior constrictor (4), uncut marking for lateral relaxing incision (5), posterior edge of hard palate (6), and distal tip of the left-sided, posteriorly based oral musculomucosal flap being retracted by pickups (7). (*B*) Close-up view of the field depicted in (*A*). (*From* Losee JE, Smith DM. Cleft palate repair. In: Butler C, editor. Head and neck reconstruction with DVD: a volume in the procedures in reconstructive surgery series. Philadelphia: Saunders Ltd; 2008. p. 271–94; with permission.)

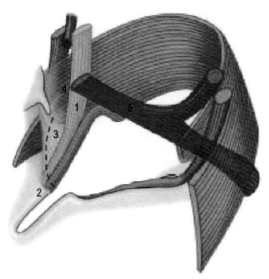

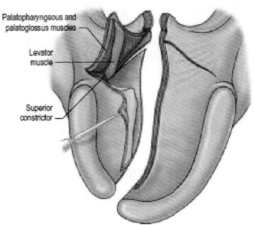

Fig. 12. The pathologic orientation and abnormal attachments of the levator (1) on the left of the figure, including the posterior edge of the hard palate (2), the tensor aponeurosis (3), and the superior constrictor (4). The dotted line illustrates the incision that will release the levator from its abnormal attachments allowing it to be radically retroposed to occupy its physiologic position and horizontal orientation in the middle 50% of the velum as drawn on the right side of the figure (5). (*From* Losee JE, Smith DM. Cleft palate repair. In: Butler C, editor. Head and neck reconstruction with DVD: a volume in the procedures in reconstructive surgery series. Philadelphia: Saunders Ltd; 2008. p. 271–94; with permission.)

Fig. 13. The incision for the right-sided, anteriorly based oral mucosal flap extends from the junction of the uvular base and the soft palate medially to the hamulus laterally. An adequate mucosal bridge must be preserved between the right-sided lateral relaxing incision and the right-sided lateral limb incision. (*From* Losee JE, Smith DM. Cleft palate repair. In: Butler C, editor. Head and neck reconstruction with DVD: a volume in the procedures in reconstructive surgery series. Philadelphia: Saunders Ltd; 2008. p. 271–94; with permission.)

incision. Blind soft tissue dissection proceeds medially, along the posterior edge of the hard palate, toward the medial cleft margin. Alternatively, this important dissection of the posterior edge of the hard palate can be made medially to laterally, by starting along the junction of the hard and soft palates medially, aiming for the region of the hamulus laterally.

Attention is next turned to the hard palate dissection. A Blair hockey-stick elevator is placed within the hard palate lateral relaxing incision, just anterior to the pedicle; the hard palate mucoperiosteal flaps are subperiosteally dissected to the midline cleft margin (Fig. 17). The dissection of the oral, hard palate flaps continues posteriorly to the posterior edge of the hard palate, which has been dissected previously. Dissection then proceeds medially to laterally, along the posterior edge of the hard palate, to join the previous dissection from the lateral relaxing incisions. During this blind dissection and release, the tips of the scissors must hug the posterior edge of the hard palate to protect the pedicle. Next, the nasal mucosa, along the medial cleft margin, is subperiosteally dissected from the nasal surface of the

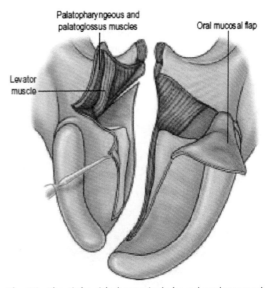

Fig. 14. The right-sided anteriorly based oral mucosal flap is elevated such that the palatopharyngeus and palatoglossus muscles are left down. (*From* Losee JE, Smith DM. Cleft palate repair. In: Butler C, editor. Head and neck reconstruction with DVD: a volume in the procedures in reconstructive surgery series. Philadelphia: Saunders Ltd; 2008. p. 271–94; with permission.)

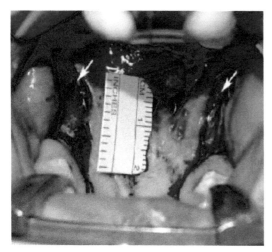

Fig. 15. View of the surgical field demonstrating the bilateral relaxing incisions (*arrows*) and the position of the reconstructed levator sling, which, after radical IVVP, resides in the middle 50% of the velum, a full 2 cm posterior to the posterior edge of the hard palate. (*From* Losee JE, Smith DM. Cleft palate repair. In: Butler C, editor. Head and neck reconstruction with DVD: a volume in the procedures in reconstructive surgery series. Philadelphia: Saunders Ltd; 2008. p. 271–94; with permission.)

foramina of the pedicle posteriorly) may be required. This ostectomy facilitates a tension-free closure at the junction of the hard and soft palates by releasing the pedicle from its bony foramina and allowing it to move posteriorly and medially.

The left-sided, anteriorly based, nasal mucosal flap is created with the left-sided oral flap retracted out of the mouth and toward the posterior pharyngeal wall (**Fig. 19**). This incision begins medially, from the junction of the base of the uvula and the velum, and continues laterally to where the left levator exits the skull base. This incision mirrors the left-sided oral incision to create a left-sided, anteriorly based nasal mucosal flap of approximately 60° and must be carried laterally all the way to the skull base.

The right-sided, posteriorly based nasal musculomucosal flap is initiated by releasing the levator from the posterior edge of the hard palate medially as well as from the tensor aponeurosis and superior constrictor laterally (**Fig. 20**). The posterior edge of the hard palate, on the right side, is subperiosteally dissected. The right-sided, posteriorly based nasal musculomucosal flap is created by an incision starting from the tip of the dissected levator medially, at the junction of the hard and soft palates, and continued laterally, aiming for the region of the hamulus. *This incision is extended only enough to release the flap and facilitate its transfer and inset to the opposite left side where the levator exits the skull base.* By limiting this incision laterally, the defect created will be smaller and more easily filled with the opposite, left-sided, anteriorly based nasal mucosal flap. Another helpful hint is

hard palate (**Fig. 18**). Further dissection in the region of the hamulus and pedicle may be required to circumferentially mobilize the pedicle and ensure tension-free closure. Circumferential subperiosteal dissection of the rim of the pedicle's bony foramina and, occasionally, a posteromedial osteotomy of the bony foramina (opening the

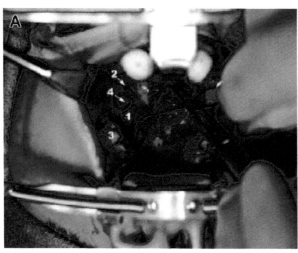

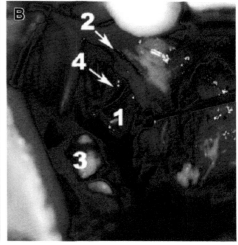

Fig. 16. (*A*) Intraoperative view of the left-sided tensor (1) coursing medially around the hamulus. This vantage is framed by the cut left lateral velar relaxing incision (2). Also visible are the first molar (3) and the space of Ernst (4), medial to the superior constrictor. (*B*) Close-up view of the field depicted in (*A*). (*From* Losee JE, Smith DM. Cleft palate repair. In: Butler C, editor. Head and neck reconstruction with DVD: a volume in the procedures in reconstructive surgery series. Philadelphia: Saunders Ltd; 2008. p. 271–94; with permission.)

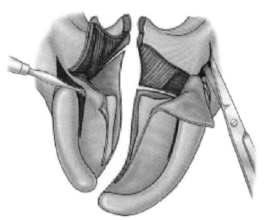

Fig. 17. Hard palate mucoperiosteal flap raised with Blair elevator inserted into lateral relaxing incision. (*From* Losee JE, Smith DM. Cleft palate repair. In: Butler C, editor. Head and neck reconstruction with DVD: a volume in the procedures in reconstructive surgery series. Philadelphia: Saunders Ltd; 2008. p. 271–94; with permission.)

as follows: 5 to 10 mm of nasal mucosa must be left at the posterior edge of the hard palate on the right side to facilitate the inset of the transposed, left-sided, anteriorly based nasal mucosal flap. Finally, 1 to 2 mm of levator is dissected free from the underlying mucosa of the right-sided, posteriorly based nasal musculomucosal

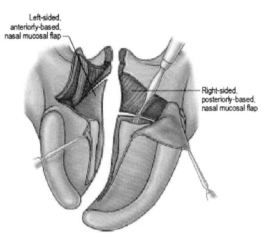

Fig. 19. A left-sided, anteriorly based nasal mucosal flap of approximately 60° and a right-sided, posteriorly based nasal musculomucosal flap of 60° to 90° are designed as illustrated. To facilitate closure of the nasal lining, several millimeters of nasal mucosa are left along the posterior edge of the hard palate on the right side. (*From* Losee JE, Smith DM. Cleft palate repair. In: Butler C, editor. Head and neck reconstruction with DVD: a volume in the procedures in reconstructive surgery series. Philadelphia: Saunders Ltd; 2008. p. 271–94; with permission.)

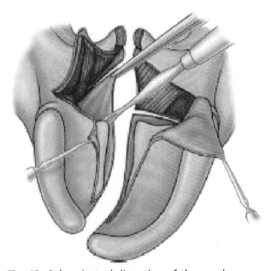

Fig. 18. Subperiosteal dissection of the nasal mucosa from the nasal side of the hard palate along its posterior edge and bilateral medial edges as they abut the cleft. (*From* Losee JE, Smith DM. Cleft palate repair. In: Butler C, editor. Head and neck reconstruction with DVD: a volume in the procedures in reconstructive surgery series. Philadelphia: Saunders Ltd; 2008. p. 271–94; with permission.)

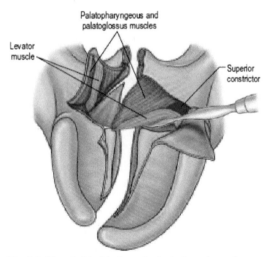

Fig. 20. The right-sided, posteriorly based nasal musculomucosal flap is designed as illustrated to include the levator, palatoglossus, and palatopharyngeus muscles. Note that the levator must be released from the posterior edge of the hard palate and the tensor aponeurosis and be swept free from the superior constrictor. (*From* Losee JE, Smith DM. Cleft palate repair. In: Butler C, editor. Head and neck reconstruction with DVD: a volume in the procedures in reconstructive surgery series. Philadelphia: Saunders Ltd; 2008. p. 271–94; with permission.)

flap so sutures can be placed in the mucosal edge, excluding muscle.

Flap inset and closure

If not already present, a nasopharyngeal (NP) airway is placed. Uvular reconstruction is achieved with 1-mm-spaced sutures on the nasal and oral sides of the uvula. Midline traction during flap inset is important in assuring that the uvula remains midline. The right-sided, posteriorly based nasal musculomucosal flap is sewn across the cleft into the corner of the left-sided, nasal lateral limb incision beneath the left-sided levator as it exits the skull base, radically transposing the right-sided levator to a horizontal lie within the middle 50% of the new velum (see **Fig. 12**). The tip of the left-sided, anteriorly based nasal mucosal flap is sewn into the corner of the defect in the nasal lining on the right side. Again, ideally, the right-sided nasal lining defect is relatively smaller in size because the nasal lining incision at the posterior aspect of the right-sided hard palate was made only as long as necessary to transpose the right-sided, posteriorly based musculomucosal flap. The limb incisions are then repaired, placing sutures *only in the mucosa* of the flaps (**Fig. 21**). The limbs of the Z-plasty are often not equal in length; repeated suture bisection optimizes the repair.

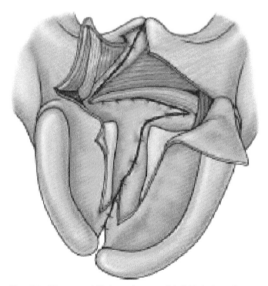

Fig. 21. The nasal lining closure, highlighting the position of the levator muscle (*yellow*). (*From* Losee JE, Smith DM. Cleft palate repair. In: Butler C, editor. Head and neck reconstruction with DVD: a volume in the procedures in reconstructive surgery series. Philadelphia: Saunders Ltd; 2008. p. 271–94; with permission.)

If a shortage of nasal lining inhibits tension-free repair at the hard and soft palate junction and/or the inset of the left-sided, anteriorly based nasal mucosal flap (**Fig. 22**), a thin piece of acellular dermal matrix (ADM) is placed as an onlay (**Fig. 23**). The ADM is limited to the region of the normal tensor aponeurosis, and *not* sewn to the levator sling. The onlay can also cover the hard palate nasal lining repair for added strength. In the bilateral cleft palate in particular, it is useful to place ADM over the nasal repair at the junction of the primary and secondary palates to reduce the risk of postoperative fistula. Nasal lining closure continues anteriorly. Vomer flaps are used as necessary.

Attention is next turned to the oral flaps. A stitch incorporating a small amount of oral mucosa with a robust bite of deeper tissue is placed into the tip of the left-sided, posteriorly based oral musculomucosal flap and inset into the corner of the right side. A small amount of oral mucosa and a healthy amount of tissue beneath are incorporated to complete the levator sling reconstruction, overlapping the levators under functional tension (**Fig. 24**). The tip of the right-sided, anteriorly based oral mucosa flap is sewn into the left-sided defect. The lateral limbs are repaired by repeatedly bisecting the limb defects with mucosal stitches.

Hard Palate

Flap design

Hard palate mucoperiosteal flaps may be unipedicled, bipedicled, or have no lateral relaxing incisions depending on the morphology of the cleft. The 2 flaps for a given case may be of different types. Unipedicled flaps, based on the greater palatine vessels, are achieved by connecting the lateral relaxing incisions to the medial cleft margin incision anteriorly (**Fig. 25**). Increased flap mobility and the ability to offset the nasal and oral repairs (avoiding overlapping incisions to reduce the chance of an oronasal fistula) come at the expense of a potentially more tenuous blood supply.

In clefts of the secondary palate only (Veau II), unipedicled flaps allow for a true push-back hard palate repair (**Fig. 26**). Bipedicled flaps require lateral relaxing incisions that do not communicate anteriorly with the cleft margin incisions. Because of decreased mobility, bipedicled flaps are limited in closing wide clefts and anterior defects. Hard palate flaps with no lateral relaxing incisions (elevated from the medial cleft margins) may be used in narrow or highly vaulted clefts. Because bipedicle flaps require less dissection, the hard palate is not as extensively denuded or exposed, and maxillary growth restriction may be minimized.

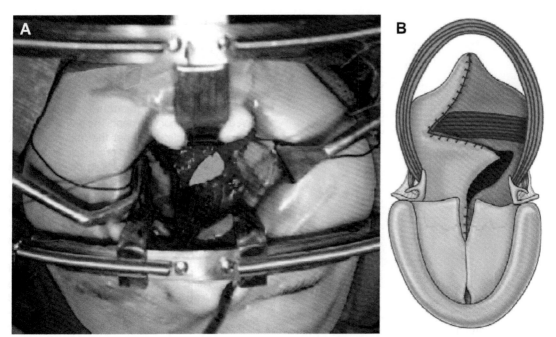

Fig. 22. (*A*) Intraoperative view demonstrating residual nasal lining defect at the junction of the hard palate and the soft palate (*green marker*) after closure of the nasal lining. (*B*) The operative field depicted in (*A*). (*From* Losee JE, Smith DM. Cleft palate repair. In: Butler C, editor. Head and neck reconstruction with DVD: a volume in the procedures in reconstructive surgery series. Philadelphia: Saunders Ltd; 2008. p. 271–94; with permission.)

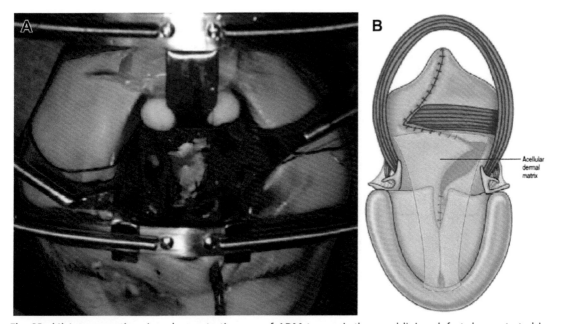

Fig. 23. (*A*) Intraoperative view demonstrating use of ADM to repair the nasal lining defect demonstrated in **Fig. 22**. (*B*) The operative field depicted in (*A*). Note also that the ADM overlays the hard palate to reinforce this repair. Anteriorly, the ADM is sutured to the alveolar mucosa. (*From* Losee JE, Smith DM. Cleft palate repair. In: Butler C, editor. Head and neck reconstruction with DVD: a volume in the procedures in reconstructive surgery series. Philadelphia: Saunders Ltd; 2008. p. 271–94; with permission.)

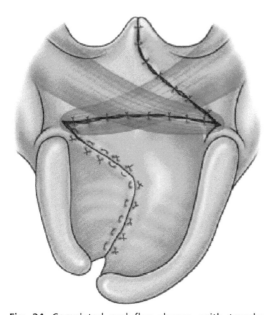

Fig. 24. Completed oral flap closure, with translucency highlighting levator sling repaired under functional tension. (*From* Losee JE, Smith DM. Cleft palate repair. In: Butler C, editor. Head and neck reconstruction with DVD: a volume in the procedures in reconstructive surgery series. Philadelphia: Saunders Ltd; 2008. p. 271–94; with permission.)

Limited mobility, increased tension, and the likelihood of overlapping nasal and oral suture lines lead the authors to avoid these flaps whenever possible.

In complete unilateral clefts of the primary and secondary palate (Veau III), a bipedicled flap is useful for the major segment; a unipedicled flap is used for the minor segment. The minor segment flap spans the cleft to meet the major segment flap, offsetting the nasal and oral incisions and assisting in anterior palate closure posterior to the alveolus. Hard palate push-back repair for Veau II clefts is achieved with unipedicled flaps (see **Fig. 26**). In complete bilateral clefts (Veau IV), the unipedicled flaps are sewn to the premaxillary mucoperiosteum to address the incisive foramen defect (**Fig. 27**).

Vomer flaps are used to assist in the closure of the nasal lining to provide a 2-layer hard palate repair. In Veau III clefts, vomer flaps are incised along the junction of the hard palate mucoperiosteum and the vomer on the unaffected side. They are turned over and inset to the nasal mucosal flap on the cleft side. In Veau IV clefts, the vomer is incised in the midline (**Fig. 28**). These flaps are also of use in closing the anterior nasal lining of the velum if the vomer extends far posteriorly.

Hard palate closure and the alveolus
The mucosal edges are everted when closing the hard palate mucoperiosteal flaps. One or

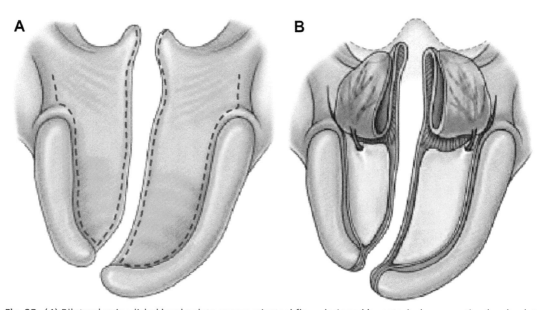

Fig. 25. (*A*) Bilateral unipedicled hard palate mucoperiosteal flaps designed by anteriorly connecting hard palate lateral relaxing incisions with medial cleft margin incisions. (*B*) Flaps designed in a raised with circumferential dissection of greater palatine neurovascular pedicles. (*From* Losee JE, Smith DM. Cleft palate repair. In: Butler C, editor. Head and neck reconstruction with DVD: a volume in the procedures in reconstructive surgery series. Philadelphia: Saunders Ltd; 2008. p. 271–94; with permission.)

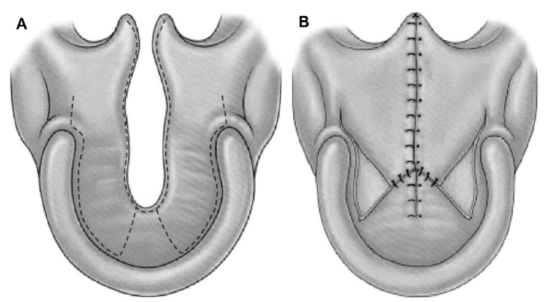

Fig. 26. (*A*) Unipedicled flaps (see **Fig. 25**) allow for push-back repair of hard palate in Veau II clefts. (*B*) Flaps designed in (*A*) are inset in V-Y fashion at the mucoperiosteum of the anterior extent of the cleft. (*From* Losee JE, Smith DM. Cleft palate repair. In: Butler C, editor. Head and neck reconstruction with DVD: a volume in the procedures in reconstructive surgery series. Philadelphia: Saunders Ltd; 2008. p. 271–94; with permission.)

two 3/0 Vicryl sutures can be placed through the hard palate flaps in the mid hard palate to secure them to the nasal lining when using bilateral unipedicled flaps. The anterior tips are secured with horizontal mattress circumdental sutures

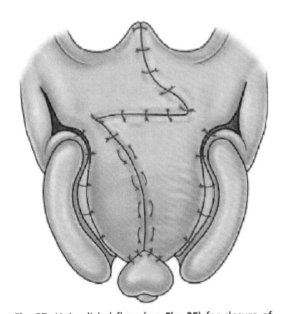

Fig. 27. Unipedicled flaps (see **Fig. 25**) for closure of the Veau IV cleft. (*From* Losee JE, Smith DM. Cleft palate repair. In: Butler C, editor. Head and neck reconstruction with DVD: a volume in the procedures in reconstructive surgery series. Philadelphia: Saunders Ltd; 2008. p. 271–94; with permission.)

and sutures anchoring the flaps to the alveolar gingiva.

Gingivoperiosteoplasty (GPP) can be performed at the time of primary lip repair if presurgical infant orthopedics had been used. Without a GPP, the primary alveolar repair, the alveolar cleft is reconstructed with an alveolar bone graft before the eruption of the primary cuspid (Editor note: Management of the alveolar cleft is discussed further in the article "Management of the Alveolar Cleft" elsewhere in this issue by Pedro E. Santiago, Lindsay A. Schuster, and Daniel Levy-Bercowski).

POSTOPERATIVE CARE

The NP airway is removed on the morning of postoperative day one if there are no airway concerns. Arm restraints are routinely used. Patients convalesce with telemetry and pulse oximetry. Clear liquids from a cup are permitted as soon as patients are recovered. After 48 hours, patients are advanced to a full liquid diet by cup for the remainder of the first week. Nothing is allowed in the mouth. Discharge occurs when oral intake is sufficient and there is no evidence of airway obstruction, which is usually on postoperative day one. Patients return to the clinic 1 week after surgery, and a soft diet is initiated. A regular diet begins 2 weeks after surgery if full healing has occurred. A cleft team visit is scheduled for a complete evaluation, including speech assessment, 3 months after surgery.

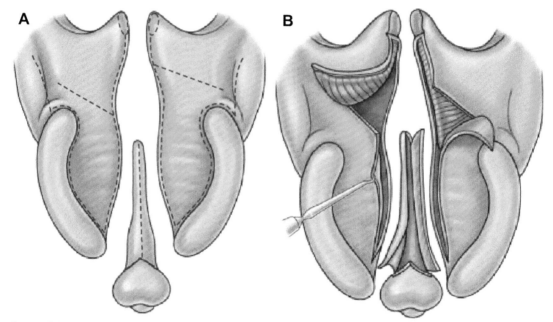

Fig. 28. (A) Markings for vomer flaps for closure of the hard palate nasal lining in Veau IV clefts; Furlow palato-plasty of the soft palate is also marked here. (B) The vomer flaps designed in (A) are elevated in preparation for inset and closure of the nasal lining. (*From* Losee JE, Smith DM. Cleft palate repair. In: Butler C, editor. Head and neck reconstruction with DVD: a volume in the procedures in reconstructive surgery series. Philadelphia: Saunders Ltd; 2008. p. 271–94; with permission.)

RECENT TRENDS AND CONTROVERSIES
Radical Intravelar Veloplasty

The distinction between an incomplete IVVP and a complete IVVP must be stressed. The levator has 3 abnormal attachments in the cleft state: pathologic insertions onto the medial aspect of the posterior hard palate, abnormal attachments to the aponeurosis of the tensor veli palatini, and aberrant associations with the superior pharyngeal constrictor laterally (see **Figs. 1**B and **3**). In an incomplete IVVP, only the first abnormal attachment is addressed: the levator is disinserted from the posterior edge of the hard palate. Although this maneuver may allow the levator to be affixed to its counterpart across the midline, the levator sling that results remains anterior to its anatomic position, and the levator maintains a largely sagittal course.

If all abnormal attachments of the levator are not completely released, the muscle sling cannot be radically retropositioned to its physiologic horizontal orientation in the middle 50% of the velum. This assertion is supported by the observation that when the authors perform conversion Furlow palatoplasties to address persistent VPI after previous straight-line palatoplasties, they visualize the original IVVP intraoperatively. The levator is almost uniformly noted to have scarred back to the

posterior edge of the hard palate. In these incomplete IVVPs, despite having reconstructed the levator sling, the levators maintain a sagittal orientation and an aberrant anterior position; persistent VPI is the result. In a series of conversion Furlow palatoplasties in patients who had previously undergone straight-line palatoplasties with reported IVVP, the authors reported a statistically significant improvement in overall Pittsburgh Weighted Speech Score (PWSS) and in every individual component of that score after the radical IVVP inherent to the Furlow.[23]

The importance of radical IVVP in achieving velopharyngeal competence has been borne out in the literature. Randall's group noted superior speech results with IVVP in his 1983 article.[24] Andrades and colleagues[25] reported significantly lower VPI and secondary speech surgery rates for patients undergoing 2-flap palatoplasty with radical IVVP as compared with those undergoing 2-flap palatoplasty without IVVP.[25] Dreyer and Trier[26] reported superior speech outcomes with IVVP in a study comparing palatoplasties performed with to those performed without the procedure; 9% of patients undergoing IVVP required secondary pharyngeal flaps for VPI as compared with 38% of those without IVVP.[26] It is instructive to note that in Marsh and colleagues'[27] series reporting no difference in VPI rates between IVVP and non-IVVP palatoplasties (both with straight-line repairs), the IVVP described was an *incomplete* IVVP.[27]

Furlow's double-opposing Z-plasty repair inherently includes a robust IVVP when the posteriorly based musculomucosal flaps are inset to reorient the cleft levators from a sagittal to horizontal orientation. Moreover, overlapping of the posteriorly based musculomucosal flaps reconstructs the levator sling under functional tension, addressing concerns that the cleft levator is too long. As the levator is not dissected free from either the nasal or oral mucosa in the Furlow repair, anterior relapse is prevented. Furlow reported that 90% of his patients had no evidence of VPI; none required secondary speech surgery (mean follow-up 44 months).[21] In Kirschner and colleagues'[28] Furlow series, "no or mild" hypernasality was reported in 93.4% of patients and 7.2% required pharyngeal flaps with extensive follow-up, averaging 7.7 years.[28]

Does Furlow Palatoplasty Reliably Lengthen the Velum?

In his initial description of the procedure, Furlow[21] wrote that the double-opposing Z-plasty would "lengthen the velum without using tissue from the hard palate."[21] The geometry of the Z-plasty has been well described,[29] and there is little doubt that the Furlow repair should indeed lengthen the soft palate at the time of surgery. Moreover, by eliminating a longitudinal scar, the Furlow procedure should minimize scar contracture and concomitant velar shortening in the postoperative period.[28] D'Antonio and colleagues[30] reported the normalization of velar length as compared with historical norms at an average of 8.6 months of follow-up.[30] Huang offered radiographic evidence of a significant increase in palatal length maintained at an average 2.9 years postoperatively as compared with historical controls.[31] Gunren and Uysal[32] documented a mean intraoperative increase in velar length of 69.05% that translated to a mean increase in length of 55.47% at an average follow-up of 4.5 years.[32] Anecdotal experience of the authors confirms the findings of palatal lengthening with the velar Z-plasty. In many cases, the shortened and clefted velum is lengthened to the point where the repaired uvula nearly approximates the poster pharyngeal wall at the end of the procedure.

Approach to Rerepair of the Cleft Palate for VPI

Rates of persistent VPI after palatoplasty range from 0% to 66% in the literature (**Table 1**). Initial attempts to address this deficiency must first be aimed at optimizing palatal anatomy because pharyngoplasty is fraught with the risk of significant morbidity, including obstructive sleep apnea, hyponasility, snoring, and mouth breathing.[33] If the primary palatoplasty was a straight-line repair, and/or there is evidence of levator muscle abnormal position, seen as a vaulted V-shaped pattern of velar elevation similar to a submucous cleft palate, an attempt to lengthen the palate and provide a more anatomic, dynamic reconstruction with conversion Furlow palatoplasty should be made. During this secondary procedure, the surgeon must be certain to perform a *complete* IVVP. If there is evidence of a symptomatic fistula, one of myriad methods of fistula repair should be used.[34] Should VPI persist despite optimized palatal anatomy, the other half of the velopharyngeal equation should be addressed with pharyngoplasty. Depending on the nature of pharyngeal closure dynamics, a detailed discussion of which is beyond the scope of this article, either a posterior pharyngeal flap or sphincter pharyngoplasty is performed (Editor note: Surgical management of VPO is discussed further in the article "Surgical Management of Velopharyngeal Insufficiency" elsewhere in this issue by Michael S. Gart and Arun K. Gosain).

ASSESSMENT OF OUTCOMES
Important Metrics

A palatoplasty is first and foremost a speech operation tasked with the creation of a competent velopharyngeal sphincter that is compatible with the development of normal elocution. The prevention of palatal fistulae is a critical goal in its own right because these recalcitrant lesions may lead to regurgitation of fluid and food as well as contribute to VPI.[35–37] It is, therefore, of critical importance to reliably assess and record speech quality and palatal integrity after palatoplasty.

Speech Outcomes

Normal speech requires a controlled balance of intraoral air pressure for oral sounds and intranasal pressure for nasal sounds. This balance is maintained by the coordinated movement of the velum and the pharyngeal walls.[38] Collectively, adequate completion of the complex functions achieved by the velopharyngeal apparatus is termed *velopharyngeal competence*. VPI is the most frequently assessed metric in globally describing the success or failure of a given palatoplasty with regard to speech outcome (see **Table 1**).

The measurement of VPI requires an assessment of multiple variables gleaned from voice samples and physical examination findings; specially trained speech pathologists are required

Table 1
Review of palatoplasty outcomes

Author	Palatoplasty Method	VPI Rate (%) or Mean Speech Score	Fistula Rate	% Secondary Speech Surgery
Brothers et al,[42] 1995	Furlow vs VWK	Furlow (20%) vs VWK (20%)	Furlow (4.8%) vs VWK (0%)	NA
Cohen et al,[43] 1991	VWK vs Furlow vs VL vs Dorrance	NA	23% overall; VWK (43%) vs Furlow (10%) vs VL (22%) vs Dorrance (0%)	NA
Dreyer & Trier,[26] 1984	VL vs palatal lengthening vs VL + IVVP	VL (38%) vs palatal lengthening (38%) vs VL + IVVP (9%)	NA	VL (38%) vs palatal lengthening (38%) vs VL + IVVP (9%)
Gunther et al,[44] 1998	Furlow vs straight line + IVVP	Reported as % difference in mean speech score; straight line + IVVP 34% higher (less desirable) than Furlow	Furlow (19%) vs straight line + IVVP (12%)[a]	Furlow (8%) vs straight line + IVVP (29%)
Khosla et al,[45] 2008	Furlow	16%	3.6%	2.1%
Kirschner et al,[46] 2000[b]	Furlow at 3–7 mo vs Furlow after 7 mo	Furlow at 3–7 mo (<5%) vs Furlow after 7 mo (<5%)[c]	NA	Furlow at 3–7 mo (10%) vs Furlow after 7 mo (6%)
Marrinan et al,[47] 1998	VL vs VWK	NA	NA	VL (14%) vs VWK (15%)
McWilliams et al,[48] 1996	Furlow vs non-Furlow	Furlow (1.7) vs non-Furlow (3.2)[d]	NA	Furlow (12.7%) vs non-Furlow (45%)[d]
Muzaffar et al,[36] 2001	2 stage	NA	8.7%	NA
Phua & de Chalain,[49] 2008	Multiple	31.8%	12.8%	13.3%
Salyer et al,[50] 2006	2 flap	8.9%[e]	10%[e]	8.9%
Sommerlad,[51] 2003	Straight line with IVVP	5.9%[e]	15%[e,f]	5.9%
Wilhelmi et al,[41] 2001	2 flap	NA	3.4%	NA
Furlow,[21] 1986	Furlow	10%	4.5%	0%
Holland et al,[52] 2007	Schweckendiek vs single stage straight line	Schweckendiek (66%) vs single stage straight line (21%)	Schweckendiek (58%) vs single stage single stage straight line (11%)	Schweckendiek (63%) vs single stage single stage straight line (20%)
Kirschner et al,[28] 1999	Furlow	3.9%	NA	7.2%
Losee et al,[35] 2008	Furlow (in 92% of cases)	1[g]	3%	0%

(continued on next page)

Table 1
(continued)

Author	Palatoplasty Method	VPI Rate (%) or Mean Speech Score	Fistula Rate	% Secondary Speech Surgery
Marsh et al[27]	Straight line vs Straight line with IVVP	Straight line (40%) vs Straight line with IVVP (31%)	Straight line (5.4%) vs straight line with IVVP (2.6%)	Straight line (5.4%) vs straight line with IVVP (7.9%)
Randall et al,[53] 2000	Furlow	1.98[h]	NA	15.2%
Rohrich et al,[10] 1996	Early vs late hard palate closure	Early (19%) vs late hard palate closure (70%)	Early (5%) vs late hard closure (35%)	0%
Bekerecioglu et al,[54] 2005	2 flap vs 4 flap	NA	2 flap (5%) vs 4 flap (9%)	NA
Helling et al,[55] 2006	Furlow with ADM	NA	3.2%	NA
Bindingnavele et al,[56] 2008	Furlow vs Furlow with islandized hemipalate	NA	Furlow (10.6%) vs Furlow with islandized hemipalate (2.1%)	NA
Sullivan et al,[57] 2009	Straight line with IVVP	14.9%	2.9%	14.9%[e]
Lu et al,[58] 2010	IVVP	NA	7%	NA
Steinbacher et al,[59] 2011	Furlow with 1-layer hard palate closure vs Furlow with 2-layer hard palate closure	Furlow with 1-layer hard palate closure (6%) vs Furlow with 2-layer hard palate closure (7%)	Furlow with 1-layer hard palate closure vs (2%) Furlow with 2-layer hard palate closure (3%)	NA

Abbreviations: NA, not available; VL, von Langenbeck.
[a] Interpreted from table.
[b] Patients with fistulas excluded.
[c] Interpreted from graph.
[d] Average PWSS.
[e] Requiring surgery.
[f] Subset from 1993–1997.
[g] Median PWSS.
[h] Calculated mean PWSS.

for collection and evaluation of these nuanced data. In addition to a qualified examiner, useful evaluation of VPI requires the child be old enough to (1) begin organized speech efforts and (2) cooperate with examination. These criteria tend to be met by between 2.5 and 3 years of age (Ford M, personal communication, 2011).

Given the complexity of measuring VPI, it is not surprising that multiple methods have arisen to quantify these measurements. The method of choice at the authors' institution is the PWSS. This validated instrument scores 5 categories of perceptual speech symptoms: nasal emission,

facial grimace, nasality, phonation, and articulation.[39] Although the individual components are qualitative assessments, the weighted composite score offers quantitative data of comparative and prognostic value, which plays an important role in determining the necessity of secondary speech surgery.[23]

Palatal Integrity

The other critical outcome of palatoplasty, integrity of the repair, is apparent on intraoral examination as the presence or absence of palatal fistulas and/or excessive scaring that would render the palate less mobile than what is required for velopharyngeal competence. Fistulas may also manifest with nasality (their most frequent symptom by some accounts[40]), halitosis caused by trapped particles of food, or nasal fluid leakage.[41] In an effort to standardize reporting, the authors described and use the Pittsburgh Fistula Classification System (PFCS) at the their center.[37] The PFCS is comprised of 7 fistula types. Type I fistulae are at the level of the uvula or may represent a bifid uvula. Fistulas in the soft palate are designated type II fistulas. Type III fistulas are at the junction of the soft palate and the hard palate. Fistulas at the hard palate are type IV. Type V fistulas are at the incisive foramen (the junction of the primary and secondary palates) and by definition occur in the context of Veau IV clefts. Type VI fistulas are lingual-alveolar; type VII fistulas are labial-alveolar. Because of the historical variability of reporting and inconsistent nomenclature, that report found it difficult to offer a concise summary of fistula rate after palatoplasty. A survey of fistula rates is offered in **Table 1**.

SUMMARY

Cleft palate repair ultimately requires an understanding of speech anatomy in its normal configuration such that a coherent approach to its pathologic variants can be formulated. At its crux, palatoplasty is about repairing the velum such that its motor, the levator, is reoriented from its pathologic sagittal to its physiologic horizontal configuration under functional tension. The dynamic levator sling suspending the soft palate from the skull base is, thus, restored, and velopharyngeal competence is optimized. It is the authors' contention that the Furlow double-opposing Z-plasty represents an elegant solution to this problem because a complete IVVP is intrinsic to the procedure.

REFERENCES

1. Friedman O, Wang TD, Milczuk HA. Cleft lip and palate. In: Cummings CW, editor. Otolaryngology: head and neck surgery. Philadelphia: Mosby; 2005. p. 4052–82.
2. Huang MH, Lee ST, Rajendran K. A fresh cadaveric study of the paratubal muscles: implications for eustachian tube function in cleft palate. Plast Reconstr Surg 1997;100:833–42.
3. Huang MH, Lee ST, Rajendran K. Anatomic basis of cleft palate and velopharyngeal surgery: implications from a fresh cadaveric study. Plast Reconstr Surg 1998;101:613–27.
4. Dayan JH, Smith DM, Oliker A, et al. A virtual reality model of eustachian tube dilation and clinical implications for cleft palate repair. Plast Reconstr Surg 2005;116:236–41.
5. Fara M, Dvorak J. Abnormal anatomy of the muscles of palatopharyngeal closure in cleft palates: anatomical and surgical considerations based on the autopsies of 18 unoperated cleft palates. Plast Reconstr Surg 1970;46:488.
6. Graivier MH, Cohen SR, Kawamoto HK, et al. A new operation for velopharyngeal insufficiency: the palatoglossus myomucosal pharyngoplasty. Plast Reconstr Surg 1992;90(4):707–10.
7. Reed GM, Sheppard VF. Basic structures of the head and neck: a programed instruction in clinical anatomy for dental professionals. Philadelphia: Saunders; 1976.
8. Huang MH, Lee ST, Rajendran K. Structure of the musculus uvulae: functional and surgical implications of an anatomic study. Cleft Palate Craniofac J 1997;34(6):466–74.
9. Rohrich RJ, Gosman AA. An update on the timing of hard palate closure: a critical long-term analysis. Plast Reconstr Surg 2004;113(1):350–2.
10. Rohrich RJ, Rowsell AR, Johns DF, et al. Timing of hard palatal closure: a critical long-term analysis. Plast Reconstr Surg 1996;98:236–46.
11. Rohrich RJ, Love EJ, Byrd HS, et al. Optimal timing of cleft palate closure. Plast Reconstr Surg 2000; 106:413–22.
12. Koberg W, Koblin I. Speech development and maxillary growth in relation to technique and timing of palatoplasty. J Maxillofac Surg 1973;1:44–50.
13. Millard DR. Cleft craft: the evolution of its surgery. Boston: Little, Brown; 1976.
14. Robertson NR, Jolleys A. The timing of hard palate repair. Scand J Plast Reconstr Surg 1974;8:49–51.
15. Musgrave RH. General aspects of the unilateral cleft lip repair. In: Grabb WC, Rosenstein SW, Bzoch KR, editors. Cleft lip and palate: surgical, dental, and speech aspects. Boston: Little, Brown and Company; 1971. p. 175–94.
16. Schaefer RB, Stadler JA III, Gosain AK. To distract or not to distract: an algorithm for airway management in isolated Pierre Robin sequence. Plast Reconstr Surg 2004;113:1113–25.
17. Randall P, Hamilton R. The Pierre Robin syndrome. In: Grabb WC, Rosenstein SW, Bzoch KR, editors. Cleft lip and palate: surgical, dental, and speech aspects. Boston: Little, Brown and Company; 1971. p. 559–70.
18. Fink SC, Hardesty RA. Craniofacial syndromes. In: Bentz ML, editor. Pediatric plastic surgery. Stanford: Appleton & Lange; 1998. p. 1–45.
19. Sadove AM, van Aalst JA, Culp JA. Cleft palate repair: art and issues. Clin Plast Surg 2004;31: 231–41.

20. LaRossa D. The state of the art in cleft palate surgery. Cleft Palate Craniofac J 2000;37:225–8.

21. Furlow LT Jr. Cleft palate repair by double opposing Z-plasty. Plast Reconstr Surg 1986;78: 724–36.

22. Flores RL, Jones BL, Bernstein J, et al. Tensor veli palatini preservation, transection, and transection with tensor tenopexy during cleft palate repair and its effects on eustachian tube function. Plast Reconstr Surg 2010;125:282–9.

23. Noorchashm N, Dudas JR, Ford M, et al. Conversion Furlow palatoplasty: salvage of speech after straight-line palatoplasty and "incomplete intravelar veloplasty". Ann Plast Surg 2006;56:505–10.

24. Brown AS, Cohen MA, Randall P. Levator muscle reconstruction: does it make a difference? Plast Reconstr Surg 1983;72:1–6.

25. Andrades P, Espinosa-de-los-Monteros A, Shell DH IV, et al. The importance of radical intravelar veloplasty during two-flap palatoplasty. Plast Reconstr Surg 2008;122:1121–30.

26. Dreyer TM, Trier WC. A comparison of palatoplasty techniques. Cleft Palate J 1984;21:251–3.

27. Marsh JL, Grames LM, Holtman B. Intravelar veloplasty: a prospective study. Cleft Palate J 1989; 26:46–50.

28. Kirschner RE, Wang P, Jawad AF, et al. Cleft-palate repair by modified Furlow double-opposing Z-plasty: the Children's Hospital of Philadelphia experience. Plast Reconstr Surg 1999;104:1998–2010.

29. Furnas DW, Fischer GW. The Z-plasty: biomechanics and mathematics. Br J Plast Surg 1971; 24:144–60.

30. D'Antonio LL, Eichenberg BJ, Zimmerman GJ, et al. Radiographic and aerodynamic measures of velopharyngeal anatomy and function following Furlow Z-plasty. Plast Reconstr Surg 2000;106: 539–49.

31. Huang MH, Riski JE, Cohen SR, et al. An anatomic evaluation of the Furlow double opposing Z-plasty technique of cleft palate repair. Ann Acad Med Singapore 1999;28:672–6.

32. Guneren E, Uysal OA. The quantitative evaluation of palatal elongation after Furlow palatoplasty. J Oral Maxillofac Surg 2004;62:446–50.

33. Kravath RE, Pollak CP, Borowiecki B, et al. Obstructive sleep apnea and death associated with surgical correction of velopharyngeal incompetence. J Pediatr 1980;96:645–8.

34. Losee JE, Smith DM, Vecchione L, et al. Post-palatoplasty fistulae: diagnosis, treatment, and prevention. In: Losee J, Kirschner R, editors. Comprehensive cleft care. New York, NY: McGraw-Hill Professional; 2008. p. 525–44.

35. Losee JE, Smith DM, Afifi AM, et al. A successful algorithm for limiting postoperative fistulae following palatal procedures in the patient with orofacial clefting. Plast Reconstr Surg 2008;122: 544–54.

36. Muzaffar AR, Byrd HS, Rohrich RJ, et al. Incidence of cleft palate fistula: an institutional experience with two-stage palatal repair. Plast Reconstr Surg 2001;108:1515–8.

37. Smith DM, Vecchione L, Jiang S, et al. The Pittsburgh Fistula Classification System: a standardized scheme for the description of palatal fistulas. Cleft Palate Craniofac J 2007;44:590–4.

38. Kummer AW. Assessment of velopharyngeal function. In: Losee J, Kirschner R, editors. Comprehensive cleft care. New York, NY: McGraw-Hill Professional; 2008. p. 1166.

39. McWilliams BJ, Morris HL, Shelton RL. Cleft palate speech. Philadelphia: B.C. Decker; 1990.

40. Amaratunga NA. Occurrence of oronasal fistulas in operated cleft palate patients. J Oral Maxillofac Surg 1988;46:834–8.

41. Wilhelmi BJ, Appelt EA, Hill L, et al. Palatal fistulas: rare with the two-flap palatoplasty repair. Plast Reconstr Surg 2001;107:315–8.

42. Brothers DB, Dalston RW, Peterson HD, et al. Comparison of the Furlow double-opposing Z-palatoplasty with the Wardill-Kilner procedure for isolated clefts of the soft palate. Plast Reconstr Surg 1995;95:969–77.

43. Cohen SR, Kalinowski J, LaRossa D, et al. Cleft palate fistulas: a multivariate statistical analysis of prevalence, etiology, and surgical management. Plast Reconstr Surg 1991;87:1041–7.

44. Gunther E, Wisser JR, Cohen MA, et al. Palatoplasty: Furlow's double reversing Z-plasty versus intravelar veloplasty. Cleft Palate Craniofac J 1998;35:546–9.

45. Khosla RK, Mabry K, Castiglione CL. Clinical outcomes of the Furlow Z-plasty for primary cleft palate repair. Cleft Palate Craniofac J 2008;45:501–10.

46. Kirschner RE, Randall P, Wang P, et al. Cleft palate repair at 3 to 7 months of age. Plast Reconstr Surg 2000;105:2127–32.

47. Marrinan EM, LaBrie RA, Mulliken JB. Velopharyngeal function in nonsyndromic cleft palate: relevance of surgical technique, age at repair, and cleft type. Cleft Palate Craniofac J 1998;35:95–100.

48. McWilliams BJ, Randall P, LaRossa D, et al. Speech characteristics associated with the Furlow palatoplasty as compared with other surgical techniques. Plast Reconstr Surg 1996;98:610–9.

49. Phua YS, de Chalain T. Incidence of oronasal fistulae and velopharyngeal insufficiency after cleft palate repair: an audit of 211 children born between 1990 and 2004. Cleft Palate Craniofac J 2008;45:172–8.

50. Salyer KE, Sng KW, Sperry EE. Two-flap palatoplasty: 20-year experience and evolution of

surgical technique. Plast Reconstr Surg 2006;118: 193–204.

51. Sommerlad BC. A technique for cleft palate repair. Plast Reconstr Surg 2003;112:1542–8.

52. Holland S, Gabbay JS, Heller JB, et al. Delayed closure of the hard palate leads to speech problems and deleterious maxillary growth. Plast Reconstr Surg 2007;119:1302–10.

53. Randall P, LaRossa D, McWilliams BJ, et al. Palatal length in cleft palate as a predictor of speech outcome. Plast Reconstr Surg 2000;106:1254–9.

54. Bekerecioglu M, Isik D, Bulut O. Comparison of the rate of palatal fistulation after two-flap and four-flap palatoplasty. Scand J Plast Reconstr Surg Hand Surg 2005;39:287–9.

55. Helling ER, Dev VR, Garza J, et al. Low fistula rate in palatal clefts closed with the Furlow technique using decellularized dermis. Plast Reconstr Surg 2006;117:2361–5.

56. Bindingnavele VK, Bresnick SD, Urata MM, et al. Superior results using the islandized hemipalatal flap in palatoplasty: experience with 500 cases. Plast Reconstr Surg 2008;122:232–9.

57. Sullivan SR, Marrinan EM, LaBrie RA, et al. Palatoplasty outcomes in nonsyndromic patients with cleft palate: a 29-year assessment of one surgeon's experience. J Craniofac Surg 2009;20:612–6.

58. Lu Y, Shi B, Zheng Q, et al. Incidence of palatal fistula after palatoplasty with levator veli palatini retropositioning according to Sommerlad. Br J Oral Maxillofac Surg 2010;48:637–40.

59. Steinbacher DM, McGrath JL, Low DW. Is nasal mucoperiosteal closure necessary in cleft palate repair? Plast Reconstr Surg 2011;127:768–73.

Surgical Considerations in Pierre Robin Sequence

Justine C. Lee, MD, PhD[a], James P. Bradley, MD[b],*

KEYWORDS

- Pierre Robin sequence • Airway protection • Micrognathic patients • Mandibular Distraction

KEY POINTS

- A portion of Pierre Robin infants will escape surgical intervention for airway protection because of postnatal growth at the posterior ramus and condylar growth sites.
- The use of a Decision Tree Model with appropriate consultants and diagnostics studies is useful to determine the best candidates for mandibular distraction.
- There was a greater that 50% reduction in tracheostomy when mandibular distraction was included in the treatment algorhythm.
- Lower morbidity and health care costs was seen when airway protection was achieved with mandibular distraction as opposed to tracheostomy.

INTRODUCTION

In the early twentieth century, Pierre Robin described a triad of manifestations in neonates that included micrognathia, glossoptosis, and upper airway obstruction.[1] Robin's description is now considered to be a sequence of developmental events without a specific genetic basis. Reports of the incidence of Pierre Robin sequence (PRS) vary widely due to the comparative rarity of the manifestations and differences in diagnostic criteria. Specifically, the presence of cleft palate is a debatable absolute inclusion criterion for PRS among some institutions. The 2 best studies from regional or institutional data in Liverpool and Copenhagen estimate the incidence for PRS between 1 case per 8500 neonates and 1 case per 14,000 neonates.[2,3]

PRS can be seen as an isolated phenomenon or in combination with other malformations. From a compilation of data from the authors institution and other centers, isolated PRS occurs in 58% to 70% of patients.[3–6] In patients who had PRS in combination with syndromes, Stickler, 22q deletion, and Treacher Collins syndrome have been the most prevalent. When PRS occurs in isolation, in utero deformational factors such as intrauterine growth restriction are generally considered to be important.[7]

ANATOMIC CHANGES IN PIERRE ROBIN SEQUENCE

The approach to a patient with PRS begins with a complete understanding of the anatomic basis of the sequence. The mandible is a first pharyngeal arch derivative and formed by the primordium of migrating neural crest cells that appear during the fourth week of gestation.[8] At 6 weeks of gestation, the trigeminal nerve stimulates endochondral osteogenesis from Meckel cartilage, forming the major structures of the mandible. When genetic syndromes or deformational factors disrupt prenatal growth, micrognathia ensues and causes the retropositioning of the tongue. If this process occurs before the eighth week of gestation, closure of the palatal shelves is prevented, thereby resulting in the formation of a U-shaped cleft palate.[9]

Postnatal mandibular growth occurs via the coordination of appositional and endochondral growth at 2 major sites. The increase in mandibular length is largely accomplished by appositional forces at the symphysis, resulting in the formation of bone at the posterior border of the ramus and the anterior border of the body during the first year of life.[10] Subsequently, chondrogenic proliferation at the condyles precedes endochondral

[a] Division of Plastic Surgery, University of California, 200 UCLA Medical Plaza, Suite 460, Los Angeles, CA 90095, USA; [b] Section of Plastic and Reconstructive Surgery, Temple University, 3440 N. Broad Street, Philadelphia, PA 19140, USA
* Corresponding author.
E-mail address: jpbradley4@mac.com

Clin Plastic Surg 41 (2014) 211–217
http://dx.doi.org/10.1016/j.cps.2013.12.007
0094-1298/14/$ – see front matter © 2014 Elsevier Inc. All rights reserved.

ossification and increase in vertical ramus height. Although neonates born with PRS may have clinically significant symptoms, a portion of children may escape surgical intervention due to postnatal mandibular catch-up growth. This phenomenon is generally more common to patients with isolated PRS, likely due to the release of interference by deformational intrauterine factors after delivery. Work by Randall and colleagues[11] emphasized that the catch-up effect is limited to only a subset of patients. They conducted a longitudinal evaluation of a cohort of patients with neonatal micrognathia with mild-to-severe respiratory obstruction and discovered 3 patterns of mandibular growth. One group of patients eventually showed an almost normal size and position of the mandible. A second group of patients showed persistent micrognathia throughout childhood. A third group of patients had a similar type of underdevelopment of the mandible but with compensatory mechanisms that allowed a fairly normal anterior relationship. Clinically, Monasterio and Figueroa, in separate studies, observed that some patients who were treated conservatively continued to have respiratory disturbances throughout life.[12,13] Thus, it is clear that specific criteria are necessary to systematically identify patients who need definitive intervention versus those who need expectant management.

GENERAL CONCEPTS FOR TREATMENT

The most critical consequence of PRS is upper airway obstruction in the neonatal period. The severity of airway obstruction is largely defined by the interventions necessary to maintain patency. In the mildest of circumstances, side or prone positioning may be sufficient to prevent respiratory compromise. In patients who cannot maintain airway patency with positioning alone, intubation using a nasopharyngeal tube or an endotracheal tube may be necessary. In neonates who require intubation for survival, a surgical procedure is virtually universal in order to extubate the child. The current armamentarium of airway interventions includes glossopexy, mandibular distraction, or tracheostomy.

The nature of the upper respiratory problems has been defined by several investigators. Using fiber optic endoscopy, Sher sought to delineate the causes for airway obstruction in PRS. With the criteria of micrognathia, cleft palate, and airway obstruction, Sher found that obstruction can occur via

1. Retropositioning of the tongue to compress against the posterior pharyngeal wall

2. Retropositioning of the tongue to compress the soft palate to the posterior pharyngeal wall
3. Lateral pharyngeal wall collapse
4. Generalized pharyngeal wall collapse

Correlating his observational data to outcomes, Sher found that glossopexy relieved airway obstruction symptoms when retropositioning of the tongue resulted in compression of the pharyngeal wall. All 3 latter circumstances could not be relieved by glossopexy alone. Cozzi and Pierro added to the knowledge of pathologic airway obstruction by noting the oropharyngeal collapse brought about inadequate pharyngeal support to resist the force of high inspiratory negative pressures.[14] They reported that in normal breathing the pharynx does not collapse in the face of negative intrathoracic pressure, because a neuromuscular mechanism motored by the genioglossus retains patency. In PRS, retrodisplacement of the mandibular attachment of the genioglossus diminishes the ability to hold the tongue out of the pharyngeal airway. Although glossopexy has the ability to temporarily relieve obstruction due to a retropositioned tongue, the procedure depends on sufficient catch-up growth for reversal. Glossopexy does not address the core anatomic disturbance. Based on this assessment of the medical literature, the preference of the authors is to either offer definitive surgical management or nonsurgical management.

In the event that a neonate demonstrates signs of critical upper airway obstruction, the authors advocates for an algorithm that emphasizes distraction osteogenesis with the caveat that other abnormalities are absent. Over the past 2 decades, mandibular distraction osteogenesis has become an important technique to reduce the proportion of children with PRS who undergo tracheostomy.

The general concept of distraction begins with an initial osteotomy followed by a mechanical linear force from the distraction device that serves to direct the formation of bone. There are 3 phases of the distraction process: latency, activation, and consolidation. Latency is the period immediately following the osteotomy, which is usually 0 to 2 days for the mandible. During the activation phase, distraction occurs at a specific rate and rhythm. A typical rate of distraction is 1 mm/d with a rhythm of turning the devices twice a day (eg, 0.5 mm in the morning and 0.5 mm at night). The length of distraction is determined by the size of the defect or the length necessary to correct a functional problem. Finally, molding the regenerate may also be a consideration during the activation phase to close an open bite, correct form, or improve symmetry while the bone remains soft. Consolidation involves the mineralization and hardening of the new bone formed by the distraction process. The time of full consolidation may vary but is generally between 6 and 12 weeks following completion of distraction.

PRS patients are precluded from mandibular distraction when they exhibit other abnormalities such as central apnea, multilevel airway obstruction, neurologic compromise, or airway edema from severe reflux. In patients who are not eligible for distraction, a tracheostomy is performed in the neonatal period. Some patients may later resolve their abnormalities and may be offered mandibular distraction to facilitate decannulation.

TREATMENT ALGORITHM: THE DECISION TREE MODEL

Prior to 1999, PRS patients were approached on a conventional case-by-case basis with tracheostomy as the standard of care for severe airway obstruction. However, the advent of mandibular distraction osteogenesis allowed a second option for the severe patient, albeit with increased complexity of decision making. To establish a systematic method for evaluation, the authors and colleagues implemented a decision tree that involves the input of a multidisciplinary team (Fig. 1). In both clinical outcomes and cost, they observed superiority of the decision tree model

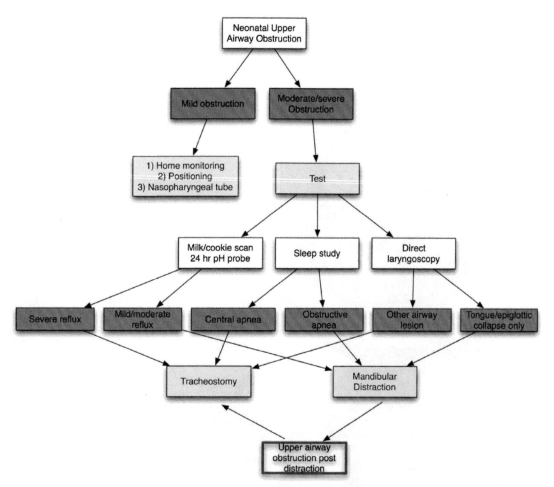

Fig. 1. Decision tree model for evaluation and treatment of Pierre Robin patients. Upon admission to the neonatal intensive care unit, patients with upper airway obstruction were stratified into either mild or moderate/severe obstruction. Patients who were mildly obstructed, defined by relief with prone or side positioning, were observed and discharged with home monitoring and instructions on positioning. For added airway protection, nasopharyngeal tube placement was performed in half of the patients. Patients with moderate or severe obstruction were subjected to 3 objective measures: (1) a sleep study to distinguish obstructive versus central apnea, (2) a milk scan or pH monitoring to document severity of reflux, (3) or direct laryngobronchoscopy to evaluate for other airway lesions. Patients were eligible for distraction provided that central apnea, severe reflux, and other airway lesions did not exist.

over unstructured care delivery. The authors and colleagues have now adopted this model as the standard of care at their institution.

In the model, newborn patients diagnosed with upper airway obstruction are admitted to the neonatal intensive care unit. The diagnosis immediately triggers the neonatologist to consult a multidisciplinary team that includes plastic surgery, otolaryngology, genetics, pulmonology, gastroenterology, and anesthesia. Comprehensive evaluation begins with a sleep study to distinguish between a central or brainstem cause for apnea and an obstructive airway cause for apnea. The study is performed with electroencephalogram (EEG), continuous pulse oximetry, and airway flow monitoring. Next, a milk scan is performed. This nuclear medicine scan is similar to the cookie swallow test used in older infants to document the prevalence and frequency of gastrointestinal reflux. In some infants, a 24-hour pH probe is used

for further documentation of reflux. The final preoperative study is a direct laryngobronchoscopy. Using a flexible endoscope, the posterior tongue and epiglottal collapse are evaluated. A rigid scope is used to rule out other airway lesions including tracheobronchial webs, vascular anomalies, or inflammation secondary to gastrointestinal reflux. At the authors institution, the direct laryngobronchoscopy is often performed just before the mandibular osteotomy and placement of internal distraction devices to contain the costs of anesthesia and the operating room.

The criteria for exclusion from mandibular distraction procedures are: (1) central apnea, (2) severe reflux, (3) other airway lesions, or (4) upper airway obstruction relieved by side or prone positioning. Neonates who demonstrate any of the first 3 criteria are subjected to tracheostomy. Neonates who demonstrate the fourth criterion are discharged with oxygen saturation and apnea

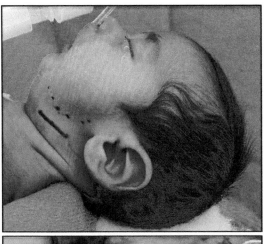
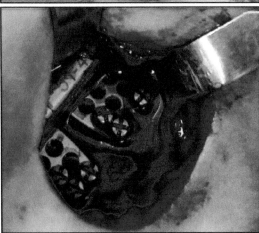
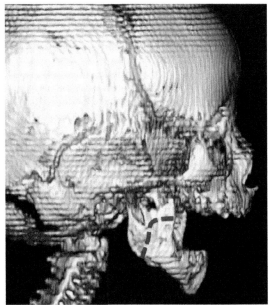

Fig. 2. Internal mandibular distractor placement. A Risdon incision is marked approximately 1 fingerbreadth below the inferior border of the mandible (*dotted line, upper left panel*). Following subperiosteal exposure of the mandible, an inverted "L" osteotomy is performed with a reciprocating saw (*right panel*). A KLS-Martin Micro Zurich internal distractor is placed on both sides of the fracture line and secured with high profile screws (*lower left panel*).

monitoring. In some discharged patients, naso-pharyngeal intubation may be performed for addi-tional security. All other patients are candidates for internal mandibular distraction.

The operative procedure for distraction is per-formed with an extraoral Risdon incision to expose the mandibular ramus in a subperiosteal plane (**Fig. 2**). An inverted "L" bicortical osteotomy is made with a reciprocating saw, and a KLS-Martin (Jacksonville, FL) Micro Zurich distractor is placed. Distraction begins after an overnight latency period at a rate of 2 mm/d and a rhythm of twice a day. The

patient may be safely extubated after 3 to 4 days of distraction. After approximately 8 days, the distrac-tion is complete, and the turning arms are removed. The distractor is removed using the same Risdon incision after 8 to 10 weeks of consolidation.

OUTCOMES OF MANDIBULAR DISTRACTION AND THE DECISION TREE MODEL

Anatomic changes following mandibular dis-traction have been evaluated with multiple modal-ities including endoscopy, videofluoroscopy, and

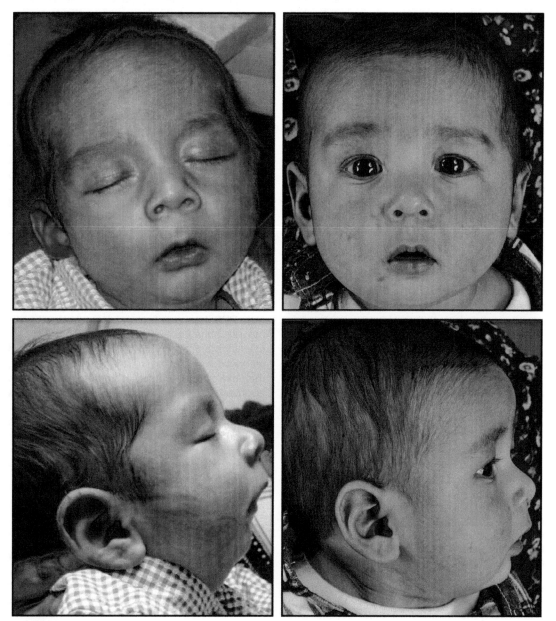

Fig. 3. Neonate with PRS who underwent mandibular distraction. Preoperative photographs (*left*) and postoper-ative photographs (*right*) are shown.

3-dimensional computed tomography.[15–17] The major changes that have correlated to improved clinical outcomes are an increase in the anterior–posterior supraglottic space, an increase in the 3-dimensional hypopharyngeal volume, and an anterior displacement of the tongue base and the hyoid (**Fig. 3**).

The authors institution and other centers have compared clinical outcomes for mandibular distraction.[4,5,18–22] These reports have documented improvements in oxygen saturation, apneic events, reflux, and feeding in neonates who received mandibular distraction. Compared with tracheostomy, patients who were treated with distraction had a shorter hospital stay, a 34-fold decreased likelihood for pneumonia, and a lower average cost per patient over the first 4 years of life ($193,128 for distraction vs $382,246 for tracheostomy).[23]

Despite the clear advantages of distraction, the number of patients who proceed to distraction and the amount of inpatient time for decision making on distraction versus tracheostomy vary between institutions. When the authors and colleagues compared the outcomes of patients at their institution treated conventionally with those treated with a decision tree model including mandibular distraction as an option, they found significant benefits from implementation of the decision tree model (**Fig. 4**).[4,18] In roughly 20% of PRS patients, prone position was sufficient for airway management in patients evaluated with either modality. With conventional treatment, most PRS neonates proceeded on to require tracheostomy. In

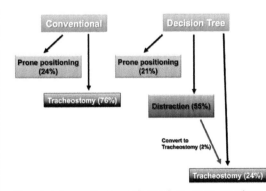

Fig. 4. Interventions performed in NICU newborns treated conventionally or with a decision tree model. Prior to the addition of mandibular distraction to the authors institutional protocol, patients were treated on a case-by-case basis. Moderate-to-severe respiratory distress obligated 76% of PRS patients to tracheostomy. Following a systematic decision tree model, tracheostomy was reserved for those patients who exhibited abnormalities beyond micrognathia-associated airway obstruction alone.

contrast, 55% of patients treated with the decision tree model received mandibular distraction with only 1 patient who required tracheostomy after distraction. Thus, the need for tracheostomy decreased from 76% to 24% of PRS patients.

Three outcomes measures were reviewed: growth, length of hospital stay, and cost.[4,23] Neonates who received conventional treatment tracheostomies averaged at the 42nd percentile for height and 28th percentile for weight. In contrast, distracted patients averaged at the 60th percentile for height and 64th percentile for weight. In terms of length of hospital stay, patients treated conventionally averaged 33 days, while patients treated with a decision tree model averaged 18 days. Finally, the total average cost per patient treated conventionally was $332,673 versus $225,998 for patients treated with a decision tree model.

The reported complications of mandibular distraction involve relapse, nerve injury, tooth injury, infection, incorrect distraction vector, and device failure.[24,25] In the neonatal population, these 6 complications are rarely detected using internal distractors. The incidence of relapse has been shown to be as high as 65%.[24] The true incidence is difficult to determine because of variabilities in growth. In patients with syndromic conditions, the authors and colleagues have noted temporomandibular joint ankylosis after distraction.[26] Elastic condylar unloading prevents most ankylosis events.

SUMMARY

The neonatal morbidity and mortality associated with PRS has significantly decreased with improved nonsurgical and surgical methods for airway protection.[27] With the introduction of distraction osteogenesis and the understanding that improved outcomes occur with a systematic approach to patient management that includes mandibular distraction for appropriate candidates, the proportion of severely micrognathic patients requiring tracheostomies can be decreased. The challenge to institutions is to implement and optimize systematic methods for evaluation and treatment of these rare neonates to achieve timely, consistent, and cost-effective outcomes.

REFERENCES

1. Robin P. Glossoptosis due to atresia and hypotrophy of the mandible. Am J Dis Child 1934;48:541–7.
2. Bush PG, Williams AJ. Incidence of the robin anomalad (Pierre Robin syndrome). Br J Plast Surg 1983; 36:434–7.
3. Printzlau A, Andersen M. Pierre Robin sequence in Denmark: a retrospective population-based

epidemiological study. Cleft Palate Craniofac J 2004;41:47–52.

4. Vyas RM, Dipple KM, Head C, et al. Management of neonatal upper airway obstruction: decreased morbidity by utilizing a decision tree model with mandibular distraction osteogenesis. J Neonatal Perinatal Med 2008;1:21–9.

5. Al-Samkari HT, Kane AA, Molter DW, et al. Neonatal outcomes of Pierre Robin sequence: an institutional experience. Clin Pediatr (Phila) 2010; 49:1117–22.

6. Cohen MM. Robin sequences and complexes: causal heterogeneity and pathogenetic/phenotypic variability. Am J Med Genet 1999;84:311–5.

7. Handley SC, Mader NS, Sidman JD, et al. Predicting surgical intervention for airway obstruction in micrognathic infants. Otolaryngol Head Neck Surg 2013; 148(5):847–51.

8. Reid RR. Facial skeletal growth and timing of surgical intervention. Clin Plast Surg 2007;34: 357–67.

9. Hanson JW, Smith DW. U-shaped palatal defect in the Robin anomalad: developmental and clinical relevance. J Pediatr 1975;87:30–3.

10. Robinson IB, Sarnat BG. Growth pattern of the pig mandible; a serial roentgenographic study using metallic implants. Am J Anat 1955;96:37–64.

11. Randall P, Krogman WM, Jahins S. Pierre Robin and the syndrome that bears his name. Cleft Palate J 1965;36:237–46.

12. Figueroa AA, Glupker TJ, Fitz MG, et al. Mandible, tongue, and airway in Pierre Robin sequence: a longitudinal cephalometric study. Cleft Palate Craniofac J 1991;28:425–34.

13. Monasterio FO, Drucker M, Molina F, et al. Distraction osteogenesis in Pierre Robin sequence and related respiratory problems in children. J Craniofac Surg 2002;13:79–83 [discussion: 84].

14. Cozzi F, Pierro A. Glossoptosis-apnea syndrome in infancy. Pediatrics 1985;75:836–43.

15. Olson TP, McMurray JS, Mount DL. Endoscopic changes in the upper airway after mandibular distraction osteogenesis. J Craniofac Surg 2011; 22:105–9.

16. Monasterio FO, Molina F, Berlanga F, et al. Swallowing disorders in Pierre Robin sequence: its correction by distraction. J Craniofac Surg 2004;15:934–41.

17. Roy S, Munson PD, Zhao L, et al. CT analysis after distraction osteogenesis in Pierre Robin Sequence. Laryngoscope 2009;119:380–6.

18. Izadi K, Yellon R, Mandell DL, et al. Correction of upper airway obstruction in the newborn with internal mandibular distraction osteogenesis. J Craniofac Surg 2003;14:493–9.

19. Genecov DG, Barceló CR, Steinberg D, et al. Clinical experience with the application of distraction osteogenesis for airway obstruction. J Craniofac Surg 2009;2(Suppl 20):1817–21.

20. Lidsky ME, Lander TA, Sidman JD. Resolving feeding difficulties with early airway intervention in Pierre Robin sequence. Laryngoscope 2008;118: 120–3.

21. Wittenborn W, Panchal J, Marsh JL, et al. Neonatal distraction surgery for micrognathia reduces obstructive apnea and the need for tracheotomy. J Craniofac Surg 2004;15:623–30.

22. Sadakah AA, Elshall MA, Farhat AA. Bilateral intraoral distraction osteogenesis for the management of severe congenital mandibular hypoplasia in early childhood. J Craniomaxillofac Surg 2009;37:216–24.

23. Kohan E, Hazany S, Roostaeian J, et al. Economic advantages to a distraction decision tree model for management of neonatal upper airway obstruction. Plast Reconstr Surg 2010;126:1652–64.

24. Master DL, Hanson PR, Gosain AK. Complications of mandibular distraction osteogenesis. J Craniofac Surg 2010;21:1565–70.

25. Mofid MM, Manson PN, Robertson BC, et al. Craniofacial distraction osteogenesis: a review of 3278 cases. Plast Reconstr Surg 2001;108:1103–14 [discussion: 1115–7].

26. Fan K, Andrews BT, Liao E, et al. Protection of the temporomandibular joint during syndromic neonatal mandibular distraction using condylar unloading. Plast Reconstr Surg 2012;129:1151–61.

27. Denny AD. Distraction osteogenesis in Pierre Robin neonates with airway obstruction. Clin Plast Surg 2004;31:221–9.

Management of the Alveolar Cleft

Pedro E. Santiago, DMD[a],*,
Lindsay A. Schuster, DMD, MS[b,c],
Daniel Levy-Bercowski, DDS, MSD[d]

KEYWORDS

• Alveolar cleft • Nasoalveolar molding • Presurgical infant orthopedics • Alveolar bone grafting

KEY POINTS

• The interdisciplinary approach to primary and secondary surgical procedures has been proven to be beneficial for patients.
• In the neonate, nasoalveolar molding has been found to optimize the aesthetic outcome of the nasal and labial repair while minimizing the extent of surgery and formation of scar tissue.
• During the mixed dentition stage, orthopedic arch preparation before the secondary alveolar bone-grafting procedure improves arch morphology, restores the functional interarch relationship, and facilitates surgical access.
• The cooperative effort between the surgeon and craniofacial orthodontist in designing strategies customized to the patient's specific needs has resulted in better esthetic and functional outcomes, minimizing surgical interventions.

INTRODUCTION

An alveolar cleft refers to the space between the maxillary segments anterior to the incisive foramen, and therefore presents a discontinuity in the dental arch. Routine cleft lip repair and subsequent cleft palate repair do not specifically address the bony deficiency at this site. Consequently, strategies specifically designed to manage the alveolar cleft must be incorporated into the complete treatment itinerary, and require a cooperative effort of the craniofacial orthodontist and surgeon. Orthopedic and orthodontic management of patients born with clefts of the lip, alveolus, and palate is based on the application of basic biomechanical principles adapted to the individualized cleft anatomy. This article focuses on orthopedic and orthodontic preparation for 2 stages of interdisciplinary orthodontic/surgical cleft care: (1) presurgical infant orthopedics

for primary lip/alveolus/nasal surgical repair; and (2) maxillary arch preparation for secondary alveolar bone grafting. These preparatory stages of orthopedic/orthodontic therapy are undertaken with the goal of restoring normal anatomic relationships to assist the surgeon in providing the best possible surgical care.

PRESURGICAL INFANT ORTHOPEDICS

The history of presurgical infant orthopedics (PSIO) dates back to 1686 when Hoffman described the use of an extraorally anchored headcap to place a retraction force on the premaxilla.[1] A similar method is described in more contemporary literature, such as in Berkowitz's 1996 article that described "a head bonnet with an external elastic that is sometimes used before surgical lip closure to ventroflex the premaxilla, thereby reducing tension at the surgical sites."[2] McNeil[3] introduced

[a] Division of Plastic Surgery, Duke University, Durham, NC, USA; [b] Cleft-Craniofacial Orthodontics, University of Pittsburgh, 4401 Penn Avenue, Pittsburgh, PA, USA; [c] Children's Hospital of Pittsburgh, Faculty Pavillion, 7th Floor, Suite 7108, Pittsburgh, PA 15224, USA; [d] Craniofacial Orthodontics, Department of Orthodontics, Georgia Regents University, 1120 15th Street, Augusta, GA 30912, USA
* Corresponding author. 3115 Academy Road, Durham, NC 27517.
E-mail address: pedro.santiago@duke.edu

Clin Plastic Surg 41 (2014) 219–232
http://dx.doi.org/10.1016/j.cps.2014.01.001
0094-1298/14/$ – see front matter © 2014 Elsevier Inc. All rights reserved.

intraorally anchored appliances in 1950, using a progressively modified feeding plate to align maxillary alveolar segments. Another popular variant of an intraoral device to mold the alveolar segments was introduced in 1980 by Latham[4]; this acrylic appliance was retained by pins to the alveolar segments and used a system of elastomeric material to move the alveolar segments in proximity. A more recent technique, nasoalveolar molding (NAM), was introduced in 1993 by Grayson and colleagues.[5] This technique not only molds the cleft alveolus as in previous PSIO protocols but also shapes and forms the nasal cartilages in preparation for the primary surgical repair.

PSIO appliances have been described as either active or passive devices. Active appliances are fixed intraorally and apply traction through mechanical means such as elastic chains, screws, and plates (eg, the Latham appliance). A passive appliance maintains the distance between the 2 maxillary segments while external force is applied to the system.[6] NAM is an example of a passive PSIO technique and is the focus of this article.

A recent study by Sischo and colleagues[7] examined the prevalence of NAM among cleft centers in the United States. Among teams interviewed via telephone survey, 37% offered NAM therapy. It was speculated that the high prevalence of NAM therapy might be due to increased insurance coverage and growing adoption of this treatment approach.

Grayson and Santiago[8] described the NAM protocol for cleft patients in 1997. NAM takes advantage of the high degree of plasticity of neonatal cartilages, molding the deformed cleft nose by incorporating a nasal stent to an alveolar molding plate. The overall goal of this presurgical orthopedic therapy is to restore the correct skeletal, cartilaginous, and soft-tissue anatomic relationships, providing the most optimal conditions for the primary lip, alveolus, and nose surgery. The intent is to create a lasting aesthetic outcome and reduce the need for, or minimize the extent of, secondary surgical revision procedures.

NAM objectives include:

1) Molding and repositioning of the alveolar processes
2) Molding and reposition of the nasal cartilages, and
3) Lengthening of the deficient columella.

Short-term (4 months to 1 year)[9-11] and long-term (4.5–9 years) studies[11-13] indicate that NAM significantly improves nasal symmetry over surgery alone.

An adjunctive surgical option, gingivoperiosteoplasty (GPP) (closure of the soft-tissue alveolar segments), is possible if there is close approximation of the cleft alveolar segments. Santiago and colleagues[14] have shown a 60% reduction in the need for a secondary alveolar bone-graft procedure in cases where a combined approach of PSIO and a GPP was performed. This combination was less expensive than a traditional protocol (lip repair, primary nasal repair, and secondary alveolar bone graft).[15] It is important to note that GPP is a separate therapeutic option from NAM, associated with its own risks and benefits.

Timing of Cleft Surgical Preparation

Referral to the cleft team before birth is now commonplace if there is diagnosis of the cleft on ultrasonography. This timing affords an opportunity for the family to become acquainted with the concept of team care and learn the generalities of the treatment options. Early consultation with the treating surgeon and NAM provider to discuss the logistics of NAM therapy in preparation for the primary lip and nose surgical repair is an important first step toward the parents' informed decisions regarding the collaborative care options.

Ideally, the interdisciplinary cleft team evaluates the neonate 1 week after birth. The cleft surgeon and craniofacial orthodontist perform a clinical examination, photos are taken, and an impression of the intraoral cleft defect is taken in a hospital setting with the surgeon as part of the impression team. This noninvasive procedure, during which the infant is fully awake and not anesthetized, is done using a premade acrylic impression tray and an elastomeric material (**Fig. 1**).

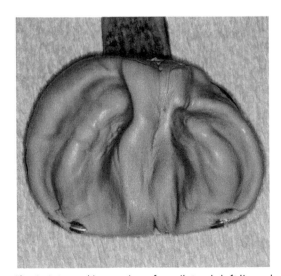

Fig. 1. Intraoral impression of a unilateral cleft lip and palate infant taken with polyvinylsiloxane material to capture the alveolar and palatal anatomy. The impression is used to create a precise stone cast model.

The impression is then used to create a stone cast and a conventional acrylic molding plate. The molding plate is made of clear orthodontic resin, and 1 or 2 (depending of the deformity) buttons or extensions are added to the anterior part of the appliance. These buttons are made of stainless-steel orthodontic wire covered with clear resin material, and grooved to hold orthodontic elastics and surgical tapes used to control the force applied to the alveolar segments (**Fig. 2**). The intraoral acrylic plate is examined for rough areas, polished, and inserted within a week of the initial visit. The molding plate is then modified on a weekly basis to approximate the intraoral segments and reduce the alveolar cleft. Once the segments are in close proximity, a nasal stent is added to mold the distorted nasal cartilages.

CORRECTING THE UNILATERAL DEFORMITY

The unilateral cleft lip and palate anomaly presents a significant nasal deformity; a detailed description of the cleft nasal deformity at infancy is provided in the article "Correction of the Cleft Nasal Deformity: From Infancy to Maturity" elsewhere in this issue by Marcus and colleagues. In brief, the lower lateral cartilage is depressed and concave on the cleft side and is separated from the contralateral cartilage located high in the nasal tip.[16] This configuration results in depression and displacement of the nasal tip and lateralization of the nostril apex. The columella and nasal septum are inclined over the cleft with the base deviated toward the noncleft side (**Fig. 3**).[17]

The goals of NAM in patients with unilateral cleft lip and palate are to reduce the severity of the cleft deformity by approximating the alveolar and lip segments and correcting malposition of the nasal cartilages, nasal tip, philtrum, and columella. These corrections are achieved through periodic

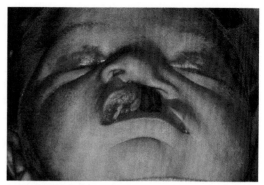

Fig. 3. The unilateral cleft lip and palate anomaly presents a significant nasal deformity. Note the depression and displacement of the nasal tip, with the columella and nasal septum inclined over the cleft with the base deviated toward the noncleft side.

modifications of the intraoral molding plate and adjustments of the extraoral nasal stent.

At the NAM appliance insertion visit, the intraoral molding plate is seated, adjusted, and activated to provide alveolar movement. Intraorally the plate is activated by the selective addition and/or removal of hard and soft acrylic. Correction of the alveolar malposition and associated soft-tissue structures is achieved by weekly modifications of the molding plate, which allows for gradual and controlled approximation of the alveolar segments.

The extraoral activation system consists of 2 surgical tapes individually folded inside the lumen of 2 orthodontic elastics, which are placed on the channel of the acrylic button. The 2 strips are then stretched and taped over a wider facial tape used to protect the neonate from skin irritation, which helps to secure the molding plate to the palate and alveolar processes. Therefore, the tape and elastic construct is usually more active on the side toward the intended movement. As the effectiveness of the NAM therapy depends on the

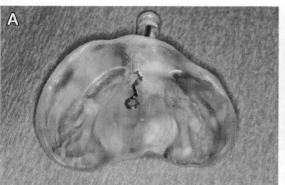
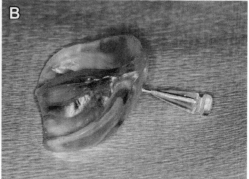

Fig. 2. (*A*) Acrylic molding plate made from a stone cast model. The plate is polished, rough surfaces removed, and a layer of soft acrylic added to the borders to avoid soft-tissue irritation. (*B*) An anterior wire and acrylic extension (button) is added and channeled to support the elastic bands attached to the tape system.

stability of the plate on the transported segment, some clinicians prefer to use a small amount of denture adhesive only on the segment to be mobilized (**Fig. 4**).

Once the alveolar segments are in close approximation (around 4 mm), lip taping and a nasal stent are added to the system (**Fig. 5**). Taping of the cleft lip segments in tight apposition assists the elastic orthopedic forces in achieving controlled approximation of the alveolar cleft segments. In addition, it improves alignment of the nasal base region by bringing the columella toward the midsagittal plane and improving symmetry of the nostril apertures. In select patients, lip taping can be started before the nasal stent is incorporated into the molding plate.

The nasal stent is constructed from an orthodontic wire carefully bent into a gooseneck shape, which is incorporated into the anterior flange of the oral molding plate. The most superior part of the wire is covered with hard and soft acrylic to ensure that tissue breakdown does not occur when positive pressure is applied to the nasal lining. The stent is positioned inside the nose underneath the apex of the alar cartilage on the cleft side. The alar dome cartilage on the cleft side is lifted by the stent to achieve normal elevation and symmetry.

The nasal stent is gradually modified on a weekly basis. The shape of the cartilaginous septum, dome, and medial and lateral crura are carefully molded to resemble the normal shape of these structures.

At the conclusion of nasal and alveolar molding, the nasal cartilages, columella, philtrum, and alveolar segments should be properly aligned to facilitate the surgical restoration of normal anatomic relationships (**Fig. 6**).

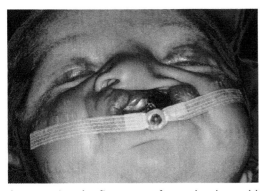

Fig. 4. During the first stage of nasoalveolar molding (NAM) therapy, the intraoral molding plate and elastics–surgical tapes system are used to differentially mobilize the alveolar segments and reduce the cleft gap.

CORRECTING THE BILATERAL DEFORMITY

The bilateral deformity presents a different set of challenges. In the bilateral cleft, the alar cartilages have failed to migrate up into the nasal tip and elongate the columella. The alar cartilages are positioned along the alar margins and are stretched over the cleft as flaring alae. In addition, the premaxilla is suspended from the tip of the nasal septum, whereas the lateral alveolar segments remain behind.[18,19] Disparate growth may occur, causing overprojection, flexion, or rotation of the premaxillary segment (**Fig. 7**).

The goal of presurgical NAM in patients born with bilateral cleft lip and palate is to lengthen the columella, reposition the nasal cartilages toward the tip, and align the alveolar segments.

As in the unilateral deformity, an intraoral impression of the neonate is taken and a bilateral acrylic molding plate is fabricated. In contrast to the unilateral plate, the bilateral plate has 2 anterior wire and acrylic extensions or buttons. The first stage of treatment consists of retracting and uprighting the everted premaxilla into the space between the 2 lateral alveolar segments (**Fig. 8**). This goal is achieved by weekly modifications of the intraoral molding plate and the use of orthodontic elastics and surgical tapes, as described for unilateral deformity. In the second stage of treatment, as the alveolar segments gradually approximate one another, 2 nasal stents are incorporated into the anterior rim of the molding plate and enter the nasal apertures (**Fig. 9**). The nasal stents support the nasal tip and create tissue-expanding forces that are directed to the columella and domes internally. A surgical tape is applied to the prolabium, pulled down, and adhered to an orthodontic elastic attached to the 2 anterior buttons (**Fig. 10**). A horizontal prolabial band made of soft acrylic may also be attached across the 2 nasal stents to depress the columella base in the region normally represented by the lip-columella junction, providing countertraction force to the columellar tissue. Each functional component of the bilateral system is gradually modified to mold the hard and soft tissues and achieve the desired goals (**Fig. 11**).

Presurgical NAM has proved to be a valuable adjuvant therapy to the primary surgical repair, offering 4 major benefits:

1. The controlled presurgical alignment of the cleft alveolar and lip segments into normalized anatomic relationships and the correction of the nasal deformity reduces tension on the repair and may reduce the extent of the primary lip and nasal surgery required. Reduction of

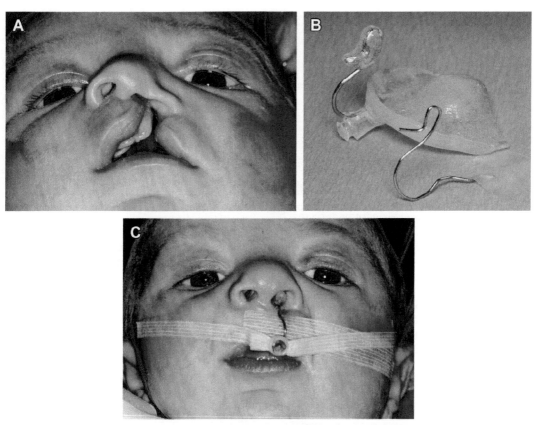

Fig. 5. (*A*) Alveolar segments in close approximation after 5 weeks of NAM therapy. (*B*) The nasal stent is constructed from an orthodontic wire carefully bent into a gooseneck shape and incorporated into the anterior flange of the oral molding plate. The most superior part of the wire is covered with hard and soft acrylic to ensure that tissue breakdown does not occur when positive pressure is applied to the nasal lining. (*C*) Taping of the cleft lip segments in tight apposition assists the elastic orthopedic forces to achieve controlled approximation of the alveolar cleft segments, and also improves alignment of the nasal base. The nasal stent molds the distorted nasal structures to resemble their normal shape.

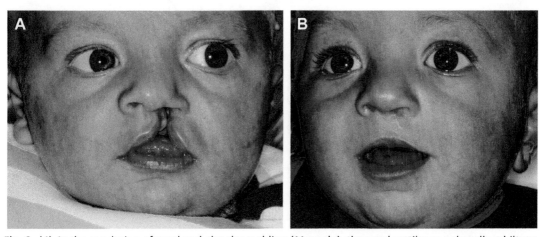

Fig. 6. (*A*) At the conclusion of nasal and alveolar molding (11 weeks), the nasal cartilages, columella, philtrum, and alveolar segments are properly aligned to facilitate the surgical restoration of normal anatomic relationships. (*B*) The goal of the combined presurgical NAM therapy and primary lip/nose surgery is to create a lasting aesthetic outcome and reduce the need or minimize the extent of secondary surgical revision procedures.

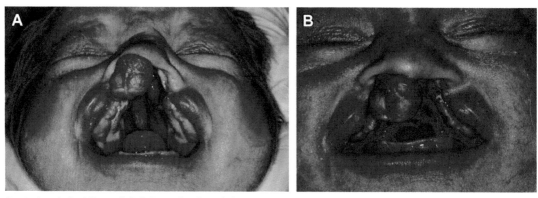

Fig. 7. (*A, B*) The bilateral cleft lip and palate deformity presents a displaced and protruded premaxilla, wide alar bases, and a deficient columella.

the primary deformity creates a more favorable and uniform starting point, which may facilitate more consistent results and diminish the residual deformity.

2. The presurgical closure of the alveolar gap provides the surgeon with the option to perform a GPP at the time of lip closure. Santiago and colleagues[14] have reported that this procedure reduces the need of a secondary bone grafting in more than 60% of the cases studied.

3. In the bilateral cleft deformity, nonsurgical columella lengthening eliminates the need for secondary surgical columella elongation and the accompanying scars at the lip-columella junction (**Fig. 12**).

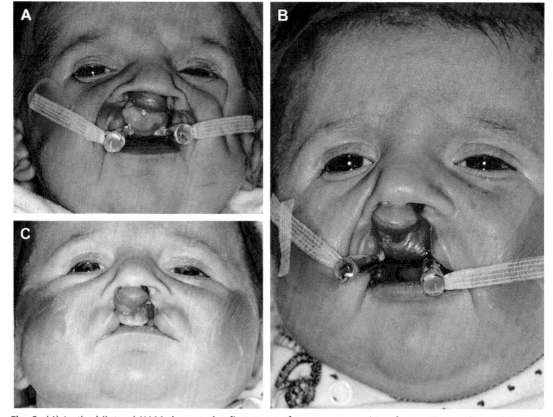

Fig. 8. (*A*) In the bilateral NAM therapy the first stage of treatment consists of retracting and uprighting the everted premaxilla into the space between the 2 lateral alveolar segments. (*B, C*) At approximately 8 weeks of NAM therapy, the premaxilla has been retracted and positioned between the lateral alveolar segments. The prolabium has been uprighted.

A

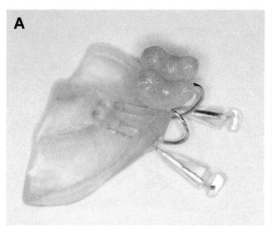

B

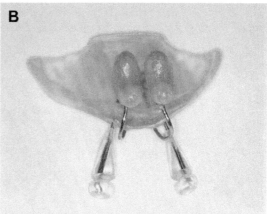

Fig. 9. (*A, B*) In the second stage of treatment, as the alveolar segments gradually approximate one another, 2 nasal stents are incorporated into the anterior rim of the molding plate to enter the nasal apertures.

4. NAM, when used in conjunction with a modified surgical approach, allows for a single initial surgical procedure to address the lip-nose-alveolus complex and its deformity. By minimizing the residual deformity, revisionary surgery may be avoided, thereby reducing the number and extent of surgeries that a cleft patient will undergo during a lifetime.

SECONDARY ALVEOLAR BONE GRAFTING IN MIXED DENTITION

In patients born with a cleft lip and palate, lip/nasal and palatal surgery are commonly performed during the first 14 months of life. If a GPP is not included at the primary surgery, the remaining bony defect in the alveolar region is addressed with a secondary alveolar bone-graft procedure during the stage of mixed dentition.

Bone grafting was introduced at the beginning of the twentieth century when Von Eiselberg used a small finger as a pedicle graft in 1901. Bone grafting using tibia and periosteum was introduced in 1914 by Drachter.[20] Secondary bone grafting using the iliac crest was introduced by Boyne in 1970. Before the advent of osseous grafting techniques to restore the bony cleft defect, prosthodontic rehabilitation was the common method of reconciling the alveolar cleft. After World War II, with the advent of antibiotic therapy, the use of bone-graft procedures for the correction of the alveolar cleft increased significantly.[21] Today, bone grafting of the alveolus has become widely accepted as the standard of care in patients with cleft lip and palate.[22–24]

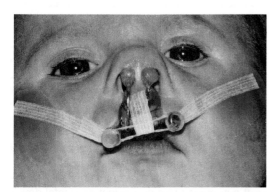

Fig. 10. A surgical tape is applied to the prolabium, pulled down, and adhered to orthodontic elastics attached to the 2 anterior buttons. This downward pull, combined with the upward and anterior force applied by the nasal stents at the tip of the nose, results in a stretching and lengthening of the columella.

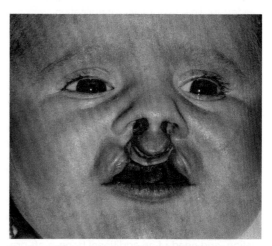

Fig. 11. At the conclusion of the bilateral NAM therapy, the alveolar and lip segments should be approximated and aligned and the columellar tissue expanded to normal anatomic values, facilitating primary lip/nose/alveolar surgery.

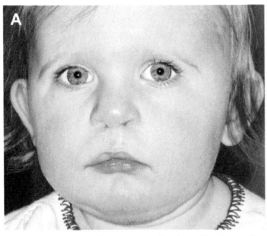
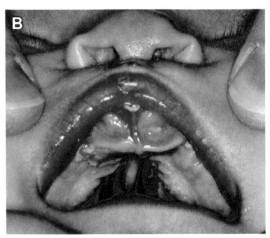

Fig. 12. (*A*) NAM with nonsurgical columella elongation may eliminate the need for surgical lengthening of the columella, minimizing the extent of scarring in the nasolabial complex. (*B*) In this patient a gingivoperiosteoplasty procedure was performed at the time of the primary surgery, providing alveolar arch continuity and a possible elimination of a secondary bone-grafting procedure.

Secondary bone grafting requires collaborative treatment planning between the members of the craniofacial team, especially the orthodontist and the surgeon. It is performed in patients born with a cleft alveolus to restore the normal architecture of the maxilla. Secondary bone grafting allows for eruption of the permanent teeth (specifically the permanent lateral incisor and the canine), closure of an oronasal fistula if present, and the stabilization of the maxillary arch by providing bone continuity between the segments. In addition, such bone grafting improves the aesthetic outcome by providing support and elevation to the alar base. Finally, it allows adequate bone support in cases where an endosteal implant is needed for final restorative rehabilitation.[22,23,25]

TIMING OF BONE GRAFTING ON THE CLEFT MAXILLA

Bone grafting in patients with cleft lip and palate can be divided into 2 main categories, primary and secondary. Primary bone grafting is performed in patients younger than 2 years with the intent to improve arch form, preserve the lateral incisor, decrease the need for orthognathic surgery, and stabilize the premaxilla in bilateral patients.[26] However, primary bone grafting has declined in popularity because of negative reports regarding compromised midfacial growth, high incidence in malocclusion, inadequate bone formation, and need of an additional bone-graft procedure later in the patient's life.[22,23,27]

Secondary bone grafting can also be classified as early, intermediate, or late. Early secondary bone grafting is performed between ages of 2 and 5 years, or at a primary dentition stage. Some advantages of this procedure have been reported, such as good quality of bone formation, allowing for the eruption or movement of the central incisor adjacent to cleft or the future eruption of the lateral incisor.[21,22,28] However, midfacial growth can be affected, as in primary bone grafting.[23] Intermediate bone grafting is carried out between 5 and 12 years old during the mixed dentition stage, with the goal of having bony support for the eruption of the permanent lateral incisor and canine without negative consequences in terms of midfacial growth.[29] Finally, late secondary bone grafting is performed in late adolescents or adult patients in the state of permanent dentition, in whom the growth of the maxilla has been completed. At this stage, the main goal is the provision of maxillary continuity in cases where orthognathic surgery is indicated, to enable a one-piece Lefort advancement and/or have adequate bone available for a future implant restoration.[22,30,31] Late bone grafting may place the teeth adjacent to the cleft at risk because of lack of bone support, and complications can occur at this stage, such as progressive root resorption caused by the direct contact of the grafted bone and the exposed root surface.[32]

In summary, timing is critical relative to the age of the patient and the stage of eruption of the teeth adjacent to the cleft.[33] The ideal timing for bone-graft surgery is more dependent on dental development than on chronologic age. Grafting during the state of primary dentition or at full dental maturity carries risks to maxillary growth and dental support, respectively. Ideally the procedure should be timed to minimize growth disturbance and detrimental effects on the adjacent dentition. The root of the permanent canine provides a guide to treatment timing; it should be formed at least to one-half or two-thirds of its definitive length at the time of the graft placement.[23,25] Numerous studies have demonstrated high success rates when the graft procedure is undertaken before the canine eruption, in comparison with delayed grafting.[28]

SOURCE OF BONE-GRAFT MATERIAL

Materials of various origins have been used to correct the maxillary alveolar cleft, including autogenous, allogeneic, and xenogeneic bone materials and, more recently, growth factors such as bone morphogenetic protein (BMP). There is a general consensus that fresh autogenous cancellous bone is the ideal bone-grafting source, because it supplies living, immunocompatible bony cells that integrate fully with the maxilla, and are indispensable for osteogenesis.[20] For autotransplantation several donor sites have been used: iliac crest, cranial bone, tibia, and mandibular symphysis.

Iliac Crest for Secondary Bone Graft

Iliac crest is used in most craniofacial centers as a source of bone for secondary bone graft.[30,34] It is easy to access, and contains a large volume of cancellous bone and a larger stem cell population that support osteogenesis after grafting.[20,21,23,28] The main concern when using iliac crest is postoperative discomfort, which can effect gait and result in a prolonged recovery. These complications can be minimized with a careful surgical approach involving limited incision, minimal elevation of the musculature on the crest, meticulous hemostasis, carefully layered wound closure with reapproximation of the cartilage cap, adequate postoperative pain control, and early ambulation.[20,28] Most surgeons favor iliac crest bone graft because it provides an adequate amount of bone and an unlimited supply of marrow rich in cellular matrix for grafting.[24,30,35]

Cranial Bone for Bone Graft

Cranial bone has been used for the last 2 decades. In comparison with iliac crest, it provides a convenient source of cortical and cancellous bone with minimal postoperative pain and a hidden scar. Grafting with calvarial bone varies with respect to the method of harvest, the area of the cranium from where it is taken, the size of the defect, and the proportion of cortical to cancellous bone available.[24,36] Potential complications include hematoma, seroma, dural tear, dural exposure,

subdural hemorrhage, cerebrospinal fluid leak, and brain injury or neurologic sequelae.[20,22,23]

Tibia Bone for Bone Graft

Tibia has been a common donor site among orthopedic surgeons, and has recently gained popularity among maxillofacial surgeons for grafting in patients with cleft lip and palate and for preprosthetic rehabilitations. Most studies using tibial bone have been conducted in adult patients, and a relatively limited quantity of bone has been obtained. For this reason, the technique is not indicated for every cleft deformity, and it is important to inform the patient about the possibility of harvesting bone from both legs. Concerns exist regarding disturbances to the epiphyseal cartilage affecting the growth of the individual, which is a disincentive to application in young patients. Some advantages have been reported, such as reduced operating time, minimal scarring, early ambulation, and reduced stay in hospital.[20,22,34]

Mandibular Symphysis for Bone Graft

The mandibular symphysis is an attractive donor site, as it involves the same operative field and has an embryonic origin analogous to that of the maxilla. Absence of visible scar, reduction of postoperative discomfort, reduced stay in hospital, faster revascularization, and an improved preservation of the graft volume have been reported as advantages of this source area.[20,34,37] As in other bone donor sites, the mandibular symphysis involves a specific set of potential complications, including the risk of damage to the canine and incisor roots and injury to the mental nerve. In addition, the quantity of bone available may be limited by the state of mandibular development.[23,34]

Rib for Bone Graft

For primary bone grafting, the Rosenstein protocol[24] uses rib as the donor source. Specific potential complications reported using rib as donor include bone resorption, atelectasis, pneumothorax, wound breakdown, scarring, and pain.[34] Other investigators have found difficulty with tooth movement during the orthodontic treatment and inconsistent tooth eruption through the graft.[21,22]

Bone Substitutes for Bone Graft

Bone substitutes such as allogeneic materials and bovine-derived hydroxyapatite have been used for secondary alveolar bone grafting. These materials share the common advantage of eliminating the morbidity of a second operative site.[22] Studies using allogeneic bone graft (freeze-dried bone) have shown the potential to achieve orthodontic movement of the canine into the grafted region, eruption of the canine, and stabilization of the segments.[38–40] Complications of infection, disease transmission from donor to host, and host incompatibility have been reported in the literature.[23,28] The consolidation of allogeneic graft seems to require a longer period of time, thereby delaying the beginning of the orthodontic treatment.[41]

BMPs are a group of growth factors that play an important role in osteogenesis and chondrogenesis. Specifically, BMP-2 and BMP-7 are known for their osteoinductive properties.[42,43] BMP has been used for several maxillofacial surgical purposes, including maxillary sinus floor for augmentation before endosteal implant placement for prosthodontic rehabilitation.[44] Several studies have shown encouraging results in alveolar cleft repair using recombinant human BMP (rhBMP). In one study performed in skeletally mature patients with cleft lip and palate, rhBMP-2 in a collagen matrix demonstrated better results when compared with autogenous iliac crest bone graft. The repaired defect had greater volume in the rhBMP-2 group; there were also reductions in hospital stay, cost, healing problems, and pain.[45] Conversely, in another study performed in skeletally immature patients, rhBMP-2 in a collagen matrix showed less bone volume measured by computed tomography (CT) when compared with the iliac crest group; however, acceptable results were obtained with both materials.[46] Despite clinical studies showing the benefits in using the rhBMP-2 for the correction of craniomaxillofacial defects, this material has been related to its own set of complications, most prominently in the orthopedic literature; significant operative-site edema has been noted, as well as resorption of vertebral bodies in spinal column repair.[43] The use of rhBMP-2 among growing patients remains off-label; the safety associated with application in this population remains uncertain. In animal models, the use of rhBMP-2 has resulted in premature fusion of sutures and growth restriction, which could be detrimental in a clinical setting.[47]

Platelet-rich Plasma Injections

Finally, among emerging experimental techniques, platelet-rich plasma injections in an animal model of the alveolar cleft has shown promise in permitting orthodontic tooth movement into the alveolar defect. The enriched blood plasma is thought to enhance new bone formation and reduce the dimensions of the alveolar bone defect.[48]

MAXILLARY ARCH PREPARATION BEFORE AN ALVEOLAR BONE-GRAFT PROCEDURE
Orthodontic Planning

Orthodontic records in patients born with a cleft lip and palate include thorough evaluation and documentation of the cleft region. Conventional records in orthodontics include facial and intraoral photographs, study models, and panoramic and cephalometric radiographs. As the cleft deformity usually presents both skeletal and dental abnormalities, it is recommended to include a 3-dimensional cone-beam CT (CBCT) of the cleft maxilla to evaluate dental development and bony architecture. CBCT facilitates the timing of decisions relative to dental eruption, and evaluation of the cleft osseous gap and adjacent dentition including supernumeraries, as well as tooth size and shape abnormalities. Moreover, CBCT may facilitate detailed and accurate postoperative outcomes analysis.[31]

There are 3 important issues to consider when performing presurgical orthodontic preparation for a secondary bone-grafting procedure: the dentition around the cleft area, the eruption of the permanent teeth through the graft, and the anteroposterior and transverse maxillary deficiencies. Supernumerary teeth, malformed permanent teeth (normally lateral incisor with poor root development), or remaining primary dentition on the cleft region should be removed before the secondary bone graft. Usually the extraction of these teeth should be performed 2 to 3 months before the surgical intervention to maintain the integrity of the palatal mucosa, cover the entire graft, and eliminate any portal for potential infection during the postoperative period.[49]

The maxillary incisors normally erupt rotated, retroclined, or in anterior cross-bite.[29] The alignment of the teeth adjacent to the cleft should not be corrected before the graft procedure, or in such a case the orthodontic movement should be limited to the available bone into which the roots of the teeth can be moved. These 2 aspects are essential in avoiding dehiscences and fenestrations.[50]

The bony and soft-tissue defects, and the presence of anomalies as well as supernumerary, missing, or malformed teeth, create an abnormal eruption pattern and increase the risk of impaction of the canine.[51] One of the most important benefits of the secondary bone graft is that the new grafted bone acts as alveolar bone, allowing the natural migration and eruption of the permanent canine. The maxillary canine can erupt spontaneously after the bone-graft procedure, with a success rate between 72% and 80%. Surgical exposure of the canine for orthodontic traction is performed in 6% to 18% of cases.[52,53] Moving the canine into the graft allows space closure and mesial movement of the posterior teeth on the affected side, eliminating the need for prosthetic replacement of the absent lateral incisor. In cases where the canine erupts before the bone-graft surgery, close evaluation of the area is necessary to reduce the possibility of a periodontal defect. Occasionally the graft can cause resorption on the cervical third of roots of the teeth adjacent to the cleft, specifically the canines. This root resorption is caused by direct contact between the grafted bone and the exposed root surface.[54]

Maxillary Expansion

Management of maxillary constriction is a ubiquitous challenge in the treatment of cleft alveolus. Patients born with a cleft of the alveolus and palate usually undergo palatal closure between 10 and 14 months of age. The surgical procedure and scar-tissue retraction often produce a collapse of maxillary alveolar segments, resulting in unilateral or bilateral posterior cross-bites. This transverse deficiency must eventually be addressed by expanding the maxillary arch to provide a functional dental occlusion. A decision has to be made on whether to expand the collapsed segments before or after the secondary bone-grafting procedure. Each case needs to be evaluated individually.

The benefits of expanding the maxillary arch before the graft procedure include improvement of the upper arch morphology, correction of posterior cross-bite, avoidance of resistance to the expansion, and increase of the upper arch perimeter in cases where dental crowding is present. Expansion of the maxilla facilitates surgery by permitting improved access for meticulous repair of the nasal floor mucosa. Presurgical expansion also increases the space for graft placement, resulting in the need for insertion of greater bone-graft volume.[23,48,55]

When bone grafting is performed before expansion, the size of the defect is smaller, which facilitates tension-free closure of the gingiva and limits the volume needed for graft material. However, access for meticulous nasal mucosal repair is limited, and the morphology postoperatively becomes stabilized in the constricted state, with less bone volume in the cleft site. Despite these shortcomings, some clinicians advocate expansion after the bone-graft procedure. Advocates report that expansion and correction of posterior cross-bite is permitted despite bone continuity at the alveolus via permission of expansile forces along the midpalatal suture in the premaxillary

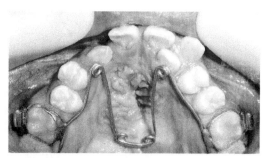

Fig. 13. Reverse quad-helix appliances provide for differential expansion in cases where more anterior than posterior expansion is needed.

region, demonstrated by the presence of a diastema between the central incisors. No radiographic alteration was observed in the grafted area during the expansion process.[56] In another study using rapid maxillary expansion after the bone graft, the midpalatal suture was opened, but the results were unpredictable.[53]

The authors' approach to maxillary constriction involves expansion before bone grafting, performed during the mixed dentition stage. The appliances may be either banded or bonded, and include the quad helix, reverse quad helix (**Fig. 13**), hyrax, fan (**Fig. 14**), and Hass expander.[30,31] In some cases, cross-bite is not observed because of the lingual tipping observed in the lower arch as a compensatory effect of the maxillary atresia.[49] Rapid maxillary expansion presents a different pattern of expansion depending on the type of the cleft. In unilateral cases the minor segment moves apart from the major segment, and in bilateral patients both segments move away symmetrically. This pattern could be affected by the moment of the graft placement,

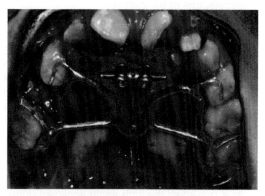

Fig. 14. A fan expander with expansion screw is a more rigid appliance by which the amount of expansion is controlled by the number of turns or activations per day. It also provides differential expansion, maintaining a stable posterior width while expanding the anterior region.

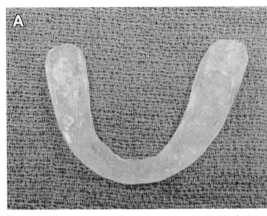
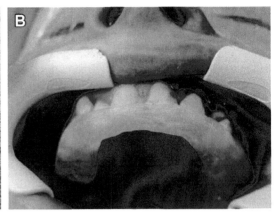

Fig. 15. (*A*) A customized acrylic surgical splint is fashioned to be placed immediately after the secondary alveolar bone-graft procedure. (*B*) The craniofacial orthodontist inserts the surgical splint while in the operating room after the surgery is performed. The splint is an integral part of the authors' protocol, as it preserves the arch width achieved during the expansion phase, protects the delicate graft area from food impaction, and reminds the patient to take proper care of the site.

because the maxillary segments move individually before the graft, and after it the palatal processes behave as a single piece.[53] Retention of the corrected cross-bite using orthodontic appliances such as the transpalatal bar with lateral projections is indicated immediately before and after the graft. The transpalatal bar can be used also as an anchorage component during comprehensive orthodontic treatment.[49]

Management Protocol

The authors' orthopedic and orthodontic protocol sequence during the bone-grafting phase includes the following.

1. A low-dose maxillary CBCT scan is ordered to evaluate dental development and skeletal architecture at the cleft site.
2. Maxillary expansion is advised if a posterior cross-bite is present.
3. After adequate expansion is achieved and a few days before surgery, the expander is removed and a maxillary retainer (Hawley) is delivered the same day to preserve arch width. An impression for a surgical splint is taken.
4. The craniofacial orthodontist inserts the surgical splint, in the operating room, after the alveolar bone graft surgery is performed (**Fig. 15**). The splint is an integral part of the protocol, as it preserves the arch width achieved during the expansion phase, protects the delicate graft area from food impaction, and reminds the patient to take proper care of the site. The splint is kept in the mouth and is evaluated by the orthodontist biweekly for 8 to 12 weeks

until radiographic evidence of bone formation is present.
5. The orthodontist removes the splint, fits bands, and makes a new impression for a transpalatal arch retainer with arms to hold the expansion and arch integrity.
6. If indicated, limited orthodontic appliances (braces) are applied to the anterior teeth to correct dental rotations or malpositions. If a maxillary hypoplasia causing a sagittal skeletal discrepancy or anterior cross-bite is present, maxillary protraction (face mask) therapy could also be incorporated into the treatment plan.

SUMMARY

The interdisciplinary approach to primary and secondary surgical procedures has proven to be beneficial for patients. In the neonate, NAM has been found to optimize the aesthetic outcome of the nasal and labial repair while minimizing the extent of surgery and scar-tissue formation. During the mixed dentition stage, orthopedic arch preparation before the secondary alveolar bone-grafting procedure improves arch morphology, restores the functional interarch relationship, and facilitates surgical access. The cooperative effort between the surgeon and craniofacial orthodontist in designing strategies customized to the patient's specific needs has resulted in better aesthetic and functional outcomes, minimizing surgical interventions.

REFERENCES

1. Grayson BG, Maule D. Cleft lip repair: trends and techniques. Semin Plast Surg 2005;19(4):294–301.

2. Berkowitz S. A comparison of treatment results in complete bilateral cleft lip and palate using a conservative approach versus Millard-Latham PSOT procedure. Semin Orthod 1996;2(3):169–84.

3. McNeil CK. Orthodontic procedures in the treatment of congenital cleft palate. Dent Records 1950;70:126–32.

4. Latham RA. Orthopedic advancement of the cleft maxillary segment: a preliminary report. Cleft Palate J 1980;17:227.

5. Grayson BH, Cutting CB, Wood R. Preoperative columella lengthening in bilateral cleft lip and palate. Plast Reconstr Surg 1993;92:1422–3.

6. Laub D, Meyers A, Peterson B. Presurgical orthopedic therapy for cleft lip and palate. Medscape Reference. 2011.

7. Sischo L, Chan J, Stein M, et al. Nasoalveolar molding: prevalence of cleft centers offering NAM and who seeks it. Cleft Palate Craniofac J 2012;49(3):270–5. Available at: http://emedicine.medscape.com/article/2036547-overview.

8. Grayson BH, Santiago PE. Presurgical orthopedics for cleft lip and palate. In: Aston SJ, Beasly RW, Thorne CH, editors. Grabb and Smith's plastic surgery. 5th edition. Philadelphia: Lippincott-Raven; 1997. p. 237–44.

9. Ezzat CF, Chavarria C, Teichgraeber JF, et al. Presurgical nasoalveolar molding therapy for treatment of unilateral cleft lip and palate: a preliminary study. Cleft Palate Craniofac J 2007;44(1):8–12.

10. Jaeger M, Braga-Silva J, Gehlen D, et al. Correction of the alveolar gap and nostril deformity by pre-surgical passive orthodontia in the unilateral cleft lip. Ann Plast Surg 2007;59(5):489–94.

11. Singh GD, Levy-Bercowski D, Santiago PE. Three-dimensional nasal changes following nasoalveolar molding in patients with unilateral cleft lip and palate: geometric morphometrics. Cleft Palate Craniofac J 2005;42(4):403–9.

12. Maull DJ, Grayson BH, Cutting CB, et al. Long-term effects of nasoalveolar molding on three-dimensional nasal shape in unilateral clefts. Cleft Palate Craniofac J 1999;36:391–7.

13. Chang CS, Por YC, Liou EJ, et al. Long-term comparison of four techniques for obtaining nasal symmetry in unilateral complete cleft lip patients: a single surgeon's experience. Plast Reconstr Surg 2010;126(4):1276–84.

14. Santiago PE, Grayson BH, Cutting CB, et al. Reduced need for alveolar bone grafting by pre-surgical othopedics and primary gingivoperiosteoplasty. Cleft Palate Craniofac J 1998;35(1):77–80.

15. Pfeifer TM, Graysonn BH, Cutting CB. Nasoalveolar molding and gingivoperiosteoplasty versus alveolar bone graft: an outcome analysis of costs in the treatment of unilateral cleft alveolus. Cleft Palate Craniofac J 2002;39(1):26–9.

16. Huffman WC, Lierle DM. Studies on the pathologic anatomy of the unilateral harelip nose. Plast Reconstr Surg 1949;4:225–34.

17. Hogan VM, Converse JM. Secondary deformity of unilateral cleft lip and nose. In: Grabb WC, Rosenstein SE, Bzoch KR, editors. Cleft lip and palate-surgical, dental, and speech aspects. Boston: Little, Brown; 1971. p. 245–64.

18. Broadbent TR, Woolf RM. Cleft lip nasal deformity. Ann Plast Surg 1984;12:216–34.

19. Millard DR. Embryonic rationale for the primary correction of classical congenital clefts of the lip and palate. Ann R Coll Surg Engl 1994;76:150–60.

20. Rawashdeh M, Telfah H. Secondary alveolar bone grafting: the dilemma of donor site selection and morbidity. Br J Oral Maxillofac Surg 2008;46:665–70.

21. Steinberg B, Padwa B, Boyne P, et al. State of the art in oral and maxillofacial surgery: treatment of maxillary hypoplasia and palatal and alveolar cleft. Cleft Palate Craniofac J 1999;36:283–91.

22. Bajaj A, Wongworawat A, Punjabi A. Management of alveolar cleft. J Craniofac Surg 2003;6:840–6.

23. Vig KW, Turvey T, Fonseca R. Orthodontic and surgical considerations in bone grafting in the cleft maxilla and palate. In: Turvey T, Vig K, Fonseca R, editors. Facial cleft and craniosynostosis. Philadelphia: WB Saunders; 1996. p. 399–411.

24. Kelly K. Alveolar cleft management. In: Guyuron B, Eriksson E, Persing J, editors. Plastic surgery indications and practice, vol. 1. Philadelphia: WB Saunders; 2008. p. 523–34.

25. Vig KW. Alveolar bone grafts: the surgical/orthodontic management of the cleft maxilla. Ann Acad Med Singapore 1999;28:721–7.

26. Rosenstein S, Dado DV, Kernahan D, et al. The case for early bone grafting in cleft lip and palate: a second report. Plast Reconstr Surg 1991;111:1–11.

27. Randall P, LaRossa D. A short history of prepalatal clefts. In: Berkowitz S, editor. Cleft lip and palate. Diagnosis and management. 2nd edition. New York: Springer; 2006. p. 275–9.

28. Cho-Lee GY, Garcis-Diez EM, Nunes RA, et al. Review of secondary alveolar cleft repair. Ann Maxillofac Surg 2013;3:46–50.

29. Abyholm F. Secondary bone grafting of alveolar clefts. In: Berkowitz S, editor. Cleft lip and palate. Diagnosis and management. 2nd edition. New York: Springer; 2006. p. 601–11.

30. Yu J, Glover A, Levy-Bercowski D, et al. Cleft-orthognathic surgery. In: Guyuron B, Eriksson E, Persing J, editors. Plastic surgery indications and practice. Philadelphia: Saunders Elsevier; 2008. p. 563–675.

31. Levy-Bercowski D, Deleon E, Stockstill J, et al. Orthognathic cleft-surgical/orthodontic treatment. Semin Orthod 2011;17:197–206.

32. Da Silva Filho OG, Teles SG, Ozawa TO, et al. Secondary bone graft and eruption of the permanent canine in patients with alveolar clefts: literature review and case report. Angle Orthod 2000; 70:174–8.

33. Meyer S, Molsted K. Long-term outcome of secondary alveolar bone grafting in cleft lip and palate patients: a 10-year follow-up cohort study. J Plast Surg Hand Surg 2013;26:1–6.

34. Al Harbi H, Al Yamani A. Long-term follow up of tibial bone graft for correction of alveolar cleft. Ann Maxillofac Surg 2012;2:146–52.

35. Fasolis M, Boffano P, Ramieri G. Morbidity associated with anterior iliac crest bone graft. Oral Surg Oral Med Oral Pathol Oral Radiol 2012;114:586–91.

36. Sadove AM, Nelson CL, Eppley BL, et al. An evaluation of calvarial and iliac donor sites in alveolar cleft grafting. Cleft Palate J 1990;27:225–8.

37. Nwoku A, Al Atel A, Al Shlash S, et al. Retrospective analysis of secondary alveolar cleft grafts using iliac of chin bone. J Craniofac Surg 2005;16: 864–8.

38. Nique T, Fonseca RJ, Upton LG, et al. Particulate allogeneic bone grafts into maxillary alveolar clefts in humans: a preliminary report. J Oral Maxillofac Surg 1987;45:386–92.

39. Kraut R. The use of allogeneic bone for alveolar cleft grafting. Oral Surg Oral Med Oral Pathol 1987;64:278–82.

40. Maxson BB, Baxter SD, Vig KW, et al. Allogeneic bone for secondary alveolar cleft osteoplasty. J Oral Maxillofac Surg 1990;48:933–41.

41. Berglan O, Semb G, Abyholm FE. Elimination of the residual alveolar cleft by secondary bone grafting and subsequent orthodontic treatment. Cleft Palate J 1986;23:175–205.

42. Van Hout W, Van der Molen M, Breugen C. Reconstruction of the alveolar cleft: can growth factor-aided tissue engineering replace autologous bone grafting? A literature review and systematic review of results obtained with bone morphogenetic protein-2. Clin Oral Investig 2011;15:297–303.

43. Chenard K, Teven C, He TC, et al. Bone morphogenetic proteins in craniofacial surgery: current techniques, clinical experiences, and the future of personalized stem cell therapy. J Biomed Biotechnol 2012;2012:1–14.

44. Boyne P, Herford A, Stringer D. Prevention of relapse following cleft bone grafting and the future use of BMP cytokines to regenerate osseous clefts without grafting. In: Berkowitz S, editor. Cleft lip and palate. Diagnosis and management. 2nd edition. New York: Springer; 2006. p. 275–9.

45. Dickinson BP, Ashley RK, Wasson KL, et al. Reduced morbidity and improved healing with bone morphogenic protein-2 in older patients with alveolar clefts defects. Plast Reconstr Surg 2008; 121:209–17.

46. Alonso N, Tanikawa D, Freitas R, et al. Evaluation of maxillary alveolar reconstruction using a resorbable collagen sponge with recombinant human bone morphogenetic protein-2 in cleft lip and palate patients. Tissue Eng Part C Methods 2010;16: 1183–9.

47. Kinsella CR, Cray JJ, Durham EL, et al. Recombinant human bone morphogenetic protein-2-induced craniosynostosis and growth restriction in the immature skeleton. Plast Reconstr Surg 2011;127:1173–81.

48. Lan Shen H, Liou E. Effect of platelet rich plasma injection on narrowing alveolar cleft through orthodontic movement. International cleft palate meeting. Orlando, May 8, 2013.

49. Freitas JA, Garib D, Oliveira T, et al. Rehabilitative treatment of cleft lip and palate: experience of the hospital for rehabilitation of craniofacial anomalies—USP (HRAC-USP)—Part-2: pediatric dentistry and orthodontics. J Appl Oral Sci 2012;20:268–81.

50. Lidral K, Vig K. Role of the orthodontist in the management of patients with cleft lip and/or palate. In: Wyszynski DF, editor. Cleft lip and palate: from origin to treatment. Oxford (England): Oxford University Press; 2002. p. 381–96.

51. Russell K, Mcleod C. Canine eruption in patients with complete cleft lip and palate. Cleft Palate Craniofac J 2008;45:73–80.

52. Matsui K, Echigo S, Kimizuka S. Clinical study on eruption of permanent canines after secondary alveolar bone grafting. Cleft Palate Craniofac J 2005;42:309–12.

53. da Silva Filho O, Boiani E, de Oliveira Cavassan A, et al. Rapid maxillary expansion after secondary alveolar bone grafting in patients with alveolar cleft. Cleft Palate Craniofac J 2009;46:331–8.

54. Rune B, Jacobsson S. Dental replacement resorption after bone grafting to the alveolar cleft. Plast Reconstr Surg 1989;23:175–205.

55. McIntyre G, Devlin M. Secondary alveolar bone grafting (CLEFTSiS) 2000-2004. Cleft Palate Craniofac J 2010;47:66–72.

56. Cavassan A, Albuquerque MA, Filho L. Rapid maxillary expansion after secondary alveolar bone graft in a patient with bilateral cleft lip and palate. Cleft Palate Craniofac J 2004;41:332–9.

Gingivoperiosteoplasty

Richard A. Hopper, MD, MS[a,b],*, Faisal Al-Mufarrej, MB BCh[a,b]

KEYWORDS

- Gingivoperiosteoplasty • Nasoalveolar molding • Alveolar cleft • POPLA

KEY POINTS

- Gingivoperiosteoplasty (GPP) replaces alveolar cleft soft tissue with a gingivoperiosteal tunnel that facilitates bone healing without the need for bone grafting.
- Skoog's descriptions of "boneless bone grafting" popularized the technique in cleft care.
- The reported negative impact of the Latham device on dentofacial growth has led to the development of nasoalveolar molding (NAM), a passive, noninvasive, molding process.
- NAM-GPP prerequisites include appropriate cleft anatomy to allow alveolar bony approximation.
- GPP seals the cleft nasally, orally, and labially by mucoperiosteal flaps.
- GPP advocates report the elimination of secondary alveolar bone grafting at mixed dentition as a benefit.
- Critics voice concerns over iatrogenic facial growth restriction and malocclusion.
- Data available on NAM-GPP (with appropriate patient selection and technique) are favorable but long-term outcome studies are required.

Gingivoperiosteoplasty (GPP) removes the soft tissue barrier within an alveolar cleft and replaces it with a gingivoperiosteal tunnel that facilitates bone healing through guided tissue regeneration (GTR) without the need for bone grafting and its associated donor site morbidity. The importance of the periosteum in bony healing has been well documented by several investigators[1,2]; however, Ollier[3] is most often credited with first emphasizing the osteogenic potential of the periosteum. This is especially true for patients at a younger age.[4] Dahlin and colleagues[5] were first to demonstrate union of critical bony defects by creating a Teflon tunnel to guide bone regeneration while impairing soft tissue in-growth and fibrous nonunion. Although the osteogenic properties of mucoperiosteum in healing a cleft palate were initially recognized by Langenbeck[6] in the 1800s, it was not until Tord Skoog's[7] descriptions of primary GPP or "boneless bone grafting" in the 1960s that the technique became popularized in cleft care. Successful GTR following a GPP depends on the integrity of the guiding tunnel to restrict fibrous in-growth, the presence of viable periosteum in the created flaps, and the age of the patient.

HISTORICAL PERSPECTIVE

Skoog[8] described the creation of local mucoperiosteal flaps with oxidized regenerated cellulose. Though not every patient grew bone initially, with repeated periosteal flaps, all patients eventually formed a bony bridge. Without presurgical molding, this method required extensive, often repeated, subperiosteal maxillary dissection to close the alveolar cleft, with an associated negative impact on facial growth. In the 1970s and 1980s, Ritsilä and colleagues,[9] and Rintala and Ranta,[10] reported the outcomes of free tibial periosteal grafts. During a 6-year period, they treated

[a] Division of Plastic Surgery, The Craniofacial Center, Seattle Children's Hospital and Regional Medical Center, 4800 Sand Point Way Northeast, Seattle, WA 98105, USA; [b] Division of Plastic Surgery, Department of Surgery, University of Washington, Seattle, WA, USA
* Corresponding author. 4800 Sand Point Way Northeast, W7847, Seattle, WA 98105.
E-mail address: richard.hopper@seattlechildrens.org

Clin Plastic Surg 41 (2014) 233–240
http://dx.doi.org/10.1016/j.cps.2013.12.006
0094-1298/14/$ — see front matter © 2014 Elsevier Inc. All rights reserved.

67 patients with Skoog's maxillary periosteal flap technique and 23 with free periosteal grafts. Although bony formation was noted in 64% of patients treated with the Skoog technique and 85% of those treated with the tibial periosteum graft technique, secondary bone grafts were required in 72% and 73% of each group, respectively. There was a lateral cross-bite in all patients. A similar finding with the Skoog technique was reported by Renkielska and colleagues.[11] They found 50% of patients had Goslon scores of 4 or 5 with need for orthognathic surgery and the technique fell out of favor.

The popularization of presurgical orthopedics ushered in the next phase in GPP care. Millard's presurgical orthopedics, periosteoplasty, and lip adhesion (POPLA) approach involved presurgical orthopedics with the "Latham device" followed by lip adhesion and GPP at 3 to 4 months of age.[12] Active mechanical presurgical approximation of the alveolar edges allowed for less subperiosteal dissection, but critics of the POPLA approach note a 40% to 42% maxillary vertical growth disturbance of the maxilla[13] and 100% of patients with cross-bites that were often difficult to correct orthodontically.[14]

NAM-GPP

The potential negative impact of the active direct force of the Latham device on dentofacial growth led to the development of a more passive molding process, nasoalveolar molding (NAM), as described by Grayson and colleagues.[15] NAM is described as guiding early alveolar growth as opposed to directly molding it. NAM-GPP differs from POPLA in the method of presurgical alveolar molding and surgical technique as well as in more rigorous selection criteria by which patients are deemed appropriate candidates for a GPP. This is partly because its advocates think NAM is a more accurate means of molding the leading edges of the alveolar cleft into a close parallel relationship to optimize flap design and osteogenesis.

PATIENT SELECTION AND EVALUATION

Prerequisites for a GPP are: (1) an informed consenting family, (2) appropriate cleft anatomy to allow alveolar bony approximation, (3) an optimally molded alveolar cleft and intact mucosa, and (4) no dental eruption. Once these criteria are met, the GPP can be scheduled at the time of the primary lip repair.

Before undergoing a GPP, the infant with a cleft must be evaluated by the practitioner administering the NAM, as well as the surgeon who will be performing the GPP. Before initiating NAM, the guardians of the infant should be introduced to the concept of a GPP, the risks and benefits reported in earlier GPP techniques, and the current data on NAM-GPP.

Variations in cleft anatomy may exclude some patients from NAM-GPP. For example, patients with isolated clefts of the primary palate are usually not good candidates for NAM-GPP. Due to the bony fusion of the secondary palate, the alveolar segments of the primary palate are more resistant to parallel presurgical molding and, in many cases, cannot be adequately aligned for a successful GPP. Another group of patients who are not candidates for a NAM-GPP are the "mesenchymal deficient" infants, with such wide unilateral clefts that the alveolar arch form would be excessively constricted should the segments be presurgically approximated. Finally, in bilateral complete clefts, it is not always possible to align both sides of the premaxilla with the lateral alveolar segments to allow for bilateral GPP. In these cases, the one aligned alveolar cleft can undergo a GPP to convert the arch form to a lesser and greater segment instead of a three-piece upper jaw. Although the contralateral cleft will need to be secondarily grafted, the premaxilla will be stabilized by the GPP to facilitate incisor mastication during early childhood.

PREOPERATIVE MANAGEMENT

During the preoperative management (NAM) process, the preoperative assessment of alveolar ridge alignment and parallel alveolar molding is subjective. Alveolar segment alignment is assessed based on the underlying bone, not on the visible gingival mucosa (**Fig. 1**). In some cases, the gingival tissue can be hypertrophied in the area of the cleft, mimicking close approximation, while the underlying bone gap is wide. In other cases, the alveolar cleft is compressed, but the bony arch forms are not in alignment, with the premaxilla wedged anterior to collapsed lesser segments or the lesser segment posterior to the greater (**Fig. 2**). If a GPP is performed in these situations, the mucoperiosteal tunnel between the exposed bone edges will be "kinked," creating a soft tissue barrier instead of GTR.

PERFORMING GPP

It is technically easiest to perform the GPP after all the primary cleft lip dissection had been completed but before repair of the lip elements is started. To understand GPP flap design, the alveolar cleft should be visualized as a pyramid on its

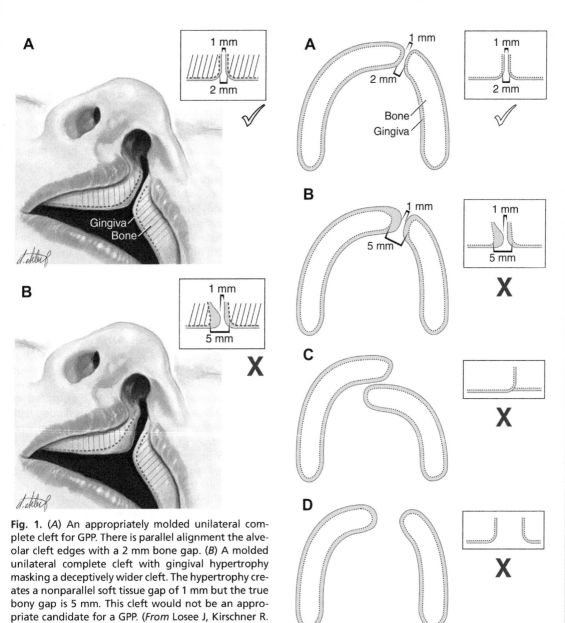

Fig. 1. (*A*) An appropriately molded unilateral complete cleft for GPP. There is parallel alignment the alveolar cleft edges with a 2 mm bone gap. (*B*) A molded unilateral complete cleft with gingival hypertrophy masking a deceptively wider cleft. The hypertrophy creates a nonparallel soft tissue gap of 1 mm but the true bony gap is 5 mm. This cleft would not be an appropriate candidate for a GPP. (*From* Losee J, Kirschner R. Comprehensive cleft care. New York: McGraw-Hill; 2008. p. 832; with permission.)

side, with a labial base and an apex located at the incisive foramen where the cephalad and caudad incisions converge (**Fig. 3**).

GPP is performed as follows:

- The goal is to seal the cleft nasally, orally, and labially by mucoperiosteal flaps, with two opposing bone surfaces on the mesial and distal walls.
- To promote GTR in this sealed tunnel, all soft tissue interference must be removed from the alveolar cleft during creation of the flaps.

Fig. 2. (*A*) An appropriately molded unilateral complete cleft for GPP. There is parallel alignment the alveolar cleft edges with a smooth arch form. (*B*) Gingival hypertrophy in the alveolar cleft can mask a bone gap that is too wide for a GPP. (*C*) A collapsed arch form is not a candidate for GPP. Although the alveolar segments are touching, the edges of the cleft are not opposing, preventing the formation of a subperiosteal tunnel. (*D*) A mesenchymal deficient cleft arch form. If this cleft was approximated by preoperative molding, it would unnaturally constrict the projection of the alveolar arch due to a deficiency in either the lesser or greater segments. (*From* Losee J, Kirschner R. Comprehensive cleft care. New York: McGraw-Hill; 2008. p. 832; with permission.)

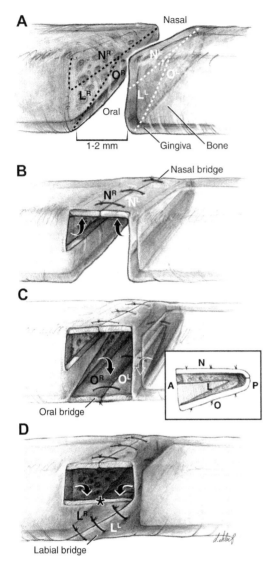

Fig. 3. (A–D) Gingivoperiosteal flap design and elevation for the Millard GPP. The dissection is limited to the tissues within the cleft. The flaps are named by the part of the periosteal tunnel they construct. A, anterior; L^L, left labial flap; L^R, right labial flap; N^L, left nasal flap; N^R, right nasal flap; O^L, left oral flap; O^R, right oral flap; P, posterior; *, Marks the mucosal edge repaired to the lip mucosa. (*From* Losee J, Kirschner R. Comprehensive cleft care. New York: McGraw-Hill; 2008. p. 833; with permission.)

- Occasionally, a deciduous tooth follicle is encountered during the flap dissection and careful sharp dissection is required to prevent disruption of dental eruption. If the flaps appear too thin or nonviable during the follicle dissection, the GPP should be aborted and the mucosa replaced.
- The "roof" of the GPP is the repair of the anterior palate, or the nasal floor, from the nasal sill back to the incisive foramen, which is typically done with most modern cleft lip repairs. This is typically achieved by suturing the inferior edge of the reconstructed lateral nasal wall to a superiorly based mucoperiosteal vomer flap.
- The vomer flap vertical dissection is kept to the bare minimum needed to achieve closure of the nasal floor, typically 1 to 2 mm at most, to avoid inadvertent damage to the premaxillary growth suture.
- The floor of the GPP is created by elevating inferiorly based mucoperiosteal flaps from the oral edges of the alveolar cleft. These flaps are raised from within the alveolar cleft itself starting from the labial surface of the alveolus back to the incisive foramen.
- The floor flaps are inferiorly rotated and sutured to each other, effectively closing the floor of the GPP.
- The mucoperiosteum that remains attached within the alveolar cleft between the cephalad roof incision and the caudad floor incision is the tissue used to close the labial (anterior) border of the GPP.
- An anteriorly based triangular flap, raised on either side of the alveolar cleft, is flipped labially and sutured to the contralateral flap.
- In designing these particular flaps, the incisions on one side of the alveolar cleft are shifted slightly superiorly relative to the other side, so that one flap covers the upper half of the anterior labial base of the cleft pyramid, while the contralateral flap covers the lower half of the base.
- To completely close off the anterior border of the GPP tunnel, the inferior edge of the lower labial flap is sutured to the anterior edge of the two oral flaps, and the superior edge of the upper labial flap is sutured to the lip mucosa.

POSTOPERATIVE CARE

The postoperative care of the GPP patient is no different than that of the cleft lip patient. The infant is resumed on normal feeding with no need for arm restraints. Postoperative flap loss may be encountered if flaps are inaccurately designed, traumatized by compressive handling, or elevated in a thin submucosal (rather than subperiosteal) plane.

TRENDS AND CONTROVERSIES

Although the international cleft community agrees that the primary goal of cleft care is to optimize function, appearance, and self-image with a minimum of surgical intervention, the community continues to debate on how best to attain it. One of the most controversial topics of debate in current cleft care is the indication for primary GPP. Advocates of GPP report the elimination of secondary alveolar bone grafting at the time of mixed dentition, hence minimizing the number of secondary surgeries (and associated morbidity and cost) by optimizing results of primary cleft lip surgery. However, GPP critics voice concerns about iatrogenic facial growth restriction and subsequent malocclusion due to early closure of the alveolar arch. Such restriction could actually increase the need for orthodontic and orthognathic treatment at time of skeletal maturity. The history and evolution of GPP, from Skoog, to Rintala, to Millard, teaches us that it can take up to 20 years before the risks and benefits of a surgical technique, performed on an infant with a cleft, can be fully appreciated. As more centers outside of the originating institution practice the technique, preliminary objective evaluation of NAM-GPP is starting to be available to the cleft care community and, it is hoped, definitive results will soon be available to define the appropriate place of the technique in the arsenal of cleft care.

Compared with studies on earlier variations of GPP, the current data on the benefits of NAM-GPP are so far more favorable. The earliest data became available through the continued work of Grayson,[15] Cutting, and Brecht from New York University (NYU), the developers of the NAM-GPP technique. In addition to their studies on the improved nasal morphology associated with the NAM technique, they have also evaluated their outcomes to date with the NAM-GPP. They have reported bone formation in 80% of unilateral clefts treated with a primary NAM-GPP, with 40% requiring secondary bone grafting (**Fig. 4**).[16] More recently, the Chang Gung Memorial Hospital group reported similar results with a 28% rate of secondary alveolar bone grafting.[17] The also critically evaluated bone quality, noting least bone formation on the palatal apical portion of the previous alveolar cleft following GPP.[17]

For bilateral clefts, unilateral primary GPP is associated with a 63% success rate; however, bilateral primary GPP has a dependent probability of 52% and conditional probability of 82% of bilateral successful dentoalveolar bone formation.[18] Bilateral GPP is recommended by the NYU group as "it results in greater stability of the premaxilla and functional occlusion of the central incisors. Furthermore, secondary bone grafting when required after GPP is technically easier with the presence of bone along the occlusal surface of the dentoalveolar ridge."[18] In support of that argument, the group demonstrated superior radiographic bone levels and alveolar anatomy in patients undergoing GPP alone or combined with secondary alveolar bone grafting as compared with conventional alveolar bone grafting alone.[19] "Failed GPP" that require secondary bone grafting have more favorable outcomes than non-GPP secondary grafting cases at time of mixed dentition, presumably due to a bone bridge formation in 80% of GPP cases (**Fig. 5**).

In a cost comparison between the nonmolded, secondary bone graft, control group and the GPP group, a savings of $2999 was seen when a primary GPP was performed.[20] This cost analysis,

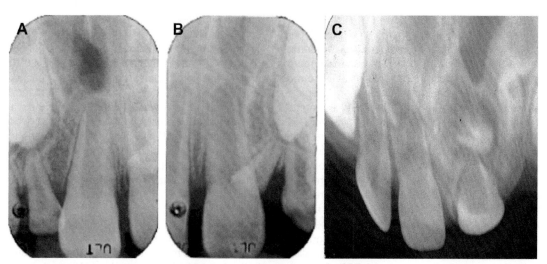

Fig. 4. (A–C) Periapical radiographs of a bilateral cleft lip and palate patient in mixed dentition with a successful previous bilateral GPP. There is adequate vertical bone height within the alveolar cleft to support tooth eruption. (*Courtesy of* Barry Grayson, DDS, New York University Medical Center.)

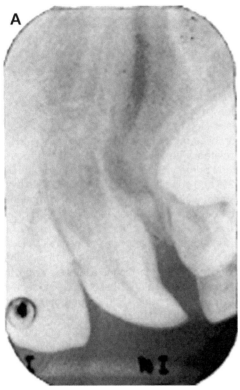
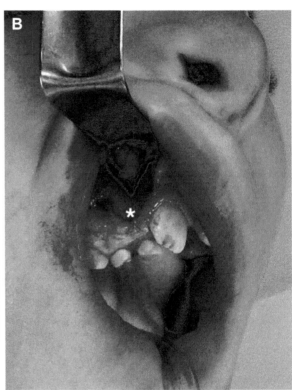

Fig. 5. A right unilateral alveolar cleft following a "failed GPP." A periapical radiograph at mixed dentition (*A*). There is formation of a bone bridge across the cleft but insufficient vertical height to support tooth eruption. At the time of secondary bone grafting, the bone bridge formation (*asterisk*) from the previous GPP provides a stable platform for the graft augmentation (*B*). (*Courtesy of* Barry Grayson, DDS, New York University Medical Center.)

however, did not take into account the potential added cost of increased orthodontic and orthognathic treatments in patients undergoing GPP. Another potential advantage of GPP is early closure of fistula. However, studies have reported fistula rates as high as 36% with GPP.[21]

In evaluating facial growth, the NYU group found no adverse effects on midface growth during mixed dentition,[22] or just before pubertal growth spurt,[23] when compared with an unmolded control group. However, Hsieh and colleagues[24] demonstrated a 2.1 and 2.9 mm deficiency in sagittal maxillary and maxillary alveolar lengths with GPP at the age of 5 years. Other investigators have also reported GPP as a stronger predictor of poor dental arch relationship outcome (Goslon 5) than initial cleft size regardless of type of presurgical orthopedics (odds ratios 2.8 and 1.3, respectively).[25] Whether delaying GPP until the time of palatal surgery improves maxillary outcome is yet to be seen.[26] Interestingly, salvage bone grafting after a failed GPP can improve vertical maxillary height compared with successful GPP. This may be due to improvement in tooth eruption at the GPP site.[27] GPP may also result in compensatory

mandibular growth disruption with decreased anteroposterior measurements. Although not studied with NAM, this has been demonstrated with patients with bilateral clefts undergoing alveolar molding with the Latham device before GPP[21] and patients undergoing primary bone grafting of unilateral clefts.[28,29]

Although early results may confirm the benefits of NAM-GPP, the effects of the technique on facial growth through skeletal maturity remain unclear. Rodent models of GPP are now available to facilitate bench-side investigations of methods to improve osteogenesis in alveolar defects while limiting adverse effects on maxillary growth.[30,31] The role of recombinant human bone morphogenic protein-2 in primary alveolar reconstruction is also under investigation.[32,33]

SUMMARY

GPP plays a central and controversial part in the cleft surgeon's mission to provide the best results in the least number of surgeries. Although it may normalize form and function at infancy and obviate secondary alveolar bone grafting at the age of mixed dentition, the technique has historically been associated with iatrogenic dentofacial restriction requiring more extensive orthodontic and orthognathic treatment at the age of skeletal maturity. Compared with previous protocols, the most recent evolution of the GPP technique associated with NAM uses passive, guided, presurgical molding of the alveolar cleft with strict patient selection criteria. At this time, the data available of the benefits of NAM-GPP are favorable but further long-term outcome studies are required before its final role in cleft care can be determined.

REFERENCES

1. Sirola K. Regeneration of defects in the calvaria. An experimental study. Ann Med Exp Biol Fenn 1960; 38(Suppl 2):1–87.
2. Breitbart AS, Grande DA, Kessler R, et al. Tissue engineered bone repair of calvarial defects using cultured periosteal cells. Plast Reconstr Surg 1998; 101:567–74 [discussion: 75–6].
3. Ollier L, editor. Traite Experimental et Clinique de la Regeneration des Os et de la Production Artificielle du Tissue Osseux. Paris: V Masson et fils; 1867.
4. Gosain AK, Santoro TD, Song LS, et al. Osteogenesis in calvarial defects: contribution of the dura, the pericranium, and the surrounding bone in adult versus infant animals. Plast Reconstr Surg 2003; 112:515–27.
5. Dahlin C, Linde A, Gottlow J, et al. Healing of bone defects by guided tissue regeneration. Plast Reconstr Surg 1988;81:672–6.
6. Langenbeck von B. Die Uranoplastik mittelst Ablosung des mucosperiostalen Gaumenuberzuges. Arch klin Chir 1861;2:205–87.
7. Skoog T. The use of periosteum and Surgicel for bone restoration in congenital clefts of the maxilla. A clinical report and experimental investigation. Scand J Plast Reconstr Surg 1967;1: 113–30.
8. Skoog T. Repair of unilateral cleft lip deformity: maxilla, nose and lip. Scand J Plast Reconstr Surg 1969;3:109–33.
9. Ritsilä V, Alhopuro S, Gylling U, et al. The use of free periosteum for bone formation in congenital clefts of the maxilla. A preliminary report. Scand J Plast Reconstr Surg 1972;6:57–60.
10. Rintala AE, Ranta R. Periosteal flaps and grafts in primary cleft repair: a follow-up study. Plast Reconstr Surg 1989;83:17–24.
11. Renkielska A, Wojtaszek-Slominska A, Dobke M. Early cleft lip repair in children with unilateral complete cleft lip and palate: a case against primary alveolar repair. Ann Plast Surg 2005;54:595–7 [discussion: 98–9].
12. Millard D. Presurgical maxillary orthopedics. In: Millard D, editor. Cleft craft. Boston: Little, Brown; 1980. p. 263.
13. Henkel KO, Gundlach KK. Analysis of primary gingivoperiosteoplasty in alveolar cleft repair. Part I: facial growth. J Craniomaxillofac Surg 1997;25: 266–9.
14. Berkowitz S, Mejia M, Bystrik A. A comparison of the effects of the Latham-Millard procedure with those of a conservative treatment approach for dental occlusion and facial aesthetics in unilateral and bilateral complete cleft lip and palate: part I. Dental occlusion. Plast Reconstr Surg 2004;113: 1–18.
15. Grayson BH, Santiago PE, Brecht LE, et al. Presurgical nasoalveolar molding in infants with cleft lip and palate. Cleft Palate Craniofac J 1999;36:486–98.
16. Santiago PE, Grayson BH, Cutting CB, et al. Reduced need for alveolar bone grafting by presurgical orthopedics and primary gingivoperiosteoplasty. Cleft Palate Craniofac J 1998;35:77–80.
17. Wang YC, Liao YF, Chen PK. Outcome of gingivoperiosteoplasty for the treatment of alveolar clefts in patients with unilateral cleft lip and palate. Br J Oral Maxillofac Surg 2013;51(7):650–5.
18. Dec W, Shetye PR, Davidson EH, et al. Presurgical nasoalveolar molding and primary gingivoperiosteoplasty reduce the need for bone grafting in patients with bilateral clefts. J Craniofac Surg 2013; 24:186–90.
19. Sato Y, Grayson BH, Garfinkle JS, et al. Success rate of gingivoperiosteoplasty with and without secondary bone grafts compared with secondary alveolar bone grafts alone. Plast Reconstr Surg 2008;121: 1356–67 [discussion: 68–9].
20. Pfeifer TM, Grayson BH, Cutting CB. Nasoalveolar molding and gingivoperiosteoplasty versus alveolar bone graft: an outcome analysis of costs in the treatment of unilateral cleft alveolus. Cleft Palate Craniofac J 2002;39:26–9.
21. Power SM, Matic DB. Gingivoperiosteoplasty following alveolar molding with a Latham appliance versus secondary bone grafting: the effects on bone production and midfacial growth in patients with bilateral clefts. Plast Reconstr Surg 2009;124: 573–82.
22. Wood RJ, Grayson BH, Cutting CB. Gingivoperiosteoplasty and midfacial growth. Cleft Palate Craniofac J 1997;34:17–20.
23. Lee CT, Grayson BH, Cutting CB, et al. Prepubertal midface growth in unilateral cleft lip and palate following alveolar molding and gingivoperiosteoplasty. Cleft Palate Craniofac J 2004;41:375–80.
24. Hsieh CH, Ko EW, Chen PK, et al. The effect of gingivoperiosteoplasty on facial growth in patients with complete unilateral cleft lip and palate. Cleft Palate Craniofac J 2010;47:439–46.

25. Hsieh YJ, Liao YF, Shetty A. Predictors of poor dental arch relationship in young children with unilateral cleft lip and palate. Clin Oral Investig 2012;16: 1261–6.

26. Berkowitz S. Gingivoperiosteoplasty as well as early palatal cleft closure is unproductive. J Craniofac Surg 2009;20(Suppl 2):1747–58.

27. Matic DB, Power SM. The effects of gingivoperiosteoplasty following alveolar molding with a pin-retained Latham appliance versus secondary bone grafting on midfacial growth in patients with unilateral clefts. Plast Reconstr Surg 2008;122:863–70 [discussion: 71–3].

28. Ross RB. Treatment variables affecting facial growth in complete unilateral cleft lip and palate. Cleft Palate J 1987;24:5–77.

29. Trotman CA, Long RE Jr, Rosenstein SW, et al. Comparison of facial form in primary alveolar bone-grafted and nongrafted unilateral cleft lip and palate

patients: intercenter retrospective study. Cleft Palate Craniofac J 1996;33:91–5.

30. Mehrara BJ, Saadeh PB, Steinbrech DS, et al. A rat model of gingivoperiosteoplasty. J Craniofac Surg 2000;11:54–8.

31. Nguyen PD, Lin CD, Allori AC, et al. Establishment of a critical-sized alveolar defect in the rat: a model for human gingivoperiosteoplasty. Plast Reconstr Surg 2009;123:817–25.

32. Fallucco MA, Carstens MH. Primary reconstruction of alveolar clefts using recombinant human bone morphogenic protein-2: clinical and radiographic outcomes. J Craniofac Surg 2009;20(Suppl 2): 1759–64.

33. Nguyen PD, Lin CD, Allori AC, et al. Scaffold-based rhBMP-2 therapy in a rat alveolar defect model: implications for human gingivoperiosteoplasty. Plast Reconstr Surg 2009;124:1829–39.

Speech Evaluation for Patients with Cleft Palate

Ann W. Kummer, PhD, CCC-SLP

KEYWORDS

- Velopharyngeal insufficiency • Velopharyngeal incompetence • Velopharyngeal mislearning
- Velopharyngeal dysfunction • Hypernasality • Nasal emission • Nasopharyngoscopy • Nasometry

KEY POINTS

- Resonance disorders are common in children with a history of cleft palate. There may be hypernasality caused by velopharyngeal insufficiency (VPI). There may also be hyponasality or cul-de-sac resonance caused by obstruction in the vocal tract.
- Speech disorders are common in children with a history of cleft palate. There may be compensatory articulation productions caused by VPI or even caused by malocclusion if there was also a cleft of the primary palate.
- Differential diagnosis of the cause of hypernasality and/or nasal emission and also of abnormal speech sound production is critical in determining appropriate treatment (eg, surgery, speech therapy, or both).
- VPI is a structural abnormality and therefore requires surgical management.
- Velopharyngeal mislearning (including the use of compensatory productions caused by VPI or a history of VPI) is a functional disorder that requires speech therapy.

 Videos of a speech sample, evaluation of nasal emission using a straw, oral examination, nasometry, and nasopharyngoscopy accompany this article

ANATOMY AND PHYSIOLOGY OF THE VELOPHARYNGEAL VALVE

The velopharyngeal valve consists of the velum (soft palate), the lateral pharyngeal walls, and the posterior pharyngeal wall. These structures work in concert to open and close the velopharyngeal valve during speech.

During nasal breathing, the velopharyngeal valve is open. The velum rests against the base of the tongue and the lateral pharyngeal walls are wide apart (**Fig. 1**). This arrangement provides a patent upper airway for unobstructed nasal breathing. During oral speech, the velum moves in a superior and posterior direction to close firmly against the posterior pharyngeal wall (or adenoids in young children) (**Fig. 2**). At the same time, the lateral pharyngeal walls move medially to close against the velum, or in some cases just behind the velum. Complete closure of the velopharyngeal valve is required for all vowels and most consonants. The exception is with the production of nasal sounds (m, n, ng), for which the velopharyngeal valve is completely open to allow nasal resonance. In connected speech, the velopharyngeal valve therefore opens and closes throughout an utterance based on the type of speech sound (oral or nasal) that is produced.

Disclosures: The author receives royalties for the following textbook: Kummer A.W. Cleft palate and craniofacial anomalies: effects on speech and resonance. 3rd edition. Clifton Park, NY: Cengage Learning; 2014. The author receives royalties for the Nasoscope clinical device, marketed as the Oral & Nasal Listener, Super Duper, Inc.

Division of Speech-Language Pathology, Cincinnati Children's Hospital Medical Center, MLC 4011, 3333 Burnet Avenue, Cincinnati, OH 45229-3039, USA
E-mail address: ann.kummer@cchmc.org

plasticsurgery.theclinics.com

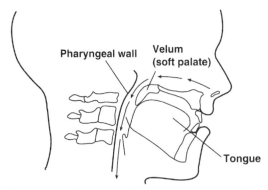

Fig. 1. Normal velar position during nasal breathing. (*From* Kummer AW. Cleft Palate & Craniofacial Anomalies, 3E. © 2014 Delmar Learning, a part of Cengage Learning, Inc. Reproduced by permission.)

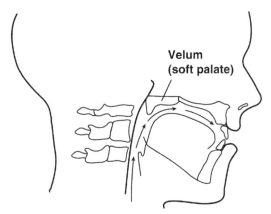

Fig. 2. Normal velopharyngeal function during oral speech. (*From* Kummer AW. Cleft Palate & Craniofacial Anomalies, 3E. © 2014 Delmar Learning, a part of Cengage Learning, Inc. Reproduced by permission.)

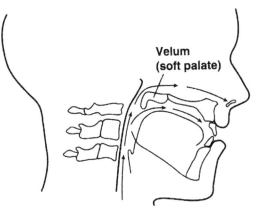

Fig. 3. Velopharyngeal insufficiency. Velopharyngeal insufficiency is caused by a structural cause. In this case, the velum has normal movement, but is too short to achieve velopharyngeal closure. (*From* Kummer AW. Cleft Palate & Craniofacial Anomalies, 3E. © 2014 Delmar Learning, a part of Cengage Learning, Inc. Reproduced by permission.)

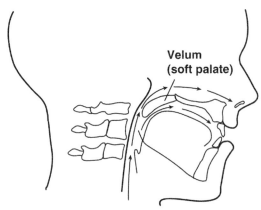

Fig. 4. Velopharyngeal incompetence. Velopharyngeal incompetence is caused by a neuromotor disorder. In this case, the velum is normal in structure, but does not move well enough to achieve velopharyngeal closure. (*From* Kummer AW. Cleft Palate & Craniofacial Anomalies, 3E. © 2014 Delmar Learning, a part of Cengage Learning, Inc. Reproduced by permission.)

VELOPHARYNGEAL DYSFUNCTION

Normal velopharyngeal function depends on 3 basic components: normal structure (anatomy), normal movement (neurophysiology), and normal articulation learning.[1]

When the velopharyngeal valve does not close consistently or completely during the production of oral sounds, this is often called velopharyngeal dysfunction (VPD). VPD is used as a general term that encompasses disorders of any of the 3 basic components of velopharyngeal function (structure, function, and learning).[1,2] Other terms are used for more specificity as to the type and causation of

VPD.[1–5] For example, velopharyngeal insufficiency (VPI) is most often used to describe a structural defect that prevents complete velopharyngeal closure (**Fig. 3**). Velopharyngeal insufficiency is the most common type of VPD because it can be caused by a history of cleft palate or submucous cleft. In contrast, velopharyngeal incompetence (also abbreviated as VPI) is used to refer to a neurophysiologic disorder in which poor movement of the velopharyngeal structures results in incomplete velopharyngeal closure (**Fig. 4**). Finally, velopharyngeal mislearning refers to an articulation disorder in which speech sounds are inappropriately produced in the pharynx. As a result of this placement, the velopharyngeal valve is open, thus mimicking VPI during attempted production of certain speech.

PERCEPTUAL EVALUATION OF VELOPHARYNGEAL FUNCTION

A speech pathology evaluation is indicated for all children with a history of cleft palate, particularly to rule out VPI.[2,6–11] Although language development is assessed at a younger age, the speech evaluation for VPI is best done when the child has some connected speech and also at a time when the airway is adequate for secondary surgery, if needed. For most children, this is around the age of 3 years. A speech evaluation is also indicated both before and after secondary surgery for VPI.

The assessment of velopharyngeal function begins with a perceptual evaluation of the patient's speech. During this evaluation, the examiner analyzes the acoustic product of velopharyngeal function in order to make inferences about the function of the velopharyngeal valve.

Speech Samples

When assessing speech, resonance, and velopharyngeal function, it is important to select an appropriate speech sample in order to obtain adequate information for a definitive diagnosis.[7,9,10] The speech samples used to assess children with suspected VPD need to be developmentally appropriate in terms of both articulation and language. Standardized (norm-referenced) articulation tests are available for comprehensive assessment of speech sound errors. In addition, the examiner usually elicits a variety of other speech samples, based on the child's language developmental level and what is suspected. These samples may include repetitive syllables (with pressure-sensitive consonants combined with both low and high vowels), rote speech (ie, counting), phonetically loaded sentences (eg, Take teddy to town), and spontaneous speech. When errors are noted, the examiner typically does more focused testing, including tests of stimulability.

What is Assessed

The perceptual evaluation includes an analysis of various components of speech, including resonance, oral air pressure and nasal emission, speech sound production, and phonation.[7,9–11] These components are further described later.

Resonance

Resonance is typically evaluated by listening to connected speech. If there is abnormal resonance,

the speech pathologist must determine the type (eg, hypernasal, hyponasal, cul-de-sac, or mixed). This distinction is of utmost importance because the type of resonance determines appropriate treatment.[9,10]

Patients with cleft palate often have hypernasal speech. Hypernasality is characterized by excess sound in the nasal cavity during the production of oral sounds. The speech is perceived as low in intensity, muffled, and unclear. Hypernasality is most perceptible on vowels, which are normally produced by altering oral resonance. There may also be nasalization of voiced consonants, so that oral phonemes (speech sounds) are perceived to be more like their nasal cognates (eg, m/b, n/d, ng/g). As a general rule, if nasal phonemes are heard more frequently than normal, or if nasal phonemes are substituted for oral phonemes, the resonance is hypernasal and VPI should be strongly suspected.

Because resonance disorders are not mutually exclusive, the speech pathologist assesses for other types of resonance deviations, which are also common in patients with cleft palate. For example, there may be hypernasality on oral sounds caused by VPI but also hyponasality on nasal sounds caused by a blockage in the pharynx. Hypernasality caused by VPI can also occur in combination with cul-de-sac resonance, which is the result of blockage at the exit of one of the resonating cavities (pharyngeal, oral cavity, or nasal cavity).

Although hypernasality is most commonly caused by VPI, it can also be caused by other factors, including a thin velum or a large oronasal fistula. Hypernasality can even be phoneme-specific because of the substitution of nasal sounds for oral sounds (ie, ng/l or ng/r) or habitual use of a high posterior tongue position on certain vowels.

Hyponasality is also commonly noted in patients with cleft lip/palate. This condition may be caused by a maxillary retrusion, a narrow pharynx, or even enlarged adenoids. Postoperative hyponasality is also a risk of surgeries to correct VPI.

Nasal emission

Patients with a history of cleft palate often have nasal emission. Nasal emission can occur with hypernasality, if the velopharyngeal gap is large, or without hypernasality, if the gap is small.[1,6–10,12,13]

The relative audibility of the nasal emission can give a clue as to the size of the velopharyngeal opening. Nasal emission that is barely audible (or inaudible but causes consonants to be weak in intensity or omitted) suggests a large velopharyngeal gap. A smaller velopharyngeal opening causes more audible nasal emission than a large one because there is more resistance to the flow, and therefore more friction. Air that flows through a small velopharyngeal opening is released with increased pressure, which causes bubbling of secretions on top of the valve. The result is a loud and distorting nasal rustle (also called nasal turbulence).[1,10,12,14]

If present, the examiner notes the occurrence of a nasal snort, which is produced most often with /s/ blends, and/or a nasal sniff, which is a friction sound that is produced by forcible inspiration. A nasal grimace commonly accompanies nasal air emission. This observation is important because it reflects the patient's extra effort in attempting to close the velopharyngeal port.

The consistency of the nasal air emission is also tested. Nasal emission that occurs during the production of all pressure-sensitive phonemes suggests a large velopharyngeal opening, particularly if it is associated with hypernasality. Nasal emission that occurs inconsistently, but on all pressure-sensitive phonemes, suggests a smaller opening because the patient can close the gap with short utterances or with effort. In contrast, nasal emission that occurs consistently on certain speech phonemes, but not on all pressure-sensitive sounds, indicates that the cause is faulty articulation placement rather than VPI. This finding is sometimes noted in patients with no history of cleft or VPI. It is also common in patients with a history of VPI who used pharyngeal fricatives as a compensatory production for certain phonemes. Despite surgical correction of the VPI, nasal emission (and sometimes hypernasality) persists because of the abnormal placement.

Speech sound production

In assessing articulation (speech sound production), the speech pathologist records all speech sound errors, including substitutions, omissions, and distortions. The potential cause of the errors is also identified (eg, abnormal structure, apraxia [a motor speech sound disorder], phonological disorder, delayed development, or normal developmental error). When there are structural anomalies, such as VPI or occlusal anomalies secondary to cleft lip and palate, the speech pathologist also determines whether there are any obligatory distortions or compensatory articulation errors.[1,9,10]

- Obligatory distortions occur when the articulation placement (the function) is normal, but the abnormality of the structure causes distortion of speech. Obligatory distortions secondary to VPI include hypernasality, nasal emission, and nasalized consonants.

- Compensatory articulation errors occur when the placement of production is altered in response to the abnormal structure. When VPI causes inadequate oral airflow for consonants, the patient may compensate by producing the sounds in the pharynx, where there is airflow.[11]

It is important to determine the cause of each error or distortion, and particularly to identify obligatory distortions versus compensatory errors. This is important because the treatment is different depending on causality. For example, obligatory distortions do not require speech therapy. Once the structure is corrected, the distortion disappears. In contrast, compensatory errors require speech therapy, preferably after correction of the structure.

Phonation

Dysphonia is common in individuals with VPI. In particular, vocal nodules often occur in patients with a small velopharyngeal gap or a nasal grimace. This condition is thought to be caused by strain in the entire vocal tract with attempts to achieve velopharyngeal closure. In addition, breathiness is sometimes used as a compensatory strategy to mask the hypernasality or to mitigate the nasal emission. In addition, patients with VPI secondary to a craniofacial syndrome are at higher risk for laryngeal anomalies. Therefore, the speech pathologist listens for characteristics of dysphonia, including hoarseness, breathiness, roughness, glottal fry, hard glottal attack, strain, inappropriate pitch level, restricted pitch range, diplophonia, or inappropriate loudness. When present, these findings are often rated on a severity scale from mild to severe using the Consensus Auditory-Perceptual Evaluation of Voice (CAPE-V).[15]

Low-technology Tools for the Assessment

There are a few low-technology tools that can be used to assist with the evaluation.[7,9,10] The most common are discussed here.

Mirror

The examiner can place a dental mirror under the child's nares while the child produces pressure-sensitive oral sounds (**Fig. 5**). If the mirror fogs, it indicates nasal air emission. A problem with this test is that the mirror needs to be placed under the nose after the individual starts speaking and removed before the individual stops speaking to avoid fogging as a result of nasal breathing. Another disadvantage is that there is no way to know whether the nasal emission was consistent or just occurred on one phoneme. In addition, the clinician must be aware that when certain

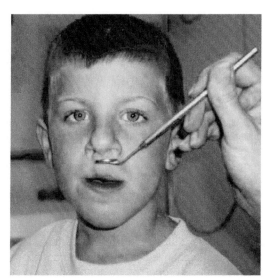

Fig. 5. Mirror test of nasal emission. (*From* Kummer AW. Cleft Palate & Craniofacial Anomalies, 3E. © 2014 Delmar Learning, a part of Cengage Learning, Inc. Reproduced by permission.)

compensatory productions (eg, nasal fricatives) are present, mirror fogging may also result.

Straw

A straw is perhaps the best tool in assessing hypernasality and nasal emission. (It is also cheap, always available, and disposable.) One end of the straw is placed in the patient's nostril and the other end is placed near the examiner's ear (**Fig. 6**). The child is asked to repeat syllables or sentences with oral consonants only. Even slight hypernasality or nasal emission can be heard easily through the straw. The straw amplifies the

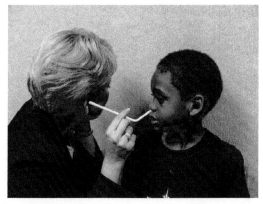

Fig. 6. Straw test of hypernasality, nasal emission, and hyponasality. (*From* Kummer AW. Cleft Palate & Craniofacial Anomalies, 3E. © 2014 Delmar Learning, a part of Cengage Learning, Inc. Reproduced by permission.)

sound, similar to a stethoscope. If hyponasality or upper airway obstruction is suspected, the child is asked to repeat syllables with nasal phonemes (ie, ma, ma, ma) or prolong an /m/ while the examiner listens through the straw. A muffled sound suggests obstruction.

Ratings

There are many perceptual rating methods to describe speech disorders associated with cleft palate. These methods include categorical judgments (eg, mild, moderate, severe); equal-appearing interval scales; direct magnitude estimation; paired comparison; and, more recently, visual analog scaling.[14] There are also some standardized protocols for rating different parameters of speech and velopharyngeal function that can be used to compare speech outcomes in intercenter studies. These protocols include the Cleft Audit Protocol for Speech-Augmented (CAPS-A)[16,17] and the Universal Parameters.[18] Speech parameters that are typically rated include hypernasality, hyponasality, audible nasal air emission and/or nasal turbulence, consonant production errors, and voice. Although severity ratings can be helpful in reporting and comparing intercenter outcomes, ratings of severity do not usually affect management decisions or the type of surgery selected for correction.

Video Recordings

Because outcomes are usually determined based on auditory perception, it is important to obtain a high-quality digital video recording (or at least an audio recording) of a representative speech sample as part of each assessment. These recordings should be retained in the patient's medical record. They can also be used for pretreatment and posttreatment comparisons, or for outcome studies and intercenter comparisons.

INTRAORAL EVALUATION

Although the status of velopharyngeal function cannot be determined through an intraoral examination, an oral examination has some importance in the evaluation of VPI and abnormal resonance in patients with a history of cleft palate.[19] A very thin velum is noteworthy because hypernasality can be caused by transmission of sound through thin tissue. During phonation, the position of the velar dimple and uvula are examined. If the velar dimple is skewed to one side or the uvula points to one side, the muscle function on the opposite side may be inadequate, causing a lateral velopharyngeal gap. If the uvula is consistently deviated to the side of a large tonsil, this indicates that the tonsil is pushing against the posterior faucial pillar and probably extends into the oropharynx. Large tonsils should be noted because they can cause pharyngeal cul-de-sac resonance and even affect articulation. In addition, dental occlusion is noted because malocclusion can have a significant effect on speech sound production.

INSTRUMENTAL EVALUATION OF VELOPHARYNGEAL FUNCTION

Instrumental procedures can provide valuable information to augment the perceptual evaluation results.[20–22] There are 2 basic categories of instrumental procedures for evaluation of velopharyngeal function: those that give indirect but objective information (eg, nasometry and aerodynamic instrumentation), and those that give direct but subjective information (eg, videofluoroscopy and nasopharyngoscopy).

Nasometry

Nasometry is a computer-based procedure used to measure the acoustic correlates of resonance and audible nasal emission. As such, nasometry provides indirect information regarding the function of the velopharyngeal valve (**Fig. 7**).[20–23] During production of the speech passage, the Nasometer II (KayPENTAX, Montvale, NJ) captures data regarding acoustic energy from both the nasal cavity and the oral cavity during speech in real time. It then calculates the average ratio of nasal/total (nasal plus oral) acoustic energy and converts this to a percentage value for the nasalance score. This score gives the examiner information about the relative percentage of nasality (hypernasality and audible nasal emission) in speech. Because nasometry measures both hypernasality and audible nasal emission, there is not a good correlation between velopharyngeal gap size and the nasalance score (because nasal emission is more audible with a small opening than a large opening). However, with the knowledge of the speech characteristics, the speech pathologist can use the nasalance results to confirm clinical impressions, and to do presurgical and postsurgical comparisons.

Speech Aerodynamics

Speech aerodynamics is a procedure to measure the mechanical properties of airflow and air pressure during speech production (**Fig. 8**).[20–22,24] The aerodynamic procedure involves the use of oral and nasal catheters that are connected to pressure transducers, and a flow tube that is connected to a heated pneumotachograph. The transducers convert the detected air pressure or flow into electrical signals. The pneumotachograph determines the rate of airflow.

Aerodynamic instrumentation can be used by the speech pathologist to provide objective documentation of intraoral air pressure levels and the amount of nasal air emission. With these data, the examiner can calculate an estimate of velopharyngeal orifice size during consonant-vowel production. Aerodynamic instrumentation can also provide evidence of airway obstruction through measurements of nasal airway resistance.

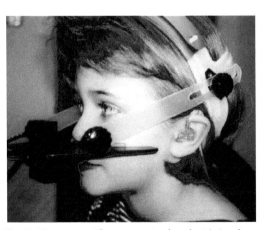

Fig. 7. Nasometry. The nasometer headset is in place. The nasometer collects acoustic data from the oral and nasal cavities during speech. (*From* Kummer AW. Cleft Palate & Craniofacial Anomalies, 3E. © 2014 Delmar Learning, a part of Cengage Learning, Inc. Reproduced by permission.)

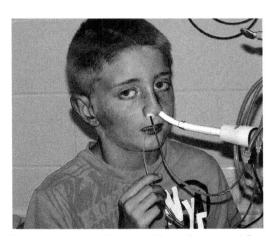

Fig. 8. Speech aerodynamics. The catheters and flow tube in place for measurement of the aerodynamics during speech production. (*From* Kummer AW. Cleft Palate & Craniofacial Anomalies, 3E. © 2014 Delmar Learning, a part of Cengage Learning, Inc. Reproduced by permission.)

Videofluoroscopic Speech Study

Once the diagnosis of VPI has been made by the speech pathologist, a videofluoroscopic speech study may be done to evaluate velopharyngeal movement and identify the structural deficiencies in velopharyngeal closure. This information may be useful for surgical planning.[20–22,25]

Because videofluoroscopy involves two-dimensional imaging, a speech study requires several views in order to see all aspects of the velopharyngeal port (**Fig. 9**). These views typically include a lateral (sagittal) view, an anteroposterior (AP) view, and a base view. The speech pathologist selects the speech sample, based on the results of the perceptual evaluation. The speech pathologist is involved in the interpretation of the results, based on knowledge of the speech characteristics and the probable cause.

Nasopharyngoscopy

Nasopharyngoscopy (also called nasendoscopy or videonasendoscopy) allows direct observation of the velopharyngeal port during speech.[20–22,26] In many centers, nasopharyngoscopy is done in addition to or instead of videofluoroscopy[27] because nasopharyngoscopy has several advantages compared with videofluoroscopy. The bird's-eye view, as seen through nasopharyngoscopy, has been found to provide more accurate information about the severity of VPI than videofluoroscopy.[28] Nasopharyngoscopy is superior to videofluoroscopy in finding the location of a velopharyngeal gap and confirming the size of the

opening, which is important in surgical planning. Even small, pin-hole-sized openings can be seen through nasopharyngoscopy, but are not visible through videofluoroscopy (**Fig. 10**). The effect of the adenoids (positive or negative) on velopharyngeal function can be directly visualized. The nasal surface of the velum can be examined for evidence of an occult submucous cleft. In addition, nasopharyngoscopy is effective in the assessment of the results of surgery for VPI.

In performing the nasopharyngoscopy procedure, it is important to observe the relative contributions of the velopharyngeal structures to closure because these vary among normal and abnormal speakers. Distinct patterns of velopharyngeal closure can be identified, based on the extent of movement of the velum and pharyngeal walls (**Fig. 11**).[29,30] The most common pattern of closure is the coronal pattern. In this case, closure is accomplished primarily by movement of the velum, which closes against a broad area of the posterior pharyngeal wall. The lateral pharyngeal walls close against the velum on both sides. When viewed from above through nasopharyngoscopy, a coronal slit is noted during complete closure. The next most common pattern of closure is the circular pattern. With this pattern, all the velopharyngeal structures contribute equally to closure so that this pattern resembles a sphincter. From a nasopharyngoscopy view, a small midline circle is seen with complete closure. The circular pattern is often associated with a Passavant because the superior constrictor

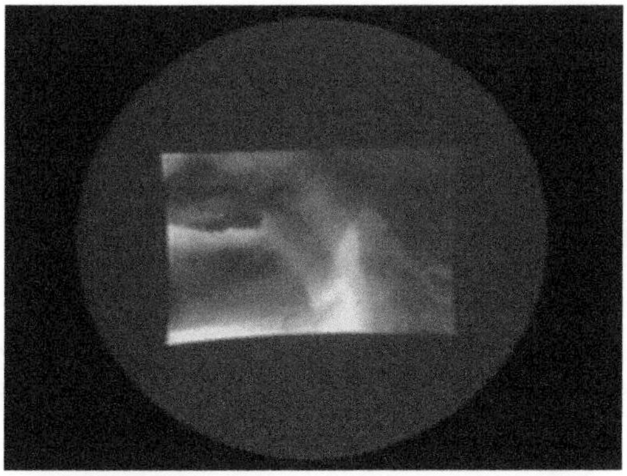

Fig. 9. Videofluoroscopy. Lateral view showing the velum and posterior pharyngeal wall during speech. In this case, the velum is normal in structure, but has poor movement. As a result, there is a large velopharyngeal gap caused by velopharyngeal incompetence. (*From* Kummer AW. Cleft Palate & Craniofacial Anomalies, 3E. © 2014 Delmar Learning, a part of Cengage Learning, Inc. Reproduced by permission.)

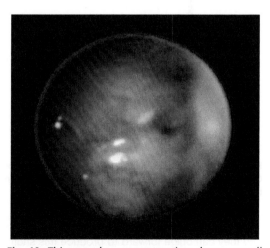

Fig. 10. This nasopharyngoscopy view shows a small but symptomatic velopharyngeal opening on the (patient's) left. It is important to ne aware of this opening for surgical planning. (*From* Kummer AW. Cleft Palate & Craniofacial Anomalies, 3E. © 2014 Delmar Learning, a part of Cengage Learning, Inc. Reproduced by permission.)

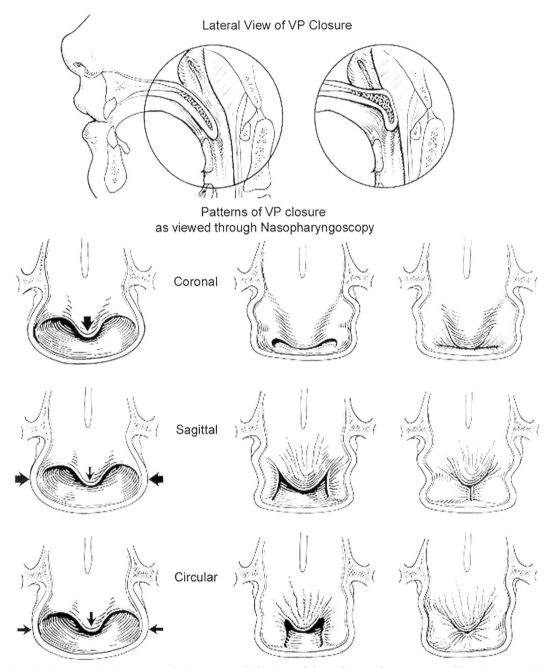

Fig. 11. Patterns of velopharyngeal closure as could be viewed through nasopharyngoscopy. (*From* Kummer AW. Cleft Palate & Craniofacial Anomalies, 3E. © 2014 Delmar Learning, a part of Cengage Learning, Inc. Reproduced by permission.)

muscles are particularly active with this pattern and they can bulge forward to produce this shelf-like structure during phonation. The least common pattern of closure is the sagittal pattern. With this pattern, the lateral pharyngeal walls are primary contributors to closure as they move medially to meet in midline behind the velum. The velum has a less active role. A sagittal slit is noted with complete closure when viewed through nasopharyngoscopy.

These natural variations in closure are important to recognize and understand during the nasopharyngoscopy procedure because the basic pattern of closure may have an impact on the type of surgical intervention that is ultimately recommended for correction of VPI.[31]

Passing the scope to perform this examination is within the scope of practice for speech pathologists. However, what is most important is that the speech pathologist is at least present during the examination and takes part in the interpretation of the results. As with videofluoroscopy, knowledge of the speech sample and speech characteristics is essential in interpretation of the results because a velopharyngeal opening during speech does not necessarily indicate VPI.

DIFFERENTIAL DIAGNOSIS

Based on the speech characteristics, the examiner can make a diagnosis of VPD, and can even predict the approximate size of the velopharyngeal opening (**Table 1**). The examiner must determine whether there are obligatory distortions and/or compensatory errors. Both can be the result of VPI or even malocclusion, which is also common in patients with cleft lip and/or palate. In addition, the type and consistency of nasal emission can help to determine causality (ie, oronasal fistula, VPI, or velopharyngeal mislearning). Most importantly, the examiner must determine the type of VPI and the cause of the speech characteristics because this information forms the basis for determination of the appropriate treatment modality (surgery, prosthetic device, and/or speech therapy).

Both types of VPI (velopharyngeal insufficiency or incompetence) require physical management for correction.[1] Physical management usually involves surgery, but may include prosthetic management if surgery is not an option. If surgical correction of VPI is indicated, nasopharyngoscopy can be particularly helpful in finding the location of the velopharyngeal opening (although this may be most important in patients with noncleft VPI). In contrast, if there is velopharyngeal mislearning, this requires speech therapy only.

It is common for a patient to show both velopharyngeal insufficiency and velopharyngeal mislearning. For example, children with velopharyngeal insufficiency (a structural disorder) often develop compensatory productions (a form of velopharyngeal mislearning). In these cases, surgical correction is required first in order to correct the VPI and normalize the velopharyngeal function. After structural correction, speech therapy is necessary to correct the faulty articulation productions in the pharynx that continue to result in characteristics of nasality.

The primary purpose of the speech pathology evaluation is to make this diagnosis through a perceptual and instrumental assessment. If surgical correction is needed, the speech pathologist can also assist in determining the type of surgery that has the best chance of success for the patient, based on the size and location of the velopharyngeal gap. If a prosthetic device is indicated, the speech pathologist can assist in fitting the device for maximum benefit. In addition, if speech therapy is needed, the evaluation results are used for development of an individualize treatment plan and determination of specific therapy strategies.

INDICATIONS FOR SPEECH THERAPY

There is a common misconception about the role of speech therapy in the management of what is often termed "cleft palate speech". Speech therapy cannot change abnormal structure and therefore cannot correct hypernasality or nasal emission caused by VPI, even if there is only a small gap.[32] There are no exercises that can change abnormal structure. Therefore, VPI (both types) requires physical management (surgery, or a prosthetic device if surgery is not an option).

Table 1
Prediction of velopharyngeal gap size based on perceptual features

Perceptual Characteristics	Predict	Relative Gap Size
Severe hypernasality Inaudible nasal emission Weak consonants Short utterance length Compensatory productions	⟹	(large oval)
Moderate hypernasality Audible nasal emission Slightly weak consonants May be compensatory productions	⟹	(medium oval)
Mild hypernasality Audible nasal emission	⟹	(small oval)
Nasal rustle (turbulence)	⟹	(very small oval)

From Kummer AW. Cleft Palate & Craniofacial Anomalies, 3E. © 2014 Delmar Learning, a part of Cengage Learning, Inc. Reproduced by permission.

In contrast, speech therapy can correct placement errors (abnormal function) that cause nasal emission or hypernasality, specifically the compensatory productions that persist after the correction of VPI.[28] Because compensatory productions typically involve articulation production somewhere in the pharynx (where there is airflow), they are produced with the velopharyngeal valve open. As a result, the airflow is released through the nose and there is nasal emission. Correction of the velopharyngeal valve through surgery does not change this placement so the nasal emission persists after surgery. It is at this time that speech therapy is effective in eliminating the nasality. In general, if there is VPI, it is important to correct the structure as soon as possible. Once the structure is corrected, speech therapy is effective in correcting the articulation placement errors that remain. The evaluation data form a basis for the development of an individualized treatment plan.

SUMMARY

All children with a history of cleft palate should undergo a speech evaluation around the age of 3 years in order to rule out VPI. Through the perceptual evaluation, the speech pathologist is able to determine whether there is VPI, and also whether there are obligatory distortions and/or compensatory productions as a result. Instrumental procedures can provide objective data for pretreatment and posttreatment comparisons. Nasopharyngoscopy is helpful in identifying the location of the opening for surgical planning. VPI always requires surgical correction. Speech therapy is often required after surgery to correct the compensatory productions that continue to cause nasality.

SUPPLEMENTARY DATA

Supplementary data related to this article can be found online at http://dx.doi.org/10.1016/j.cps.2013.12.004.

REFERENCES

1. Kummer AW. Resonance disorders and velopharyngeal function. In: Kummer AW, editor. Cleft palate and craniofacial anomalies: the effects on speech and resonance. 3rd edition. Clifton Park (NY): Cengage Learning; 2014.
2. Smith BE, Kuehn DP. Speech evaluation of velopharyngeal dysfunction. J Craniofac Surg 2007;18(2):251–60.
3. Trost-Cardamone JE. Coming to terms with VPI: a response to Loney and Bloem. Cleft Palate J 1989; 26(1):68–70.
4. Loney RW, Bloem TJ. Velopharyngeal dysfunction: recommendations for use of nomenclature. Cleft Palate J 1987;24(4):334–5.
5. Folkins JW. Velopharyngeal nomenclature: incompetence, inadequacy, insufficiency, and dysfunction. Cleft Palate J 1988;25(4):413–6.
6. Kuehn DP, Henne LJ. Speech evaluation and treatment of patients with cleft palate. Am J Speech Lang Pathol 2003;12:103–9.
7. Kummer AW. Assessment of velopharyngeal function. In: Lossee JE, Kirschner RE, editors. Comprehensive cleft care. New York: McGraw-Hill; 2009.
8. Smith B, Guyette TW. Evaluation of cleft palate speech. Clin Plast Surg 2004;31(2):251–60.
9. Kummer AW. Perceptual assessment of resonance and velopharyngeal function. Semin Speech Lang 2011;32(2):159–67.
10. Kummer AW. Speech and resonance assessment. In: Kummer AW, editor. Cleft palate and craniofacial anomalies: the effects on speech and resonance. 3rd edition. Clifton Park (NY): Cengage Learning; 2014.
11. American Cleft Palate–Craniofacial Association (ACPA). Parameters for evaluation and treatment of patients with cleft lip/palate or other craniofacial anomalies. Cleft Palate Craniofac J 2009; 30(Suppl):1–16.
12. Kummer AW. Disorders of resonance and airflow secondary to cleft palate and/or velopharyngeal dysfunction. Semin Speech Lang 2011;32(2): 141–9.
13. Baylis AL, Munson B, Moller KT, et al. Perceptions of audible nasal emission in speakers with cleft palate: a comparative study of listener judgments. Cleft Palate Craniofac J 2011;48(4):399–411.
14. Kummer AW, Briggs M, Lee L. The relationship between the characteristics of speech and velopharyngeal gap size. Cleft Palate Craniofac J 2003; 40(6):590–6.
15. Kempster B, Gerratt B, Verdolini Abbott K, et al. Consensus auditory-perceptual evaluation of voice: development of a standardized clinical protocol. Am J Speech Lang Pathol 2009;18:124–32.
16. John A, Sell D, Sweeney T, et al. The cleft audit protocol for speech-augmented: a validated and reliable measure for auditing cleft speech. Cleft Palate Craniofac J 2006;43(3):272–88.
17. Sell D, John A, Harding-Bell A, et al. Cleft audit protocol for speech (CAPS-A): a comprehensive training package for speech analysis. Int J Lang Commun Disord 2009;44(4):529–48.
18. Henningsson G, Kuehn DP, Sell D, et al. Universal parameters for reporting speech outcomes in individuals with cleft palate. Cleft Palate Craniofac J 2008;45(1):1–17.
19. Kummer AW. Orofacial examination. In: Kummer AW, editor. Cleft palate and craniofacial anomalies: the

effects on speech and resonance. 3rd edition. Clifton Park (NY): Cengage Learning; 2014.

20. Hinton VA. Instrumental measures of velopharyngeal function. In: Lossee JE, Kirschner RE, editors. Comprehensive cleft care. New York: McGraw-Hill; 2009.

21. Karnell MP. Instrumental assessment of velopharyngeal closure for speech. Semin Speech Lang 2011;32(2):168–78.

22. Kummer AW. Overview of instrumental procedures. In: Kummer AW, editor. Cleft palate and craniofacial anomalies: the effects on speech and resonance. 3rd edition. Clifton Park (NY): Cengage Learning; 2014.

23. Kummer AW. Nasometry. In: Kummer AW, editor. Cleft palate and craniofacial anomalies: the effects on speech and resonance. 3rd edition. Clifton Park (NY): Cengage Learning; 2014.

24. Zajac DJ. Speech aerodynamics. In: Kummer AW, editor. Cleft palate and craniofacial anomalies: the effects on speech and resonance. 3rd edition. Clifton Park (NY): Cengage Learning; 2014.

25. Kummer AW. Videofluoroscopy. In: Kummer AW, editor. Cleft palate and craniofacial anomalies: the effects on speech and resonance. 3rd edition. Clifton Park (NY): Cengage Learning; 2014.

26. Kummer AW. Nasopharyngoscopy. In: Kummer AW, editor. Cleft palate and craniofacial anomalies: the

effects on speech and resonance. 3rd edition. Clifton Park (NY): Cengage Learning; 2014.

27. Kummer AW, Clark SL, Redle EE, et al. Current practice in assessing and reporting speech outcomes of cleft palate and velopharyngeal surgery: a survey of cleft palate/craniofacial professionals. Cleft Palate Craniofac J 2011;49(2):146–52.

28. Lam DJ, Starr JR, Perkins JA, et al. A comparison of nasendoscopy and multiview videofluoroscopy in assessing velopharyngeal insufficiency. Otolaryngol Head Neck Surg 2006;134(3):394–402.

29. Croft CB, Shprintzen RJ, Rakoff SJ. Patterns of velopharyngeal valving in normal and cleft palate subjects: a multi-view videofluoroscopic and nasendoscopic study. Laryngoscope 1981;91(2):265–71.

30. Skolnick ML, Shprintzen RJ, McCall GN, et al. Patterns of velopharyngeal closure in subjects with repaired cleft palate and normal speech: a multi-view videofluoroscopic analysis. Cleft Palate J 1975;12: 369–76.

31. Armour A, Fischbach S, Klaiman P, et al. Does velopharyngeal closure pattern affect the success of pharyngeal flap pharyngoplasty? Plast Reconstr Surg 2005;115(1):45–52 [discussion: 53].

32. Kummer AW. Speech therapy. In: Kummer AW, editor. Cleft palate and craniofacial anomalies: the effects on speech and resonance. 3rd edition. Clifton Park (NY): Cengage Learning; 2014.

Surgical Management of Velopharyngeal Insufficiency

Michael S. Gart, MD[a],*, Arun K. Gosain, MD[b]

KEYWORDS

- Velopharyngeal insufficiency • Hypernasal speech • Cleft palate • Surgical technique
- Sphincter pharyngoplasty • Pharyngeal flap • Furlow palatoplasty

KEY POINTS

- Speech assessment, including nasoendoscopy and multiview video fluoroscopy are essential tools in identifying patients who will benefit from surgical management of velopharyngeal insufficiency and guiding procedure selection.
- Although there is no current consensus on the best available technique, many centers select the corrective procedure based on velopharyngeal closure pattern and pharyngeal gap.
  - With sagittal closure patterns, double-opposing Z-palatoplasty (DOZ) is effective with small pharyngeal gaps; pharyngeal flaps are used if the gap is large.
  - For coronal closure patterns, dynamic sphincter pharyngoplasty (DSP) can be used with small gaps; a combination of DOZ and DSP can be used with large gaps.
- Patients with velocardiofacial syndrome often do well with a high-inset, wide pharyngeal flap procedure. However, alternative surgical techniques are being investigated in these patients.

OVERVIEW

The primary goal of cleft palate repair is to create an anatomically and functionally intact palate to improve feeding and achieve normal speech while minimally impacting maxillary growth and development.[1] In order to produce normal speech, a child must have velopharyngeal competence, defined as the ability to completely close the velopharyngeal sphincter that separates the oro- and nasopharynx. The absence of this ability, termed velopharyngeal insufficiency (VPI), is seen in a wide range of patients following primary cleft palate repair, with approximately 20-30% requiring secondary surgical correction.[2–5]

The velopharyngeal mechanism is a muscular valve extending from the posterior bony palate to the posterior pharynx. With the exception of three sounds in the English language (/m/, /n/, /ng/), all speech is produced with a closed velopharyngeal port.[6] The muscles involved in velopharyngeal closure are depicted in **Fig. 1**. While understanding the normal anatomy and physiology of this mechanism is essential to appropriate care of the patient with VPI, a full description is beyond the scope of this chapter.

The following will discuss the patient assessment, treatment options, and the surgical management of VPI. Recent trends and future directions in management are also presented. After reading, one should be able to describe the approach to a patient with suspected VPI, including the selection and execution of the appropriate surgical procedure.

Disclosures: The authors have nothing to disclose relevant to this article.
[a] Division of Plastic & Reconstructive Surgery, Northwestern University Feinberg School of Medicine, 675 North Saint Clair Street, Galter Pavilion, Suite 19-250, Chicago, IL 60611, USA; [b] Division of Plastic & Reconstructive Surgery, Ann & Robert H. Lurie Children's Hospital of Chicago, 225 East Chicago Avenue, Chicago, IL 60611, USA
* Corresponding author.
E-mail address: michael-gart@northwestern.edu

Clin Plastic Surg 41 (2014) 253–270
http://dx.doi.org/10.1016/j.cps.2013.12.010
0094-1298/14/$ — see front matter © 2014 Elsevier Inc. All rights reserved.

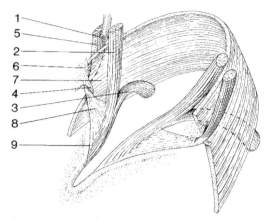

Fig. 1. Anatomy of the velopharyngeal mechanism. 1, eustachian tube orifice; 2, levator veli palatini; 3, palatopharyngeus; 4, hamulus; 5, tensor veli palatini; 6, medial pterygoid; 7, superior pharyngeal constrictor; 8, palatal aponeurosis; 9, posterior margin of bony palate. (*From* Furlow LT Jr. Cleft palate repair by double-opposing Z-plasty. In: Vistnes LM, editor. How they do it: procedures in plastic and reconstructive surgery. Boston: Little, Brown and Company; 1991; with permission.)

HISTORICAL PERSPECTIVE

Surgical manipulation of the velopharyngeal port dates back to the nineteenth century. The first recorded attempt by Passavant[7] in 1865 was direct adhesion of the soft palate to the posterior pharyngeal wall. Shoenborn later described the familiar pharyngeal flap operation in 1875,[8] which was popularized in the United States by Padgett[9] in 1930. Subsequent modifications to flap design and orientation have focused on minimizing nasal air emission while preventing airway obstruction.[10,11] The importance of pharyngeal flap design and orientation continues to be debated in the literature.[12–16]

In 1950, Wilfred Hynes[17,18] described an operation to address failed cleft palate repair whereby he secured myomucosal flaps, containing salpingopharyngeus and palatopharyngeus muscles, to the posterior pharyngeal wall. His technique has since undergone several modifications, most notably by Orticochea[19] in 1968, who advocated lower flap inset and inclusion of a third, inferiorly based posterior pharyngeal flap; Jackson and Silverton[20] in 1977, who advocated a combination of palatopharyngeal flaps and a superiorly based pharyngeal flap; and Riski and colleagues[21] in 1984, who advocated higher fixation of the myomucosal flaps to the posterior pharyngeal wall, at or near the point of velar contact. Several additional modifications have been made to each

procedure, with various outcomes studies available for each technique.[22–24]

Augmentation of the posterior pharynx to decrease velopharyngeal port size dates back to the early twentieth century. Beginning with Vaseline in 1900,[25] various materials, including paraffin,[26] cartilage,[27] silicone,[28] porous polyethylene,[29] Proplast,[30] collagen,[31] calcium-hydroxyapatite,[32,33] Teflon,[34] GoreTex,[30] dermis-fat flaps,[35] and, more recently, autologous fat grafts[36] have all been used to augment the posterior pharyngeal wall. Several of these techniques have shown considerable success in treating velopharyngeal insufficiency (VPI); however, all materials have advantages and disadvantages. With recent advances in autologous fat grafting techniques, there has been increasing focus on the potential for this modality in the treatment of VPI.

PATIENT ASSESSMENT
Patient History

As with all surgical patients, the assessment of a patient presenting with evidence of VPI should begin with a thorough history and physical examination. In particular, the onset of speech anomalies, previous history of cleft lip and/or cleft palate (CLP), as well as any previous palatopharyngeal surgery (tonsillectomy, adenoidectomy, and so forth) or neurologic disorders should be elucidated.

A history of repaired or unrepaired cleft palate is the most common cause of VPI.[37] The most common causes of VPI in children with a history of repaired cleft palate are inadequate lengthening of the velum at the time of primary palatoplasty, abnormal function of the levator musculature, and cicatricial contracture of the velum.[38] Other causes include submucous cleft palate; neurogenic VPI caused by central or peripheral insults to the cranial nerves innervating the velopharyngeal mechanism; and iatrogenic VPI following maxillary resection, uvulopalatopharyngoplasty, or adenoidectomy.[37,39–49] Although physiologic involution of the adenoid pads can result in VPI, these structures are not thought to function in normal velopharyngeal closure.[50,51] Patients with progressive pubertal VPI in the absence of adenoidectomy are rare and are thought to have underlying velopharyngeal disproportion.[52] The causes of structural, functional, and dynamic VPI are summarized in **Table 1**. For a more comprehensive discussion of the multiple causes of VPI, including their diagnosis and management, readers are directed to several excellent review articles.[37,40–42,52–56]

Table 1
Causes and Classification of velopharyngeal insufficiency

Mechanism	Diagnosis	
	Congenital	Acquired
Structural Abnormalities		

Palatopharyngeal disproportion	1. Short soft palate
	  a. Repaired cleft palate
	  b. Submucous cleft palate
	  c. Noncleft palate
	2. Deep nasopharynx
	3. Combination
		1. After tonsillectomy and adenoidectomy
		2. Resection for tumor
		3. After infectious palate slough

Abnormal anatomy of levator palati muscles	1. Unrepaired cleft of primary and secondary palate
	  a. Unilateral
	  b. Bilateral
	2. Unrepaired cleft of secondary palate only
	  a. Isolated cleft
	  b. Associated with syndromes (branchial arch, Klippel-Feil, mandibular hypoplasia, Pierre-Robin, frontonasal, craniostenosis, orofacial digital, and so forth)
	3. Repaired cleft palate, without levator sling reconstruction or palatal pushback
	4. Submucous cleft palate
	  a. Isolated
	  b. Associated with other abnormalities (congenital hard palate fistula, mental retardation, maxillary hypoplasia, hearing disorders, and so forth)	

Functional Abnormalities		
	1. Deafness 2. Mental retardation	1. Persistent habit patterns after correction of anatomic and physiologic defects 2. Mimicry 3. Psychoneurosis 4. Hearing disorder (vascular, tumor, infection, degenerative)
Dynamic Abnormalities		
Palatal Paresis		
Upper motor neuron	1. Cerebral palsy 2. Dystonias	1. Cerebral vascular accident 2. Brain tumors 3. Meningitis, encephalitis 4. Pseudobulbar palsy
Nuclear	1. Facial paralysis	1. Spinal muscular atrophy 2. Poliomyelitis 3. Amyotrophic lateral sclerosis
Peripheral nerve	—	1. After diphtheria 2. Polyneuritis (alcoholic, toxic)
Myoneural junction	—	1. Myasthenia gravis

Primary muscular abnormality	1. Hypoplasia
	  a. Repaired cleft palate
	  b. Moebius syndrome
	  c. Branchial arch syndrome including Treacher-Collins
	2. Myotonic dystrophy
	3. Arthrogryposis
		1. Muscular dystrophy (fascioscapulohumeral)
		2. Collagen diseases
		  a. Dermatomyositis
		  b. Scleroderma
		3. Polymyositis

(continued on next page)

Table 1		
(continued)		
	Diagnosis	
Mechanism	Congenital	Acquired
Nonspecific or undetermined cause	1. Minor coordination problems (fine motor sequencing) 2. Ectodermal dysplasia 3. Neurofibromatosis	—
Obstructive and Restrictive Causes	1. Hamartomas (eg, neurofibromas)	1. Tumor 2. Large tonsils 3. Tonsillar pillar scars 4. Scars after cleft palate repair 5. Restrictive pharyngeal flaps

From Minami RT, Kaplan EN, Wu G, et al. Velopharyngeal incompetence without overt cleft palate. Plast Reconstr Surg 1975;55:574–5; with permission.

Speech Assessment

A detailed discussion on speech assessment is provided by Kummer and colleagues elsewhere in this issue.

It is of paramount importance for the child with suspected VPI to undergo formal evaluation by a speech-language pathologist before considering surgical intervention. This evaluation begins with a perceptual speech evaluation to assess articulation, resonance, nasal airway emission, and voice.[57]

Multiple scales exist for evaluation of velopharyngeal function. In our practice, we use the Pittsburgh Weighted Speech Score (PWSS)[58] to grade VPI on a quantitative scale. This scale uses a standardized scoring system to evaluate a patient based on nasal air emission, facial grimace, resonance, voice quality, and articulation. A sample patient assessment worksheet is shown in **Fig. 2**. The individual scores are summed, and the total scores are used to classify patients into one of 4 categories of velopharyngeal function (in increasing order of dysfunction): competence, borderline competence, borderline incompetence, and incompetence.

If the formal speech evaluation indicates borderline or frank velopharyngeal incompetence (PWSS score of 3 or greater), adjunctive studies are available to guide the selection of the best intervention.

Instrumental Assessment of the Velopharyngeal Mechanism

There are several diagnostic modalities available to image the dynamic function of the velopharyngeal mechanism and determine its pattern of closure. The 3 basic closure patterns are described as:

1. Coronal, in which movement of the velum is primarily responsible for velopharyngeal closure, with little contribution from the lateral pharyngeal walls
2. Sagittal, in which medial displacement of the lateral pharyngeal walls is primarily responsible for closure, with little posterior movement of the velum
3. Circular, in which movement of the velum and the pharyngeal walls contribute to a sphincteric or purse-string closure of the velopharyngeal port

The most common diagnostic evaluations of velopharyngeal function and closure pattern are nasoendoscopy and multiview video fluoroscopy.[59] Nasoendoscopy uses a flexible endoscope inserted through the middle meatus to the posterior pharynx to visualize the velopharyngeal mechanism from a bird's-eye view while the patient phonates a speech sample. Nasoendoscopy provides visualization of the size and location of the velopharyngeal opening and relative contributions of the velum, lateral pharyngeal walls, and posterior pharynx during attempted velopharyngeal closure. Nasoendoscopy is also useful to assess for palatal scarring, oronasal fistulae, submucous clefting, and the status of the tonsils and adenoids.[59,60]

Multiview video fluoroscopy (MVF) involves imaging of the same speech sample through multiple views, including lateral and anterior-posterior views to evaluate the relative contributions of the velum and lateral pharyngeal walls in attempted closure, respectively. Although MVF can be useful in identifying the point of attempted velar contact, it is limited in its ability to measure multiple variables in a single view.[61] Therefore, most clinicians prefer to use MVF in conjunction with nasoendoscopy.

PITTSBURG WEIGHTED SPEECH SCALE (PWSS)
Weighted Values for Speech Symptoms Associated with Velopharyngeal Incompetence

NASAL AIR EMISSION	RIGHT	LEFT
Score most patent nostril and provide only the highest value. Maximum Score = 3		
Not Present	0	
Inconsistent, Visible	1	
Consistent, Visible	2	
Nasal escape on nasals appropriate	0	
Reduced	0	
Absent	0	
Audible	3	
Turbulent	3	

Presence of **FACIAL GRIMACE**	2

NASALITY / RESONANCE	
Normal	0
Mild Hypernasality	1
Moderate Hypernasality	2 (- 3)
Severe Hypernasality	4
Mixed: Hyponasality - Hypernasality	2
Cul de Sac	2
Hyponasality	0

PHONATION / VOICE	
Normal	0
Hoarseness OR Breathiness	
Mild	1
Moderate	2
Severe	3
OR:	
Reduced Loudness	2
Tension in System	3
Other:	

ARTICULATION	
Normal	0
Developmental Errors	0
Errors from other causes not related to VPI	0
Errors related to anterior dentition	0
Reduced intraoral pressure for sibilants	1
Reduced intraoral pressure for other fricatives	2
Reduced intraoral pressure for plosives	3
Omission of fricatives or plosives	2
Omission of fricatives or plosives plus hard glottal attack for vowels	3
Lingual-Palatal sibilants	2
Pharyngeal fricatives, plosives, backing, snorts, inhalations, or exhalation substitutions	3
Glottal stops	3
Nasal substitutions for pressure sounds	4

Probable Nature of Velopharyngeal Valve:		TOTAL
Competent	0	
Boderline Competent	1 – 2	
Borderline Incompetent	3 – 6	
Incompetent	7 and Up.	

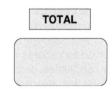

Fig. 2. VPI assessment worksheet. (*Adapted from* McWilliams BJ, Phillips BJ. Velopharyngeal incompetence: audio seminars in speech pathology. Philadelphia: WB Saunders; 1979; with permission.)

MVF is also useful with children who do not tolerate nasoendoscopy.[11,37] Although these modalities provide complementary information in assessing the velopharyngeal closure pattern, nasoendoscopy has been shown to correlate more strongly with VPI severity.[59]

Magnetic resonance imaging (MRI) has gained popularity in recent years as an imaging modality that may provide better-tolerated and more precise information regarding the anatomy of the velopharyngeal mechanism. Clear benefits of this technology include its noninvasive nature and avoidance of ionizing radiation in a mostly pediatric population.[62] Although several centers have reported success with this technique, limitations remain in its ability to obtain clear images with short enough exposure time to limit motion-related artifact during dynamic speech.[62,63] With the further development and refinement of MRI technology, this may offer a more precise and better-tolerated assessment of the velopharyngeal mechanism during speech.

Nasometry is a technique that can provide objective measurement of the acoustic energy emitted from the nasal cavity relative to that of the combined oral and nasal cavities.[64] To achieve this, the nasometer consists of a headset with 2 microphones positioned in front of the nose and mouth with an intervening metallic plate to isolate acoustic energy from each cavity. The headset is connected to a computer that interprets and graphically represents the proportion of nasal/total acoustic energy emission as nasalance scores (0–100) for comparison with available normative data.[65] Although this modality provides a purely objective assessment of acoustic energy distribution, it is best used as an adjunctive measure to perceptual speech assessment to provide the most comprehensive speech assessment.[60]

CURRENT PRACTICE

Available treatment options for VPI include speech therapy, prosthetic devices, and surgical management. Although prosthetic devices are usually reserved for patients who are considered poor surgical candidates, or for whom surgical treatment is not available, they have shown a high success rate in the treatment of VPI.[55,66,67] The most commonly used techniques for the surgical management of VPI are:

1. Furlow palatoplasty, or double-opposing Z-plasty, for palatal lengthening
2. Pharyngeal flap
3. Dynamic sphincter pharyngoplasty (DSP)

Although some investigators have also advocated the use of posterior pharyngeal augmentation, by means of injectable or implantable alloplastic and autologous materials,[30,32,36] these techniques are not currently in widespread use and are not discussed in detail in this article. The reader is directed to the references provided for additional information regarding these modalities.

AUTHORS' PREFERRED TECHNIQUE
Preoperative Planning

A detailed knowledge of the patient's history and mechanics of attempted velopharyngeal closure usually suffice in determining the best course of surgical treatment. As mentioned previously, closure of the velopharyngeal mechanism depends primarily on the elevation and posterior motion of the velum; however, important contributions are made by movement of the lateral pharyngeal walls toward the midline as well as anterior bulging of the posterior pharyngeal wall.[6] The success of surgical correction of VPI depends as much or more on the selection of the appropriate procedure than on technical expertise. In our experience, a perfectly performed procedure cannot correct VPI in an improperly selected patient and may increase upper airway complications. To that end, any surgical procedure performed to address VPI should take into consideration the existing pattern of velopharyngeal closure.

Algorithmic Approach to Procedure Selection

Our surgical approach is selected based on the pattern of velopharyngeal closure and the pharyngeal gap, or size of the aperture present with attempted closure. For patients with a sagittal pattern of closure, the deficiency lies in a lack of posterior velar movement or in palatal length; therefore, for patients with this closure pattern and a pharyngeal gap of less than 9 mm, palatal lengthening alone is often sufficient, and we prefer using a double-opposing Z-palatoplasty (DOZ). In patients with a sagittal closure pattern and a gap of greater than 9 mm, a superiorly based pharyngeal flap is a good solution. The airway concerns commonly associated with pharyngeal flaps are less likely to occur in these patients because the lateral pharyngeal wall mobility allows opening of the lateral velopharyngeal ports.

In patients with poor lateral wall motion (coronal closure pattern), the velum is the primary contributor to velopharyngeal closure. In such patients, with a velopharyngeal gap of 9 mm or less, DSP is preferred rather than a pharyngeal flap. In these patients, the poor motion of the lateral walls may contribute to nasal airway obstruction should a pharyngeal flap be attempted.

Patients who have a coronal closure pattern with a pharyngeal gap of more than 9 mm present a challenging problem. Based on a review of 13 patients with such velopharyngeal mechanics, we have found that the combination of DOZ and DSP works well to lengthen the palate, which, combined with the sphincteric motion of the DSP, can effect velopharyngeal competence.[68] In this series, 15% of patients had persistent hypernasality, which was corrected in all cases with secondary placement of a narrow pharyngeal flap. The combination of DOZ and DSP was shown to significantly improve speech and voice ratings on a standardized scale.[68]

For patients with a circular, or sphincteric, closure pattern, but persistent pharyngeal gap, the procedure of choice depends on the gap size. If there is a small gap (<9 mm), our procedure of choice is the DOZ; for large gaps, narrow pharyngeal flaps are used, because the adequate lateral wall motion allows closure of the lateral ports and minimizes risk of airway obstruction.

In general, our preference is to use a pharyngeal flap as a last resort, except in cases of velocardiofacial syndrome (VCFS), as described later.

OPERATIVE TECHNIQUES
Furlow Palatoplasty/DOZ

Leonard Furlow[69] first described his eponymous double-opposing Z-plasty technique for primary palatoplasty in 1986. This technique transposed the abnormally inserted levator musculature into a more anatomic, posterior, and transverse orientation, thus recreating the levator sling and simultaneously lengthening the velum and constricting the velopharyngeal port.[69,70] To distinguish this technique of primary palatoplasty from secondary double-opposing Z-plasty performed secondarily for management of VPI, this article uses the term Furlow palatoplasty to refer to primary cleft palate repair and DOZ for secondary palatoplasty for VPI management.

The DOZ begins with marking of the oral mucosa as shown in **Fig. 3**. By convention, a posteriorly based oromuscular (oral mucosa and muscle) flap is elevated on the left side and an anteriorly based oral mucosal (mucosa only) flap is elevated on the right side, as shown in **Fig. 4**A. Flap elevation in the absence of previous intravelar veloplasty is shown in **Fig. 4**B.

Care must be taken to preserve the greater palatine arterial pedicles supplying the levator veli

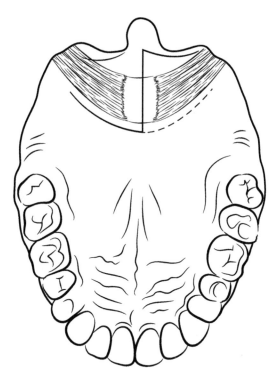

Fig. 3. Oral mucosal markings.

palatini muscles in both the oromuscular and nasomuscular flaps.

Once the oral dissection is completed, nasal mucosal flaps are elevated as mirror images of the oral flaps, with a left-sided, anteriorly based mucosal flap and right-sided, posteriorly based nasomuscular flap.

In secondary palatoplasty, the levator musculature is encased in scar. It is essential to remove all scar tissue to promote better postoperative function of the levator sling. We use a muscle stimulator to differentiate functional muscle in the oromuscular and nasomuscular flaps from scar tissue.

The nasomuscular flap is then transposed to the patient's left-posterior side, and the nasal mucosal flap transposed right-anterior (**Fig. 5**). Transposition of the oromuscular flap left-anterior and the oral mucosal flap right-posterior reconstructs the levator sling and completes the DOZ (**Fig. 6**).

One distinct advantage of the DOZ technique is that it can be applied in all patients, regardless of whether or not an intravelar veloplasty was performed at the time of primary palatoplasty. The Z-plasty lengthens the velum at the expense of palatal width. This loss of width functions to tighten the velopharyngeal port and is a secondary benefit of this technique. Moreover, this technique leaves several options available should VPI persist after surgery.

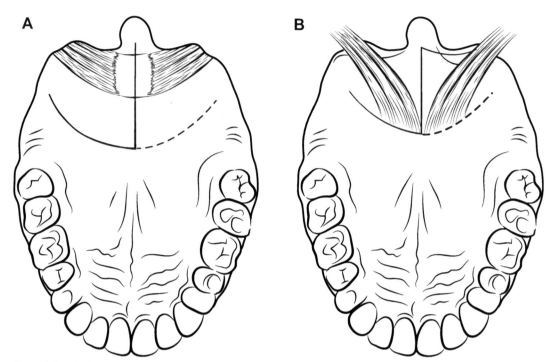

Fig. 4. (A) Palatal incisions, with left-sided oromuscular flap and right-sided mucosal flap. (B) An absence of previous intravelar veloplasty.

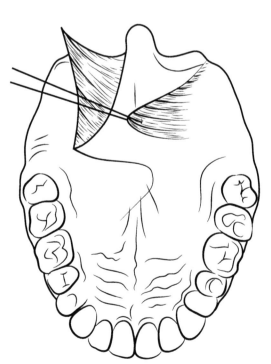

Fig. 5. Transposition of the nasomuscular (left-posterior) and nasal mucosal flaps (right-anterior) into their new positions.

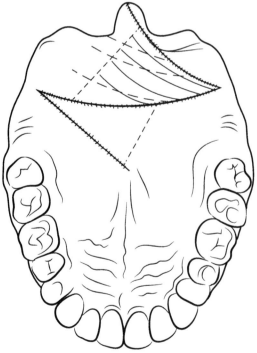

Fig. 6. Transposition of the oromuscular (right-posterior) and oral mucosal (left-anterior) flaps into their new positions. Lines indicate the direction of the transposed muscle fibers.

High-inset Pharyngeal Flap

As mentioned earlier, the pharyngeal flap is our last resort for surgical management of VPI, except in cases of VCFS. Our modification to the pharyngeal flap procedure for treatment of these patients is discussed here.[71] In the past, multiple factors have contributed to poor outcomes and persistent VPI following secondary palatoplasty in these patients, including poor lateral wall motion caused by pharyngeal hypotonia; abnormal muscular action; and an obtuse basicranium, which contributes to the pharyngeal gap.[72] Although DSP has been advocated, patients with VCFS have shown twice the revision rate of patients without VCFS (22% vs 11%).[73] The high, wide pharyngeal flap, proposed by Shprintzen and colleagues,[74–76] has become an accepted form of treatment of these patients; however, the success of this operation depends on high flap inset, which is technically demanding because of limited visualization. The senior author has developed a technique for high pharyngeal flap inset that avoids such difficulties, as described later.

The palate and posterior pharyngeal wall are marked and preinfiltrated with 0.25% bupivacaine with 1:200,000 epinephrine before placement of a Dingman retractor suspended on a Mayo stand.

A superiorly based myomucosal flap containing the superior pharyngeal constrictor muscle is elevated in a plane anterior to the pharyngobasilar fascia (**Figs. 7** and **8**). A fishmouth incision is created on the nasal side of the velum, superior to the uvula (**Fig. 9**A), and a counterincision is made on the oral surface of the velum immediately posterior to the junction of the hard and soft palates (see **Fig. 9**B). A 3-cm-wide pocket is then dissected from the nasal side through the levator musculature, connecting these two incisions (see **Fig. 9**C). The pharyngeal flap is then passed through this pocket using an angled clamp or forceps (see **Fig. 9**D). Once successfully passed through this tunnel, the flap is inset into the oral mucosa using 5 interrupted 4-0 Vicryl (Ethicon, Inc, Somerville, NJ) horizontal mattress sutures. The fishmouth incision on the nasal side of the soft palate is left to heal secondarily. An attempt can be made to close the donor site with 4-0 Vicryl sutures (**Fig. 10**); however, if a wide flap was designed, the donor site can similarly be left to heal secondarily. In order to prevent postoperative synechiae formation between the lateral aspect of the pharyngeal flap and the lateral pharyngeal walls, a 3-Fr endotracheal tube is placed in each naris and passed through the corresponding lateral port.

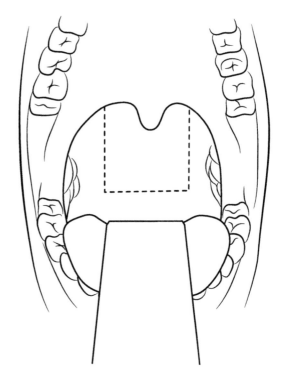

Fig. 7. Marking of the pharyngeal flap.

Patients are discharged home once oral intake is adequate to maintain hydration, usually on the first or second postoperative day, and the endotracheal tubes are removed in clinic 1 week after surgery.

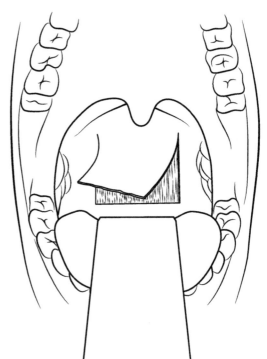

Fig. 8. Elevation of pharyngeal flap anterior to prevertebral fascia.

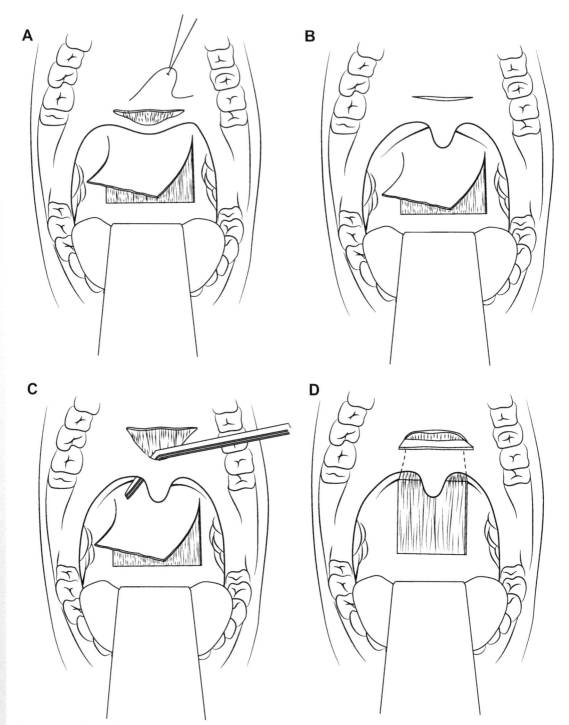

Fig. 9. (*A*) Fishmouth incision on the nasal surface of the soft palate; (*B*) Counter incision on the oral surface of the soft palate, immediately posterior to the hard-soft palate junction; (*C*) Flap transposition; (*D*) Flap in place.

Sphincter Techniques

We perform the DSP as described by Ortico-chea.[19] An incision is made along the anterior border of the posterior tonsillar pillar, extending inferiorly to the base of the tonsil. The palatophar-yngeus muscle is then freed from the pharyngeal constrictor musculature before incising the inferior and posterior aspects of the posterior tonsillar pillar. This myomucosal flap is raised superiorly

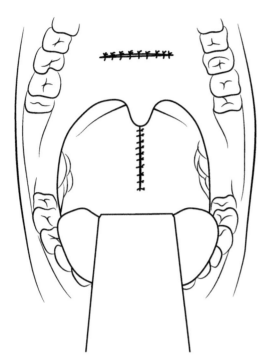

Fig. 10. Final postoperative appearance, showing primary closure of flap donor site.

to allow the flap to pivot approximately 90° into the desired position at the base of the adenoid pad, as high as possible in the posterior pharynx, without undue tension on the flap. The flaps are then sutured together in an overlapping or end-to-end fashion, and secured to the posterior pharyngeal wall, completing the sphincter pharyngoplasty. The flap donor sites are closed primarily whenever possible using a running 4-0 chromic suture.

Fig. 11 shows the operative technique for the combined DOZ and DSP, described earlier for patients with poor lateral pharyngeal wall motion and large pharyngeal gaps.

When performing a DSP in the absence of DOZ, the velum is simply retracted rather then opened to provide exposure to the base of the adenoid pad along the posterior pharyngeal wall.

The highest point that the myomucosal flaps can be inset is the base of the adenoid pad, because the adenoid tissue does not hold suture. Therefore, if the patient has low-lying adenoid tissue, otolaryngology referral should be made for inferior adenoidectomy to a level just superior to the desired inset of the myomucosal flaps. This referral should be done at least 6 weeks before DSP to allow adequate healing of the posterior pharyngeal wall.

The sphincter pharyngoplasty has several advantages as a corrective treatment of VPI. First, it creates a dynamic structure, which alleviates the

concerns for the persistent hypernasality or hyponasality seen with an improperly sized pharyngeal flap. Moreover, this procedure can easily be revised if hypernasality persists by reelevation and further overlap of the two myomucosal flaps, further narrowing the velopharyngeal port. If hypernasality persists despite revision, the option exists for secondary placement of a narrow pharyngeal flap.

Prosthetics

Although more commonly used in the setting of iatrogenic or neurogenic VPI,[43–49] prosthetic management of velopharyngeal dysfunction has been shown in several studies to be equivalent to surgical management.[77–81] The most commonly used prosthetic devices are palatal lifts and palatopharyngeal obturators/pharyngeal bulbs. These devices are anchored to the dentition and allow closure of the velopharyngeal port, either by altering the position of the velum (palatal lift prosthesis) or by occupying the pharyngeal gap (pharyngeal bulb). A comprehensive discussion of prosthetic management of VPI is beyond the scope of this article, but readers are directed to several comprehensive reports.[43–47,66,77–79,81]

Advantages of this technique include avoidance of surgery for patients who are poor surgical candidates or who refuse surgery, and reduced costs. In a randomized trial comparing palatal prostheses with pharyngeal flaps, Marsh and Wray[78] showed equivalent speech outcomes with a cost savings of 60% using prosthetics.

COMPLICATIONS AND AVOIDANCE
Furlow Palatoplasty/DOZ

Aside from inherent complications associated with any palatal surgery, including partial flap loss and/or development of oronasal fistulae, there are no inherent complications in a DOZ. The most common pitfall in this technique is inadequate gain in palatal length or levator muscle function. Levator muscle function can be optimized by removal of all scar tissue encasing the velar musculature.

Pharyngeal Flap

Early complications
The static nature of the pharyngeal flap remains its primary functional drawback. A flap designed too narrow fails to close the velopharyngeal port and results in persistent nasal airway emission and hypernasal speech, whereas a flap designed too wide obstructs the nasopharyngeal passage, resulting in hyponasality or airway compromise with obstructive sleep apnea (OSA).

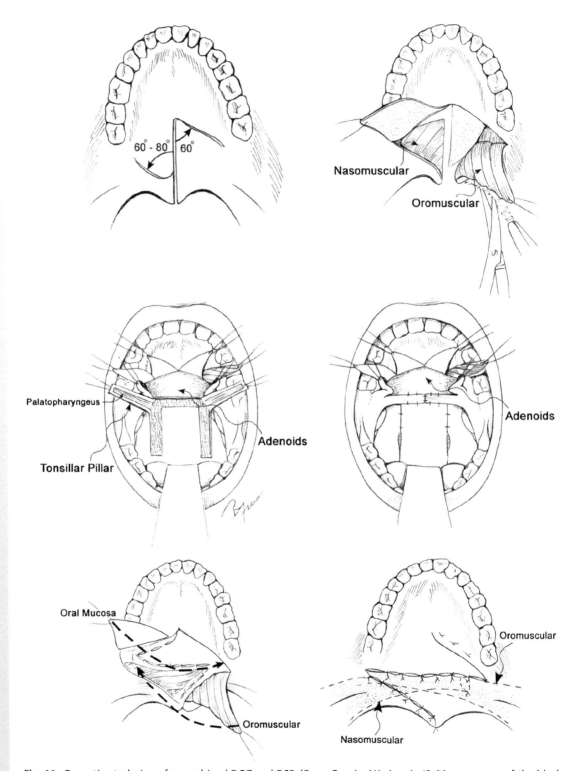

Fig. 11. Operative technique for combined DOZ and DSP. (*From* Gosain AK, Arneja JS. Management of the black hole in velopharyngeal incompetence: combined use of a Furlow palatoplasty and sphincter pharyngoplasty. Plast Reconstr Surg 2007;119(5):1540; with permission.)

The most serious complication with pharyngeal flap surgery is upper airway obstruction. There have been several reports in the literature of airway obstruction and even death following pharyngeal flaps.[82–88] Intraoperative corticosteroid administration is a simple measure that can reduce postoperative edema, and only requires advance communication with the anesthesiology staff.

We recommend that these patients are observed overnight and discharged home the next day if there are no signs and symptoms of airway compromise. Many surgeons prefer the use of a tongue stitch; however, we have found that intraoperative release of the Dingman retractor every 90 minutes obviates a tongue stitch by minimizing postoperative edema of the tongue.

In addition, patients with a history of VCFS may have medial displacement of the internal carotid arteries. This condition may dictate the dimensions of a proposed pharyngeal flap[89–91] or lead to unanticipated and significant intraoperative complications. It is our practice to obtain preoperative vascular imaging, by means of computed tomography angiography, magnetic resonance angiography, or both for surgical planning in patients with VCFS. For further discussion of this topic, the reader is referred to the article by Kirschner and colleagues elsewhere in this issue.

Late complications

OSA Any surgery for VPI has the risk of making the pharyngeal port too narrow, which results clinically in signs and symptoms of OSA. In the case of the pharyngeal flap, the reported incidence of postoperative sleep apnea is as high as 38%.[92] Moreover, the incidence and severity of OSA is greater with pharyngeal flap surgery than sphincter pharyngoplasty.[93] Signs of upper airway obstruction (ie, snoring) in the immediate postoperative setting are common, but are usually mild and resolve as surgical edema subsides.

For OSA that persists beyond the immediate postoperative period and/or is symptomatic, there are several treatment options available, including continuous positive airway pressure (CPAP) therapy, prosthetic, and surgical treatment. The focus here is on the specific population of patients presenting with OSA following surgical correction of VPI with pharyngeal flap.

Diagnosis In the proper setting, the diagnosis is often clear when the symptoms are elicited from the patients or patient's family members. New-onset snoring, drooling, daytime sleepiness, difficulty sleeping, hypertension, headaches, or frequent waking following VPI surgery are signs of possible OSA. If clinical suspicion warrants

further work-up, patients are formally evaluated with polysomnography (an overnight sleep study). In OSA, there is either complete (apneic) or incomplete (hypopneic) closure of the upper airway despite sustained efforts to breathe. This condition leads to coughing and disturbance of the sleep cycle. In polysomnography, brain activity (electroencephalogram), eye movements, heart rate/rhythm, and respiration rate are monitored continuously during sleep. Apneic and hypopneic episodes are recorded and expressed as the Apnea-Hypopnea Index (AHI), which measures the number of events per hour. An AHI of 5 or more indicates OSA; 5 to 15 represents mild disease, 16 to 30 moderate disease, and more than 30 represents severe disease.[94]

Treatment Nighttime CPAP therapy is sufficient in most cases to treat OSA; however, for those patients who do not improve with CPAP, surgical treatment is available. A previous study of 12 patients undergoing pharyngeal flap division for OSA found that dividing the flap as it joins the soft palate is effective in treating OSA.[92] Division of this flap did not produce any changes in velopharyngeal function based on preoperative and postoperative perceptual speech assessment.[92] The investigators hypothesized that this is caused either by retained flap bulk in the posterior pharynx, or by learned compensations that persist despite flap division.

Sphincter Pharyngoplasty

Positioning of the transposed myomucosal flaps at the time of sphincter pharyngoplasty is critical to the resolution of hypernasality. Orticochea's[19] original description of this procedure did not take full advantage of the lateral pharyngeal and velar motion occurring high in the nasopharynx.[4,19] One of the most common early causes of failure of this technique was low flap inset along the posterior pharyngeal wall.[4,95] Attempts should be made to inset the flaps high in the pharynx, at or near the point of velar contact, which can be determined preoperatively with imaging studies.

Over time, several investigators suggested more superior placement of these flaps, with Riski and colleagues[21] first showing the success of this modification in 1984.[96,97] One limitation to achieving high flap inset, as pointed out by Hynes,[98] is the presence of the adenoid pad at or near the point of velar contact with the posterior pharyngeal wall. In this case, many investigators have moved to partial or complete resection of the adenoid pads to allow for high flap inset, with resultant improvements in speech outcomes.[4,95]

Cicatricial contracture of the vertical donor site scars can similarly result in inferior displacement of the myomucosal flaps; therefore, primary closure of the donor sites is recommended to limit contracture.[4]

Although airway compromise has not been as common historically with sphincter pharyngoplasty compared with pharyngeal flaps, there have been documented cases of acute postoperative sleep apnea.[99]

Prosthetics

The primary drawbacks to prosthetics are acceleration of dental carries with concomitant poor dental hygiene, noncompliance, and emotional distress associated with wearing the prosthesis.[78] Noncompliance may be exacerbated by the need for frequent device adjustments and the number of follow-up visits necessary for proper fitting.

CONTROVERSIES AND RECENT TRENDS
Controversies

Despite several publications comparing different flap types, there is no current consensus regarding optimal management of patients with VPI. The pharyngeal flap remains the most commonly performed surgical procedure for management of VPI, although some clinicians express a strong preference for avoiding this flap and its potential complications. Much has been written about the relative advantages and disadvantages of inferiorly versus superiorly based flaps, with many investigators concluding that outcomes are equivalent.[12–14,16] In the past, the concerns with inferiorly based flaps have been inferior traction on the velum and/or inadequate length of the flap.[9]

The number of modifications to the sphincter pharyngoplasty similarly indicates the lack of consensus in this operation.[17–25,68,96,100] Although there have been few studies comparing outcomes between sphincter pharyngoplasty methods and pharyngeal flaps, the available data suggest that, with the exceptions of a possible trend toward more revisional surgery for pharyngoplasty and an increased risk of airway obstruction with pharyngeal flaps, excellent speech outcomes can be obtained with either method.[101,102] A recent multicenter, randomized controlled trial comparing these two operations showed no difference in any measured outcome at 1-year follow-up.[103]

Recent Trends

There has recently been a revival in the use of autologous fat grafting to augment the posterior pharyngeal wall. Fat grafting techniques have improved in recent years, which may account for the reported success in several series.[36,104–106] This technique offers the advantages of considerably less morbidity and ease of repeatability. Augmentation of the posterior pharyngeal wall with autologous fat has the potential to avoid the need to alter the pharyngeal anatomy in patients with mild VPI,[104–106] and may serve as a useful adjunct to palatal lengthening in more severe cases of VPI.[36]

MEASURING OUTCOMES

Measuring outcomes following surgical management of VPI proceeds in an identical fashion to the preoperative assessment, which provides a means of direct comparison to evaluate the efficacy of therapeutic interventions. We recommend that patients undergo repeat perceptual speech assessment with a trained speech-language pathologist at 3 months after surgery. If hypernasal speech or concern for VPI persists, subsequent evaluation proceeds according to the preoperative work-up, with nasoendoscopy/MVF and nasometry measurements guiding any secondary therapeutic measures.

As mentioned previously, there currently is no standardized scale for perceptual speech assessment. Available scales in use include the PWSS, Cleft Audit Protocol for Speech-Augmented (CAPS-A),[107] and the universal parameters.[108] Use of a reliable scale in all patients allows comparison of treatment protocols across patients, surgeons, and centers.

SUMMARY

VPI is a common complication following primary palatoplasty. The decision to operate, as well as the selection of operative procedure, depends on a multimodal patient assessment, including speech evaluation and imaging studies of the pharyngeal mechanism. A thorough understanding of velopharyngeal anatomy and physiology is crucial to understanding the deficits in patients with VPI as well as the myriad methods of surgical correction. Although many techniques are available, there are no conclusive data to guide procedure choice, and newer techniques of imaging and treating patients with VPI continue to evolve.

REFERENCES

1. Fisher DM, Sommerlad BC. Cleft lip, cleft palate, and velopharyngeal insufficiency. Plast Reconstr Surg 2011;128(4):342e–60e.

2. Bicknell S, McFadden LR, Curran JB. Frequency of pharyngoplasty after primary repair of cleft palate. J Can Dent Assoc 2002;68(11):688–92.

3. Morris HL. Velopharyngeal competence and primary cleft palate surgery, 1960-1971: a critical review. Cleft Palate J 1973;10:62–71.

4. Pryor LS, Lehman J, Parker MG, et al. Outcomes in pharyngoplasty: a 10-year experience. Cleft Palate Craniofac J 2006;43(2):222–5.

5. Riski JE. Articulation skills and oral-nasal resonance in children with pharyngeal flaps. Cleft Palate J 1979;16(4):421–8.

6. Perry JL. Anatomy and physiology of the velopharyngeal mechanism. Semin Speech Lang 2011; 32(2):83–92.

7. Passavant G. Ueber die Beseitigung der naselnden Sprache bei angeborenen Splaten des harten und weichen Gaumens (Gaumensegel-Schlundnacht und Rucklagerung des Gaumensegels). Arch Klin Chir 1865;6:333–49.

8. Sloan GM. Posterior pharyngeal flap and sphincter pharyngoplasty: the state of the art. Cleft Palate Craniofac J 2000;37(2):112–22.

9. Padgett EC. The repair of cleft palates after unsuccessful operations, with special reference to cases with an extensive loss of palatal tissue. Arch Surg 1930;20:453–72.

10. Hogan VM. A clarification of the surgical goals in cleft palate speech and the introduction of the lateral port control (L.P.C.) pharyngeal flap. Cleft Palate J 1973;10:331–45.

11. Shprintzen RJ, Lewin ML, Croft CB, et al. A comprehensive study of pharyngeal flap surgery: tailor made flaps. Cleft Palate J 1979;16(1):46–55.

12. Hamlen M. Speech changes after pharyngeal flap surgery. Plast Reconstr Surg 1970;46(5): 437–44.

13. Karling J, Henningsson G, Larson O, et al. Comparison between two types of pharyngeal flap with regard to configuration at rest and function and speech outcome. Cleft Palate Craniofac J 1999; 36(2):154–65.

14. Skoog T. The pharyngeal flap operation in cleft palate. A clinical study of eighty-two cases. Br J Plast Surg 1965;18:265–82.

15. Wattanawong K, Tan YC, Lo LJ, et al. Comparison of outcomes of velopharyngeal surgery between the inferiorly and superiorly based pharyngeal flaps. Chang Gung Med J 2007;30(5):430–6.

16. Whitaker LA, Randall P, Graham WP, et al. A prospective and randomized series comparing superiorly and inferiorly based posterior pharyngeal flaps. Cleft Palate J 1972;9:304–11.

17. Hynes W. Pharyngoplasty by muscle transplantation. Br J Plast Surg 1950;3(2):128–35.

18. Hynes W. The results of pharyngoplasty by muscle transplantation in failed cleft palate cases, with special reference to the influence of the pharynx on voice production; Hunterian lecture, 1953. Ann R Coll Surg Engl 1953;13(1):17–35.

19. Orticochea M. Construction of a dynamic muscle sphincter in cleft palates. Plast Reconstr Surg 1968;41(4):323–7.

20. Jackson IT, Silverton JS. The sphincter pharyngoplasty as a secondary procedure in cleft palates. Plast Reconstr Surg 1977;59(4):518–24.

21. Riski JE, Serafin D, Riefkohl R, et al. A rationale for modifying the site of insertion of the Orticochea pharyngoplasty. Plast Reconstr Surg 1984;73(6): 882–94.

22. James NK, Twist M, Turner MM, et al. An audit of velopharyngeal incompetence treated by the Orticochea pharyngoplasty. Br J Plast Surg 1996; 49(4):197–201.

23. Moss AL, Pigott RW, Albery EH. Hynes pharyngoplasty revisited. Plast Reconstr Surg 1987;79(3): 346–55.

24. Witt PD, D'Antonio LL, Zimmerman GJ, et al. Sphincter pharyngoplasty: a preoperative and postoperative analysis of perceptual speech characteristics and endoscopic studies of velopharyngeal function. Plast Reconstr Surg 1994; 93(6):1154–68.

25. The classic reprint. Concerning a subcutaneous prosthesis: Robert Gersuny. (Uber eine subcutane Prothese. Zeitschrift f. Heilkunde Wien u Leipzig 21:199, 1900.). Translated from the German by Miss Rita Euerle. Plast Reconstr Surg 1980;65(4): 525–7.

26. Eckstein H. Demonstration of paraffin prosthesis in defects of the face and palate. Dermatologica 1904;11:772–8.

27. Hess DA, Hagerty RF, Mylin WK. Velar motility, velopharyngeal closure, and speech proficiency in cartilage pharyngoplasty: an eight year study. Cleft Palate J 1968;5:153–62.

28. Blocksma R. Silicone implants for velopharyngeal incompetence: a progress report. Cleft Palate J 1964;16:72–81.

29. Ulkur E, Karagoz H, Uygur F, et al. Use of porous polyethylene implant for augmentation of the posterior pharynx in young adult patients with borderline velopharyngeal insufficiency. J Craniofac Surg 2008;19(3):573–9.

30. Lypka M, Bidros R, Rizvi M, et al. Posterior pharyngeal augmentation in the treatment of velopharyngeal insufficiency: a 40-year experience. Ann Plast Surg 2010;65(1):48–51.

31. Remacle M, Bertrand B, Eloy P, et al. The use of injectable collagen to correct velopharyngeal insufficiency. Laryngoscope 1990;100(3):269–74.

32. Brigger MT, Ashland JE, Hartnick CJ. Injection pharyngoplasty with calcium hydroxylapatite for velopharyngeal insufficiency: patient selection

and technique. Arch Otolaryngol Head Neck Surg 2010;136(7):666–70.

33. Sipp JA, Ashland J, Hartnick CJ. Injection pharyngoplasty with calcium hydroxyapatite for treatment of velopalatal insufficiency. Arch Otolaryngol Head Neck Surg 2008;134(3):268–71.

34. Furlow LT Jr, Williams WN, Eisenbach CR, et al. A long term study on treating velopharyngeal insufficiency by Teflon injection. Cleft Palate J 1982; 19(1):47–56.

35. Girgis IH, Khalifa MS, Basiony A. Correction of velopharyngeal insufficiency by dermofat graft. J Laryngol Otol 1974;88(9):885–90.

36. Cao Y, Ma T, Wu D, et al. Autologous fat injection combined with palatoplasty and pharyngoplasty for velopharyngeal insufficiency and cleft palate: preliminary experience. Otolaryngol Head Neck Surg 2013;149(2):284–91.

37. Conley SF, Gosain AK, Marks SM, et al. Identification and assessment of velopharyngeal inadequacy. Am J Otolaryngol 1997;18(1):38–46.

38. Chen PK, Wu JT, Chen YR, et al. Correction of secondary velopharyngeal insufficiency in cleft palate patients with the Furlow palatoplasty. Plast Reconstr Surg 1994;94(7):933–41 [discussion: 942–3].

39. Kaplan EN. The occult submucous cleft palate. Cleft Palate J 1975;12:356–68.

40. Lewin ML, Croft CB, Shprintzen RJ. Velopharyngeal insufficiency due to hypoplasia of the musculus uvulae and occult submucous cleft palate. Plast Reconstr Surg 1980;65(5):585–91.

41. Peterson-Falzone SJ. Velopharyngeal inadequacy in the absence of overt cleft palate. J Craniofac Genet Dev Biol Suppl 1985;1:97–124.

42. Trier WC. Velopharyngeal incompetency in the absence of overt cleft palate: anatomic and surgical considerations. Cleft Palate J 1983;20(3): 209–17.

43. Bohle G 3rd, Rieger J, Huryn J, et al. Efficacy of speech aid prostheses for acquired defects of the soft palate and velopharyngeal inadequacy– clinical assessments and cephalometric analysis: a Memorial Sloan-Kettering Study. Head Neck 2005;27(3):195–207.

44. Finkelstein Y, Shifman A, Nachmani A, et al. Prosthetic management of velopharyngeal insufficiency induced by uvulopalatopharyngoplasty. Otolaryngol Head Neck Surg 1995;113(5): 611–6.

45. Rilo B, Fernandez-Formoso N, da Silva L, et al. A simplified palatal lift prosthesis for neurogenic velopharyngeal incompetence. J Prosthodont 2013; 22(6):506–8.

46. Riski JE, Gordon D. Prosthetic management of neurogenic velopharyngeal incompetency. N C Dent J 1979;62(1):24–6.

47. Shifman A, Finkelstein Y, Nachmani A, et al. Speech-aid prostheses for neurogenic velopharyngeal incompetence. J Prosthet Dent 2000;83(1): 99–106.

48. Yoshida H, Michi K, Ohsawa T. Prosthetic treatment for speech disorders due to surgically acquired maxillary defects. J Oral Rehabil 1990; 17(6):565–71.

49. Yoshida H, Michi K, Yamashita Y, et al. A comparison of surgical and prosthetic treatment for speech disorders attributable to surgically acquired soft palate defects. J Oral Maxillofac Surg 1993;51(4): 361–5.

50. Hubbard BA, Rice GB, Muzaffar AR. Adenoid involvement in velopharyngeal closure in children with cleft palate. Can J Plast Surg 2010;18(4): 135–8.

51. Mason RM, Warren DW. Adenoid involution and developing hypernasality in cleft palate. J Speech Hear Disord 1980;45(4):469–80.

52. Shapiro RS. Velopharyngeal insufficiency starting at puberty without adenoidectomy. Int J Pediatr Otorhinolaryngol 1980;2(3):255–60.

53. Dudas JR, Deleyiannis FW, Ford MD, et al. Diagnosis and treatment of velopharyngeal insufficiency: clinical utility of speech evaluation and videofluoroscopy. Ann Plast Surg 2006;56(5): 511–7 [discussion: 517].

54. Hirschberg J. Velopharyngeal insufficiency. Folia Phoniatr (Basel) 1986;38(2–4):221–76.

55. Rudnick EF, Sie KC. Velopharyngeal insufficiency: current concepts in diagnosis and management. Curr Opin Otolaryngol Head Neck Surg 2008; 16(6):530–5.

56. Shprintzen RJ, Marrinan E. Velopharyngeal insufficiency: diagnosis and management. Curr Opin Otolaryngol Head Neck Surg 2009;17(4):302–7.

57. Kummer AW. Perceptual assessment of resonance and velopharyngeal function. Semin Speech Lang 2011;32(2):159–67.

58. McWilliams BJ, Phillips BJ. Velopharyngeal incompetence: audio seminars in speech pathology. Philadelphia: WB Saunders; 1979.

59. Lam DJ, Starr JR, Perkins JA, et al. A comparison of nasendoscopy and multiview videofluoroscopy in assessing velopharyngeal insufficiency. Otolaryngol Head Neck Surg 2006;134(3):394–402.

60. Karnell MP. Instrumental assessment of velopharyngeal closure for speech. Semin Speech Lang 2011;32(2):168–78.

61. Skolnick ML. Videofluoroscopic examination of the velopharyngeal portal during phonation in lateral and base projections–a new technique for studying the mechanics of closure. Cleft Palate J 1970;7: 803–16.

62. Kao DS, Soltysik DA, Hyde JS, et al. Magnetic resonance imaging as an aid in the dynamic

assessment of the velopharyngeal mechanism in children. Plast Reconstr Surg 2008;122(2):572–7.

63. Silver AL, Nimkin K, Ashland JE, et al. Cine magnetic resonance imaging with simultaneous audio to evaluate pediatric velopharyngeal insufficiency. Arch Otolaryngol Head Neck Surg 2011;137(3): 258–63.

64. Fletcher SG, Bishop ME. Measurement of nasality with tonar. Cleft Palate J 1970;7:610–21.

65. Fletcher SG. "Nasalance" vs. listner judgements of nasality. Cleft Palate J 1976;13:31–44.

66. Pinto JH, da Silva Dalben G, Pegoraro-Krook MI. Speech intelligibility of patients with cleft lip and palate after placement of speech prosthesis. Cleft Palate Craniofac J 2007;44(6):635–41.

67. Tachimura T, Kotani Y, Wada T. Nasalance scores in wearers of a palatal lift prosthesis in comparison with normative data for Japanese. Cleft Palate Craniofac J 2004;41(3):315–9.

68. Gosain AK, Arneja JS. Management of the black hole in velopharyngeal incompetence: combined use of a Furlow palatoplasty and sphincter pharyngoplasty. Plast Reconstr Surg 2007;119(5): 1538–45.

69. Furlow LT Jr. Cleft palate repair by double opposing Z-plasty. Plast Reconstr Surg 1986; 78(6):724–38.

70. Furlow LT Jr. Flaps for cleft lip and palate surgery. Clin Plast Surg 1990;17(4):633–44.

71. Arneja JS, Hettinger P, Gosain AK. Through-and-through dissection of the soft palate for high pharyngeal flap inset: a new technique for the treatment of velopharyngeal incompetence in velocardiofacial syndrome. Plast Reconstr Surg 2008; 122(3):845–52.

72. Losken A, Williams JK, Burstein FD, et al. Surgical correction of velopharyngeal insufficiency in children with velocardiofacial syndrome. Plast Reconstr Surg 2006;117(5):1493–8.

73. Witt P, Cohen D, Grames LM, et al. Sphincter pharyngoplasty for the surgical management of speech dysfunction associated with velocardiofacial syndrome. Br J Plast Surg 1999;52(8):613–8.

74. Mitnick RJ, Bello JA, Golding-Kushner KJ, et al. The use of magnetic resonance angiography prior to pharyngeal flap surgery in patients with velocardiofacial syndrome. Plast Reconstr Surg 1996; 97(5):908–19.

75. Shprintzen RJ, Goldberg RB, Lewin ML, et al. A new syndrome involving cleft palate, cardiac anomalies, typical facies, and learning disabilities: velo-cardio-facial syndrome. Cleft Palate J 1978; 15(1):56–62.

76. Tatum SA 3rd, Chang J, Havkin N, et al. Pharyngeal flap and the internal carotid in velocardiofacial syndrome. Arch Facial Plast Surg 2002;4(2): 73–80.

77. La Velle WE, Hardy JC. Palatal lift prostheses for treatment of palatopharyngeal incompetence. J Prosthet Dent 1979;42(3):308–15.

78. Marsh JL, Wray RC. Speech prosthesis versus pharyngeal flap: a randomized evaluation of the management of velopharyngeal incompetency. Plast Reconstr Surg 1980;65(5):592–4.

79. Pinto JH, Pegoraro-Krook MI. Evaluation of palatal prosthesis for the treatment of velopharyngeal dysfunction. J Appl Oral Sci 2003;11(3): 192–7.

80. Sell D, Mars M, Worrell E. Process and outcome study of multidisciplinary prosthetic treatment for velopharyngeal dysfunction. Int J Lang Commun Disord 2006;41(5):495–511.

81. Tuna SH, Pekkan G, Gumus HO, et al. Prosthetic rehabilitation of velopharyngeal insufficiency: pharyngeal obturator prostheses with different retention mechanisms. Eur J Dent 2010;4(1):81–7.

82. Jackson P, Whitaker LA, Randall P. Airway hazards associated with pharyngeal flaps in patients who have the Pierre Robin syndrome. Plast Reconstr Surg 1976;58(2):184–6.

83. Kravath RE, Pollak CP, Borowiecki B, et al. Obstructive sleep apnea and death associated with surgical correction of velopharyngeal incompetence. J Pediatr 1980;96(4):645–8.

84. Robson MC, Stankiewicz JA, Mendelsohn JS. Cor pulmonale secondary to cleft palate repair. Case report. Plast Reconstr Surg 1977;59(5):754–7.

85. Schettler D. Intra- and postoperative complications in surgical repair of clefts in infancy. J Maxillofac Surg 1973;1(1):40–4.

86. Thurston JB, Larson DL, Shanks JC, et al. Nasal obstruction as a complication of pharyngeal flap surgery. Cleft Palate J 1980;17(2):148–54.

87. Valnicek SM, Zuker RM, Halpern LM, et al. Perioperative complications of superior pharyngeal flap surgery in children. Plast Reconstr Surg 1994;93(5): 954–8.

88. Wray C, Dann J, Holtmann B. A comparison of three technics of palatorrhaphy: in-hospital morbidity. Cleft Palate J 1979;16(1):42–5.

89. Even-Or E, Wohlgelernter J, Gross M. Medial displacement of the internal carotid arteries in velocardiofacial syndrome. Isr Med Assoc J 2005; 7(11):749–50.

90. Lai JP, Lo LJ, Wong HF, et al. Vascular abnormalities in the head and neck area in velocardiofacial syndrome. Chang Gung Med J 2004;27(8):586–93.

91. MacKenzie-Stepner K, Witzel MA, Stringer DA, et al. Abnormal carotid arteries in the velocardiofacial syndrome: a report of three cases. Plast Reconstr Surg 1987;80(3):347–51.

92. Agarwal T, Sloan GM, Zajac D, et al. Speech benefits of posterior pharyngeal flap are preserved after surgical flap division for obstructive sleep

apnea: experience with division of 12 flaps. J Craniofac Surg 2003;14(5):630–6.

93. Liao YF, Noordhoff MS, Huang CS, et al. Comparison of obstructive sleep apnea syndrome in children with cleft palate following Furlow palatoplasty or pharyngeal flap for velopharyngeal insufficiency. Cleft Palate Craniofac J 2004;41(2): 152–6.

94. Ramar K, Olson EJ. Management of common sleep disorders. Am Fam Physician 2013;88(4):231–8.

95. Riski JE, Ruff GL, Georgiade GS, et al. Evaluation of failed sphincter pharyngoplasties. Ann Plast Surg 1992;28(6):545–53.

96. Orticochea M. A review of 236 cleft palate patients treated with dynamic muscle sphincter. Plast Reconstr Surg 1983;71(2):180–8.

97. Roberts TM, Brown BS. Evaluation of a modified sphincter pharyngoplasty in the treatment of speech problems due to palatal insufficiency. Ann Plast Surg 1983;10(3):209–13.

98. Hynes W. The results of pharyngoplasty by muscle transplantation in "failed cleft palate" cases, with special reference to the influence of the pharynx on voice production. 1953. Br J Plast Surg 1993; 46(5):430–9.

99. Witt PD, Marsh JL, Muntz HR, et al. Acute obstructive sleep apnea as a complication of sphincter pharyngoplasty. Cleft Palate Craniofac J 1996; 33(3):183–9.

100. Pigott RW. The results of pharyngoplasty by muscle transplantation by Wilfred Hynes. Br J Plast Surg 1993;46(5):440–2.

101. Pensler JM, Reich DS. A comparison of speech results after the pharyngeal flap and the dynamic sphincteroplasty procedures. Ann Plast Surg 1991;26(5):441–3.

102. Sloan GM, Reinisch JR, LS N, et al. Surgical management of velopharyngeal insufficiency: pharyngoplasty vs. pharyngeal flap. Plast Surg Forum 1990;128–30.

103. Abyholm F, D'Antonio L, Davidson Ward SL, et al. Pharyngeal flap and sphincterplasty for velopharyngeal insufficiency have equal outcome at 1 year postoperatively: results of a randomized trial. Cleft Palate Craniofac J 2005;42(5):501–11.

104. Cantarella G, Mazzola RF, Mantovani M, et al. Treatment of velopharyngeal insufficiency by pharyngeal and velar fat injections. Otolaryngol Head Neck Surg 2011;145(3):401–3.

105. Cantarella G, Mazzola RF, Mantovani M, et al. Fat injections for the treatment of velopharyngeal insufficiency. J Craniofac Surg 2012;23(3):634–7.

106. Leboulanger N, Blanchard M, Denoyelle F, et al. Autologous fat transfer in velopharyngeal insufficiency: indications and results of a 25 procedures series. Int J Pediatr Otorhinolaryngol 2011;75(11):1404–7.

107. Sell D, John A, Harding-Bell A, et al. Cleft audit protocol for speech (CAPS-A): a comprehensive training package for speech analysis. Int J Lang Commun Disord 2009;44(4):529–48.

108. Henningsson G, Kuehn DP, Sell D, et al. Universal parameters for reporting speech outcomes in individuals with cleft palate. Cleft Palate Craniofac J 2008;45(1):1–17.

Surgical Considerations in 22Q11.2 Deletion Syndrome

Richard E. Kirschner, MD*, Adriane L. Baylis, PhD, CCC-SLP

KEYWORDS

- 22q11.2 deletion syndrome • Velocardiofacial syndrome • DiGeorge syndrome
- Velopharyngeal dysfunction

KEY POINTS

- The 22q11.2 deletion syndrome comprises the disorders also named DiGeorge syndrome and velocardiofacial syndrome.
- The 22q11.2 deletion syndrome is the syndrome most commonly associated with velopharyngeal dysfunction.
- Speech and language delays are common in patients with 22q11.2 deletion syndrome. The complexity of the associated speech and language disorders requires a multidisciplinary approach to management.
- Optimal surgical management of children with 22q11.2 deletion syndrome requires careful preoperative assessment, including imaging of the velopharyngeal mechanism.
- Functional and anatomic abnormalities of the velopharynx associated with 22q11.2 deletion syndrome demand that the surgical approach be tailored to each patient's individual needs.
- Medical comorbidities associated with 22q11.2 deletion syndrome require rigorous preoperative assessment and postoperative monitoring.

INTRODUCTION AND HISTORICAL PERSPECTIVE

General Overview of 22q11.2 Deletion Syndrome

The 22q11.2 deletion syndrome (22q11DS) is a common genetic disorder typically involving cardiac defects, cognitive-behavioral problems, speech-language disorders, velopharyngeal dysfunction (VPD), and dysmorphic facial appearance.[1–7] 22q11DS occurs in approximately 1 in 4000 births and is recognized as the most frequently occurring syndrome associated with VPD and palatal anomalies.[8–10]

Over the past few decades, the nomenclature associated with this syndrome has varied significantly. In 1955, velofacial hypoplasia (referred to as Sedlackova syndrome) was first described by Sedlackova,[11,12] a Czech phoniatrician, in a group of 26 children with congenital short soft palate, hypernasal speech, facial and ear dysmorphism, and muscle fiber abnormalities. In the late 1960s, Angelo DiGeorge[13] identified a new condition termed the DiGeorge anomalad, which included hypocalcemia, hypoparathyroidism, immune deficiency, and cardiac defects.[7,13–15] Later, in 1978, Shprintzen and colleagues[2] reported on a syndrome with typical facies, including a prominent nose and retruded mandible, cardiovascular anomalies, cleft palate, and learning disabilities, later named velocardiofacial syndrome. It was later discovered that these overlapping phenotypes share a common underlying genomic disorder, 22q11DS, now known to be responsible for most cases with these previously described conditions.[15,16]

Disclosures: None.
Section of Plastic and Reconstructive Surgery, Department of Plastic Surgery, Nationwide Children's Hospital, The Ohio State University College of Medicine, 700 Children's Drive, Columbus, OH 43205, USA
* Corresponding author.
E-mail address: richard.kirschner@nationwidechildrens.org

Clin Plastic Surg 41 (2014) 271–282
http://dx.doi.org/10.1016/j.cps.2013.12.002
0094-1298/14/$ – see front matter © 2014 Elsevier Inc. All rights reserved.

Inheritance of the 22q11.2 deletion is autosomal dominant with incomplete penetrance and variable expressivity, and most cases are de novo.[3,7,9,17] In 2005, it was reported that there was a bimodal distribution of age at diagnosis, with a peak at 6.5 years and remaining cases diagnosed in infancy (92% of which had a cardiac defect). For those children diagnosed after 2 years of age, most presented with a speech-language disorder and developmental delay.[18] At present, the diagnosis of 22q11DS is based on a combination of clinical features and genetic confirmation of the deletion. The presence of the 22q11.2 deletion can be confirmed with fluorescence in situ hybridization (FISH) testing as well as microarray. With advancements in genetic testing, smaller and more specific mutations in the same region of the genome can also be identified (eg, TBX1 mutations).[7,19,20]

More than 90% of children with 22q11DS present with speech and language disorders, VPD, and some degree of developmental delay.[2,5,7,21–23] Other frequent clinical findings include cardiac defects and vascular anomalies, including medial displacement and tortuosity of the internal carotid arteries.[24–31] Chiari malformation and cervical spine anomalies have also been observed.[28] Upper respiratory illnesses and feeding difficulties are frequent in infancy.[32] Typical craniofacial features (**Fig. 1**) include a long midface and vertical maxillary excess, malar flatness, and mandibular retrusion. Prominent nose with a squared nasal root, bulbous nasal tip, and hypoplastic nasal alae are also consistent. Also reported are narrow palpebral fissures, long philtrum and thin upper lip, reduced facial affect, and minor external ear anomalies, such as dysmorphic helices.[2,4,7] Endocrine, immune, and renal abnormalities are common.[8,26,27] Behavioral difficulties, as well as significant psychiatric disorders, are also frequently identified.[21,33,34] For a summary of additional phenotypic features, as well as general medical care guidelines for the syndrome, the reader is referred to Bassett and colleagues.[1]

Speech and Language Disorders in 22q11DS

Generalized speech-language delays are commonly reported in 22q11DS, with many children showing early signs of velopharyngeal (VP) inadequacy.[2,6,23,35,36] In addition to hypernasality, children may have articulation or phonological disorders, with a small percentage displaying motor speech disorders as well.[28,35,37,38,39] Flat affect, reduced emotional expression, fast rate, high pitch, and monotone speech are also observed

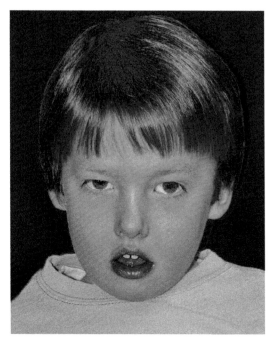

Fig. 1. Typical craniofacial features associated with 22q11DS, including long midface with vertical maxillary excess, malar flatness, prominent nose with squared nasal root and bulbous nasal tip, hypoplastic nasal alae, narrow palpebral fissures, thin upper lip, and mild craniofacial asymmetry.

in many children. A significant proportion of preschool and school-aged children with 22q11DS show glottal stop substitutions, which are the most common compensatory error in the speech of children with cleft palate.[35,36,40] The articulation skills of children with 22q11DS have been shown to be poorer than those of children with nonsyndromic cleft palate/VPD.[41] A comprehensive review of information regarding speech-language disorders in 22q11DS is given by Gorlin and Baylis.[42]

VPD in 22q11DS: Structural and Neuromuscular Considerations

VPD in patients with 22q11DS has a complex causal origin (**Fig. 2**). Although overt palate clefting is uncommon in 22q11DS, studies cite a high incidence of VPD and submucous clefting, as well as palatopharyngeal hypotonia, and obtuse cranial base or deep retropharynx (termed palatopharyngeal disproportion), all of which can compromise VP adequacy for speech.[2,4,7,19,23,43,44] Ruotolo and colleagues[45] reported that the increased pharyngeal depth associated with platybasia combines with increased pharyngeal width in affected patients to produce large increases in

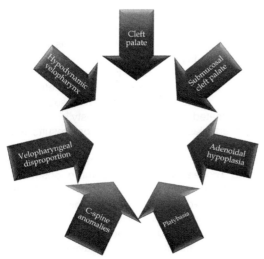

Fig. 2. The multiple factors that contribute to the presence, severity, and complexity of VPD in patients with 22q11DS.

pharyngeal volume and VP valve area. Postadenoidectomy VPD is also common in children with this syndrome.[3,44,46–49] Studies have reported an incidence of VPD in 22q11DS ranging from 64% to 87%,[50,51] and, regardless of the cause, VPD and hypernasal speech are considered hallmark features of the syndrome.[2,7,37] Children with 22q11DS tend to have hypernasal resonance of greater persistence, frequency, and severity than seen in other cleft and VPD populations. Thus, they pose a greater challenge to surgeons and speech pathologists.[24,52–54]

In addition to structural abnormalities that contribute to VPD in 22q11DS, evidence has begun to surface regarding neuromuscular problems also affecting VP closure for speech. Pharyngeal muscle hypoplasia, cranial nerve abnormalities, and comorbid neuromotor speech disorders have also been reported as factors that could influence the degree of perceived hypernasality in speech, as well as negatively affect VP closure dynamics and surgical outcome.[28,52,55]

PATIENT ASSESSMENT
Speech Assessment: Perceptual Evaluation and Instrumental Assessment

In general, the protocol for assessment of speech in patients with 22q11DS is similar to that encountered in other populations with cleft palate or VPD. For the purposes of this article, syndrome-specific considerations are highlighted. All patients with 22q11DS should be followed by a cleft/craniofacial team that is familiar with management of VPD. The speech-language pathologist should

ideally begin following the child starting in infancy, monitoring speech and language acquisition and managing therapy needs. For toddlers and preschoolers, the focus of speech assessment and treatment is articulation and language. The speech pathologist should closely monitor the child's articulation for the presence of compensatory articulation errors (eg, glottal stops), and, if present, speech therapy should aggressively target their remediation as soon as they are identified. The child needs a phonetic inventory that includes at least 1 or 2 oral pressure consonants (eg, P, B, T) with correct placement in order to participate in VP imaging during speech. In general, most children with 22q11DS are able to produce an adequate speech sample that allows perceptual and instrumental assessment of VP function by 4 to 5 years of age. The speech evaluation should include conversational speech, repetition of standard sentences, and articulation testing. An intraoral examination should always be completed and additional perceptual assessment techniques (eg, nasal mirror testing, nasal occlusion) should also be considered. When symptoms of VPD are observed, instrumental assessment may be helpful as an adjunct to the perceptual evaluation. This assessment may include use of the Nasometer (KayPENTAX), an acoustic measurement that correlates with resonance, and/or pressure-flow testing (eg, PERCI-SAR, Microtronics), which allows measurement of intraoral pressure, nasal airflow, and estimated VP orifice size. Nasopharyngoscopy and/or multiview videofluoroscopy during speech should then be completed to provide additional information on VP function during speech and assist with surgical planning.

Imaging Recommendations

Regardless of which imaging modality (or modalities) is selected, the quality of the VP imaging study is directly related to the accuracy of the speech sample produced. Only patients who are able to produce at least a minimally accurate speech sample (in terms of oral consonant production) should undergo imaging, in order to obtain the most accurate information about VP function. If children with severe compensatory articulation disorders (eg, only produce glottal stops during the speech sample) undergo imaging, the outcome of the procedure is known without even conducting the study: lack of VP closure characterized by a large gap and minimal to no VP motion. Instead, if the child is able to produce at least 1 or 2 plosive consonants (ideally P, B, T, D), even if they are weak in pressure or accompanied by nasal emission, the examiner is able to see the patient's true attempts at maximum VP closure during speech. This assessment also allows the most accurate surgical planning possible, treating only the VP gap that remains during the accurate speech attempts, and provides a more accurate characterization of movement of the VP mechanism. A well-trained craniofacial speech pathologist can determine what speech sample is most appropriate to use in the study, based on the child's phonetic inventory, articulation accuracy, and desired complexity of the sample (eg, oral-only words vs phrases or sentences). In terms of the type of imaging procedure, multiview video-fluoroscopy and nasopharyngoscopy both offer distinct advantages, as well as disadvantages, however, these are beyond the scope of discussion of this chapter.

Timing of VPD Surgery

Children with 22q11DS traditionally undergo VPD surgery at slightly later ages than their peers with cleft palate or nonsyndromic VPD. On average, surgical intervention is usually recommended at approximately 4 to 6 years of age or older. Treatment is later because of a variety of factors including, but not limited to, (1) diagnosis of VPD is often later in 22q11DS than that for children born with overt cleft palate, because children born with overt structural anomalies tend to be monitored for VPD by their craniofacial team from infancy; (2) other emergent medical issues (eg, cardiac, airway) in children with 22q11DS may take precedent over VP management; (3) many children with 22q11DS have severe articulation disorders that require a longer duration of speech therapy to correct until the diagnosis of VPD is confirmed and VP imaging can be completed successfully (ie, sufficiently accurate articulation and adequate cooperation for the study).

CURRENT SURGICAL PRACTICE

There is little consensus and scant scientific evidence supporting a specific surgical treatment algorithm for patients with VPD associated with 22q11DS. However, the literature suggests that palate repair alone often fails to restore VP competence in patients with 22q11DS with submucosal palatal clefts,[53,56,57] most likely because of the degree of VP disproportion present in most affected individuals and because of the persistence of high pharyngeal depth/palatal length ratios after cleft palate repair.

For patients with small (less than 5 mm) gaps and submucosal clefts of the palate, Furlow palatoplasty may be a reasonable surgical option,

because the degree of palatal length gained by the velar Z-plasty may be sufficient to avoid more obstructive procedures, such as posterior pharyngeal flap or sphincter pharyngoplasty in this select group. Some investigators have reported acceptable rates of VP competence in carefully selected 22q11DS with submucosal clefts treated by Furlow palatoplasty.[58]

Nevertheless, the generally poor results after submucosal cleft palate repair in many patients with 22q11DS have led some clinicians to recommend proceeding directly to more obstructive procedures in order to reduce the risk of having to perform additional surgery for persistent VPD after palatoplasty. Mehendale and colleagues[59] suggested a staged approach, noting that optimization of levator function by intravelar veloplasty may allow the creation of a less obstructive pharyngoplasty in those patients who show persistent VPD after submucosal cleft palate repair.

AUTHORS' SURGICAL APPROACH
Selection of Procedure

In patients with a submucosal cleft palate and a small (<5 mm) gap, Furlow palatoplasty is used as a first-line surgical intervention for VPD management (**Fig. 3**). Parents are counseled that secondary surgery may be required for persistent VPD in some instances. Patients without submucosal cleft palate and with similarly small gaps and coronal VP closure patterns are managed with a modified Hynes pharyngoplasty (**Fig. 4**). In order to optimize surgical outcomes, the sphincter should be placed at the level of attempted VP closure, as determined by preoperative imaging.[60] If the level of attempted closure is within the adenoid pad, preoperative adenoidectomy is performed at least 4 months earlier in order to facilitate proper placement of the sphincter on the posterior pharyngeal wall.

Patients with larger gaps, with or without submucosal cleft palate, are managed by creation of a superiorly based posterior pharyngeal flap, the width of which is determined by the degree of lateral pharyngeal wall motion. Although many techniques have been described for creation of posterior pharyngeal flaps, use of a superiorly based flap inset into a transverse incision into the posterior velum provides the surgeon with maximum flexibility in flap design and port size.[61] Flap width (and, conversely, port size) may be altered by both the width of its design on the posterior pharyngeal wall and the width of its inset along the posterior velum. The position of the base of the flap should correspond with the level of attempted VP closure as determined by

oral mucosal flap

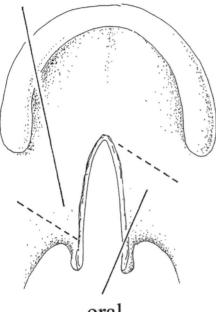

oral
musculo-mucosal flap

nasal mucosal flap

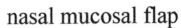

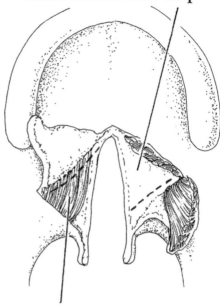

nasal
musculo-mucosal flap

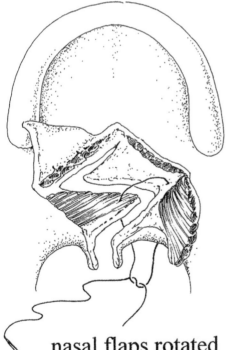

nasal flaps rotated

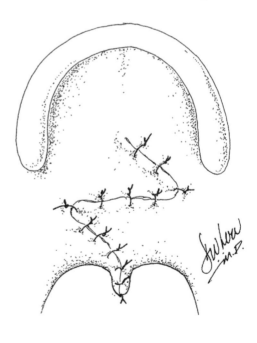

oral flaps rotated

Fig. 3. Furlow Z-palatoplasty procedure. (*From* Kirschner RE. Palatal anomalies and velopharyngeal dysfunction associated with velo-cardio-facial syndrome. In: Murphy KC, Scambler PJ, editors. Velo-cardio-facial syndrome: a model for understanding microdeletion disorders. Cambridge: Cambridge University Press; 2005; with permission.)

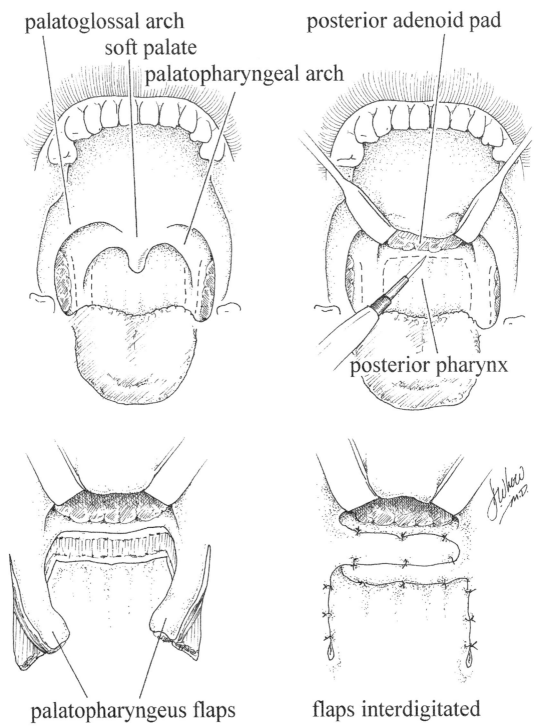

Fig. 4. Modified Hynes pharyngoplasty procedure. (*From* Kirschner RE. Palatal anomalies and velopharyngeal dysfunction associated with velo-cardio-facial syndrome. In: Murphy KC, Scambler PJ, editors. Velo-cardio-facial syndrome: a model for understanding microdeletion disorders. Cambridge: Cambridge University Press; 2005; with permission.)

preoperative imaging and is often higher in patients with 22q11DS than in nonsyndromic patients. Preoperative adenoidectomy is often performed before pharyngeal flap or sphincter procedures in order to facilitate proper flap placement when the level of attempted closure is within the adenoid pad.

Preoperative Assessment

Preoperative preparation includes a careful assessment of comorbid medical conditions. In patients with congenital heart disease, surgical management of VPD should be performed only after consultation with the patient's cardiologist. All patients are assessed for evidence of upper airway obstruction both by history and by preoperative polysomnography. Patients with tonsillar hyperplasia are also treated by preoperative tonsillectomy in order to minimize the risk of postoperative upper airway obstruction and sleep apnea.

Anatomic anomalies of the internal carotid arteries are a common feature of 22q11DS, with as many as 20% to 25% of affected individuals showing medial deviation of one or both vessels at the level of the posterior pharynx, placing them a risk for injury at the time of VPD surgery (**Fig. 5**).[4,29,30,62] Carotid pulsations noted on preoperative nasopharyngoscopy may be transmitted

from a normally placed vessel and should not be considered reliable evidence of internal carotid displacement. The authors recommend preoperative magnetic resonance imaging to define the vascular anatomy and to assist with preoperative planning and informed consent. Often, a medially displaced vessel lateralizes with cervical extension at the time of surgery. Vessels that remain within the operative field may be swept laterally and protected beneath a malleable retractor.

Surgical Technique

At surgery, the patient is positioned supine with the neck either in the neutral position or slightly extended (**Fig. 6**). Use of an oral RAE tube and a Dingman mouth gag facilitates exposure. The velum is retracted superiorly with a broad malleable retractor, and the base of the flap is marked on the posterior pharyngeal wall at the site of VP closure. A transverse incision is then marked at the distal margin of the flap, taking care to ensure that the flap is of adequate length to reach the posterior velum with minimal tension or redundancy. Flap width is tailored to the degree of lateral pharyngeal wall motion as seen on preoperative imaging studies. In patients with minimal lateral wall motion, the flap may span the width of the posterior pharynx. Flap elevation is performed with fine needlepoint electrocautery in order to

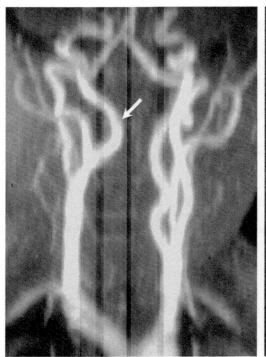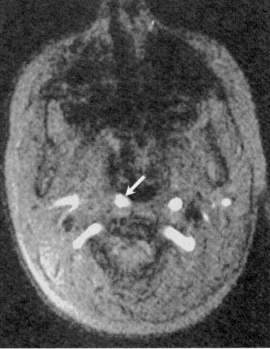

Fig. 5. Deviated right internal carotid artery (*arrows*) in a patient with 22qDS.

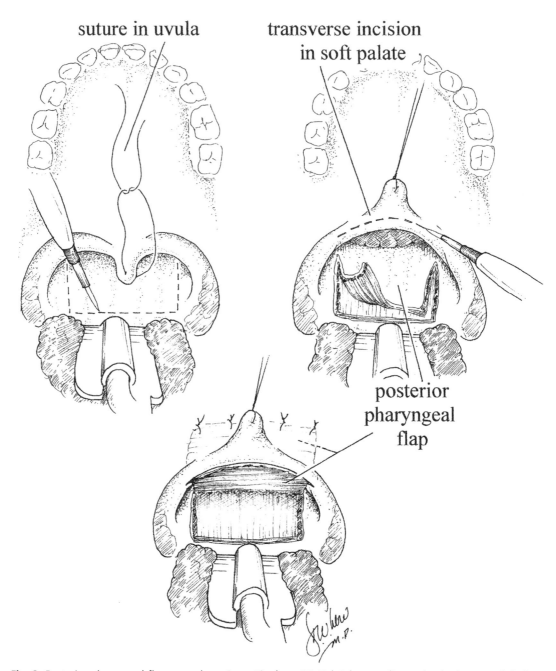

Fig. 6. Posterior pharyngeal flap procedure. *From* Kirschner RE. Palatal anomalies and velopharyngeal dysfunction associated with velo-cardio-facial syndrome. In: Murphy KC, Scambler PJ, editors. Velo-cardio-facial syndrome: a model for understanding microdeletion disorders. Cambridge: Cambridge University Press; 2005; with permission.)

ensure a dry field and optimal visualization, which is particularly important in patients with a medially deviated internal carotid artery because clear visualization is essential to avoiding vascular injury. The mucosa is incised using the cutting current in order to minimize thermal damage, and the fibers of the superior pharyngeal constrictor are divided using a blend of cutting and coagulative currents. The flap is then elevated to its base in a plane superficial to the prevertebral fascia.

Once the flap is elevated, attention is directed to the creation of a transverse pocket in the velum to accept its inset. Hooks are placed in the posterior velum, and the velum is retracted orally and anteriorly in order to expose its nasal surface. The incision is marked on the nasal surface 5 to 7 mm anterior to the base of the uvula. The width of inset corresponds with the degree of lateral pharyngeal wall motion. In patients with minimal lateral wall motion, the inset extends from the superior aspect of one posterior tonsillar pillar, across the velum, and to the superior aspect of the contralateral pillar. A shorter transverse incision is used in patients with greater degrees of lateral pharyngeal wall motion. The incision is again made with the cutting current of the electrocautery, and a pocket is dissected deep to the nasal submucosa to a depth of 5 to 7 mm. The flap is then inset with a series of 5 resorbable horizontal mattress sutures, passed through the apex of the submucosal pocket and tied on the oral side of the anterior velum.

After surgery, patients are admitted to the pediatric intensive care unit for close airway monitoring, including telemetry and pulse oximetry. Serum calcium levels are measured for the first 24 hours in order to avoid the complication of postoperative hypocalcemia. A clear liquid diet is instituted as soon as the child is awake and alert, and this is advanced to a soft diet the following day. Snoring and upper airway congestion are common in the immediate postoperative period, because the small lateral ports are often occluded secondary to postoperative secretions and edema. These symptoms usually resolve over several weeks as the edema subsides.

As noted earlier, most patients who have undergone posterior pharyngeal flap surgery experience some degree of nasal airway obstruction in the immediate postoperative period, caused primarily by the effects of postoperative edema and secretions. Although most patients show hyponasal speech soon after surgery, resonance usually improves as edema subsides. The tendency of pharyngeal flaps to narrow over time is minimized by using the technique illustrated in this article. Nevertheless, resonance may still be noted to increase over time in some patients because of flap narrowing. Because this process may evolve over a 6-month to 12-month period, surgical results are best assessed after that period of time.

Some patients may show signs and symptoms of persistent upper airway obstruction, including snoring, obligate mouth breathing, and hyponasality. All patients should undergo polysomnography after the edema has fully subsided and the flap has matured (even in the absence of obstructive symptoms) in order to ensure the absence of significant sleep disordered breathing.

MEASURING OUTCOMES

As with preoperative evaluation, surgical outcome should be assessed by the surgeon and the speech pathologist working closely together as a team. Because cicatricial changes may alter both flap width and position, outcomes are most accurately assessed 12 or more months after VPD surgery. Assessment of speech should be performed as described earlier and should include comparison of preoperative perceptual ratings and instrumental measures. Persistent evidence of VPD warrants repeat diagnostic imaging and consideration of revisional surgery.

Although the literature is replete with theory regarding the optimal surgical procedure for the management of VPD based on VP closure pattern, there is little evidence to support the notion that posterior pharyngeal flap procedures are most appropriate for use in patients with sagittal closure patterns resulting from good lateral pharyngeal wall motion and that better outcomes are achieved when patients with coronal closure patterns and poor lateral pharyngeal wall motion are treated by sphincter pharyngoplasty. Proposed surgical algorithms for VPD management in patients with 22q11DS have thus far been based on preference and intuitive reasoning and not on well-controlled clinical trials. Randomized clinical trials comparing posterior pharyngeal flaps with sphincter pharyngoplasty procedures in nonsyndromic patients have shown no difference in speech outcomes.[63] Whether or not the same results can be generalized to patients with 22q11DS undergoing surgical management of VPD remains to be established. A recent systematic review by Spruijt and colleagues[64] of all published series describing the surgical management of VPD in patients with 22q11DS revealed no significant difference in outcomes across all types of surgical procedures.

Although some series have shown similarly good outcomes in patients with 22q11DS and nonsyndromic patients,[65,66] many investigators report that persistent VPD is commonly observed after any type of surgical intervention in patients with 22q11DS.[59,67,68] Overall surgical outcomes have been observed to be more similar to those of children with other craniofacial syndromes or those with a history of neuromuscular disorders than to those of nonsyndromic patients with VPD.[53] Overall, the severity of preoperative VP dysfunction and hypernasality is reported to be greater in patients with 22q11DS than in nonsyndromic patients, likely as a result of several factors including VP hypodynamism and disproportion. It is likely that these same factors, along with others such as motor speech disorders and abnormal VP timing, may combine to impair VP closure after surgical intervention.

The disparity in reported outcomes after Furlow palatoplasty, posterior pharyngeal flap surgery, or sphincter pharyngoplasty may reflect differences in patient selection. More importantly, the disparity may be caused by significant technical variation in how the procedures were performed by each surgeon. The increased cross-sectional area and hypodynamism of the VP port in many patients with 22q11DS mandate that surgical interventions greatly reduce port size in order to eliminate hypernasality, thereby potentially increasing the risk of postoperative upper airway obstruction. In some cases, persistent hypernasality may be the result of deliberate undercorrection in an effort to prevent postoperative obstructive apnea.

SUMMARY

VPD in patients with 22q11DS is a complex disorder that remains incompletely understood. Children with 22q11DS are more likely to exhibit some residual symptoms of VPD than their peers. Therefore optimal management demands a comprehensive team approach, meticulous preoperative assessment, and individualization of surgical approach. There are currently no blinded speech outcomes studies of children with 22q11DS. Past reports have used chart reviews of speech ratings obtained by the treating clinician and thus carry the risk of bias. Future studies should use blinded multiple listener ratings of prerecorded speech samples in order to provide new information about speech outcome in children with 22q11DS compared with other craniofacial populations. In addition, there is significant need for randomized controlled trials of VP surgery techniques to determine whether one procedure is more effective or whether outcomes primarily depend on surgeon skill and experience.

REFERENCES

1. Bassett AS, McDonald-McGinn DM, Devriendt K, et al, International 22q11.2 Deletion Syndrome Consortium. Practical guidelines for managing patients with 22q11.2 deletion syndrome. J Pediatr 2011;159:332–9.
2. Shprintzen RJ, Goldberg R, Lewin ML, et al. A new syndrome involving cleft palate, cardiac anomalies, typical facies, and learning disabilities: velocardiofacial syndrome. Cleft Palate J 1978;15: 56–62.
3. Shprintzen RJ, Goldberg R, Young D, et al. The velocardiofacial syndrome: a clinical and genetic analysis. Pediatrics 1981;67:167–72.
4. Goldberg R, Motzkin B, Marion R, et al. Velocardiofacial syndrome: a review of 120 patients. Am J Med Genet 1993;45:313–9.
5. Golding-Kushner KJ, Weller G, Shprintzen RJ. Velo-cardio-facial syndrome: language and psychological profiles. J Craniofac Genet Dev Biol 1985;5:259–66.
6. McDonald-McGinn DM, LaRossa D, Goldmuntz E, et al. The 22q11.2 deletion: screening, diagnostic workup, and outcome of results; report on 181 patients. Genet Test 1997;1:99–108.
7. Gorlin RJ, Cohen MM, Hennekam R. Syndromes of the head and neck. 4th edition. New York: Oxford UP; 2001.
8. Emanuel BS, McDonald-McGinn DM, Saitta C, et al. The 22q11.2 deletion syndrome. Adv Pediatr 2001;48:39–73.
9. Devriendt K, Fryns JP, Mortier G. The annual incidence of DiGeorge/velocardiofacial syndrome. J Med Genet 1998;35:789–90.
10. Wilson D, Cross I, Wren P, et al. Minimum prevalence of chromosome 22q11.2 deletions. Am J Hum Genet 1994;55:169.
11. Sedlackova E. The syndrome of the congenital shortening of the soft palate (in Czech). Cas Lek Cesk 1955;94:1304–7.
12. Sedlackova E. The syndrome of the congenitally shortened velum—the dual innervation of the soft palate. Folia Phoniatr 1967;19:441–50.
13. DiGeorge AM. Discussion on a new concept of the cellular basis of immunology. J Pediatr 1965; 67:907.
14. Taitz LS, Zarate-Salvador C, Schwartz E. Congenital absence of the parathyroid and thymus glands in an infant (III and IV pharyngeal pouch syndrome). Pediatrics 1966;38:412–8.
15. Driscoll DA, Spinner NB, Budarf ML, et al. Deletions and microdeletions of 22q11.2 in velocardiofacial syndrome. Am J Med Genet 1992;44:261–8.
16. Scambler PJ, Kelly D, Lindsay E, et al. The velocardiofacial syndrome is associated with chromosome 22 deletions encompassing the DiGeorge locus. Lancet 1992;333:1138–9.
17. Carlson C, Sirotkin H, Pandita R, et al. Molecular definition of 22q11.2 deletions in 151 velocardiofacial syndrome patients. Am J Hum Genet 1997;61: 620–9.
18. Oskarsdottir S, Persson C, Eriksson BO, et al. Presenting phenotype in 100 children with the 22q11.2 deletion syndrome. Eur J Pediatr 2005; 164:146–53.
19. Lipson AH, Yuille D, Angel M, et al. Velocardiofacial (Shprintzen) syndrome: an important syndrome for the dysmorphologist to recognize. J Med Genet 1991;28:596–604.
20. Vorstman JA, Jalali GR, Rappaport EF, et al. MLPA: a rapid, reliable, and sensitive method for detection

and analysis of abnormalities of 22q. Hum Mutat 2006;27:814–21.

21. Niklasson L, Rasmussen P, Oskarsdottir S, et al. Neuropsychiatric disorders in the 22q11 deletion syndrome. Genet Med 2001;3:79–84.

22. Swillen A, Devriendt K, Legius E, et al. Intelligence and psychosocial adjustment in velocardiofacial syndrome: a study of 37 children and adolescents with VCFS. J Med Genet 1997;34:453–8.

23. Solot CB, Knightly C, Handler SD, et al. Communication disorders in the 22q11.2 microdeletion syndrome. J Commun Dis 2000;33:187–204.

24. D'Antonio LL, Marsh JL. Abnormal carotid arteries in the velocardiofacial syndrome. Plast Reconstr Surg 1987;80:471–2.

25. Young D. Cardiac malformations in the velocardiofacial syndrome. Am J Cardiol 1980;46:643–8.

26. Shprintzen RJ. Syndrome identification for speech-language pathology. San Diego (CA): Singular; 2000.

27. McDonald-McGinn DM. Much ado about 22q: what's new with chromosome 22? Abstract of the 10th Annual International Meeting of the Velocardiofacial Educational Foundation and 4th International Congress for 22q11.2 deletions. Atlanta (GA), July 23, 2004.

28. Hultman CS, Riski JE, Cohen SR, et al. Chiari malformation, cervical spine anomalies, and neurologic deficits in velocardiofacial syndrome. Plast Reconstr Surg 2000;106:16–24.

29. Mitnick RJ, Bello JA, Golding-Kushner KJ, et al. The use of magnetic resonance angiography prior to pharyngeal flap surgery in patients with velocardiofacial syndrome. Plast Reconstr Surg 1996;97:908–19.

30. Mackenzie-Stepner K, Witzel MA, Stringer D. Abnormal carotid arteries in velocardiofacial syndrome: a report of 3 cases. Plast Reconstr Surg 1987;80:347–51.

31. Tatum SA, Chang J, Havkin N, et al. Pharyngeal flap and the internal carotid in velocardiofacial syndrome. Arch Facial Plast Surg 2002;4:73–80.

32. Eicher PS, McDonald-McGinn DM, Fox CA, et al. Dysphagia in children with a 22q11.2 deletion: unusual pattern found on modified barium swallow. J Pediatr 2000;137:158–64.

33. Bearden CE, Jawad AF, Lynch DR, et al. Effects of a functional COMT polymorphism on prefrontal cognitive function in patients with 22q11.2 deletion syndrome. Am J Psychiatry 2004;161:1700–2.

34. Van Amelsvoort T, Daly E, Henry J, et al. Brain anatomy in adults with velocardiofacial syndrome with and without schizophrenia: preliminary results of a structural MRI study. Arch Gen Psychiatry 2004;61:1085–96.

35. Scherer NJ, D'Antonio LL, Kalbfleisch JH. Early speech and language development in children with velocardiofacial syndrome. Am J Med Genet 1999;88:714–23.

36. Golding-Kushner KJ. Speech and language disorders in velocardiofacial syndrome. In: Murphy KC, Scambler PJ, editors. Velocardiofacial syndrome: a model for understanding microdeletion disorders. Cambridge (United Kingdom): Cambridge University Press; 2005. p. 181–99.

37. Persson C, Lohmander A, Jonsson R, et al. A prospective cross-sectional study of speech in patients with the 22q11.2 deletion syndrome. J Commun Dis 2003;36:13–47.

38. Carneol SD, Marks SM, Weik L. The speech-language pathologist: key role in the diagnosis of velocardiofacial syndrome. Am J Speech Lang Pathol 1999;8:23–32.

39. Baylis AL, Jensen JN, Kirschner RE, et al. Motor speech deficits in children with 22q11.2 deletion syndrome. Abstract of the International Congress on Cleft Lip/Palate and Related Craniofacial Anomalies. Orlando (FL), May 7, 2013.

40. D'Antonio LL, Scherer NJ, Miller LL, et al. Analysis of speech characteristics in children with VCFS and children with phenotypic overlap without VCFS. Cleft Palate Craniofac J 2001;39:455–67.

41. Baylis AL, Munson B, Moller KT. Factors affecting phonetic accuracy in children with velocardiofacial syndrome and children with cleft palate or velopharyngeal dysfunction: a preliminary report. Cleft Palate Craniofac J 2008;45:193–207.

42. Gorlin RJ, Baylis AL. Developmental and genetic aspects of cleft lip and palate. In: Moller KT, Glaze LE, editors. Interdisciplinary management of cleft lip and palate: for clinicians by clinicians. Austin (TX): Pro-Ed; 2009. p. 103–69.

43. Shprintzen RJ. Palatal and pharyngeal anomalies in craniofacial syndromes. Birth Defects Orig Artic Ser 1982;18:53–78.

44. Arvystas M, Shprintzen RJ. Craniofacial morphology in the velocardiofacial syndrome. J Craniofac Genet Dev Biol 1984;4:39–45.

45. Ruotolo RA, Veitia N, Corbin A, et al. Velopharyngeal anatomy in 22q11.2 deletion syndrome: a three-dimensional cephalometric analysis. Cleft Palate Craniofac J 2006;43:446–56.

46. Glander K, Cisneros GJ. Comparison of the craniofacial characteristics of two syndromes associated with Pierre Robin sequence. Cleft Palate Craniofac J 1992;29:210–9.

47. Croft CB, Shprintzen RJ, Daniller A, et al. The occult submucous cleft palate and the musculus uvulae. Cleft Palate J 1978;15:150–4.

48. Finkelstein Y, Zohar Y, Nachmani A, et al. The otolaryngologist and the patient with velocardiofacial syndrome. Arch Otolaryngol Head Neck Surg 1993;119:563–9.

49. Witzel MA, Rich RH, Margar-Bacal R, et al. Velopharyngeal insufficiency after adenoidectomy: an 8-year review. Int J Pediatr Otorhinolaryngol 1986;11:15–20.
50. Rommel N, Vantrappen G, Swillen A, et al. Retrospective analysis of feeding and speech disorders in 50 patients with velo-cardio-facial syndrome. Genet Couns 1999;10:71–8.
51. Nayak J, Sell D. Communication disorders in velocardiofacial syndrome: a clinical audit. Abstract of the 4th Annual Meeting of the Velocardiofacial Educational Foundation. Boston, June 26, 1998.
52. Baylis AL, Watson PJ, Moller KT. Aeromechanical and auditory-perceptual speech characteristics of children with velocardiofacial syndrome (22q11.2 deletion): a preliminary analysis. Folia Phoniatr 2009;61:93–6.
53. D'Antonio LL, Davio M, Zoller K, et al. Results of Furlow z-plasty in patients with velocardiofacial syndrome. Plast Reconstr Surg 2001;107:1077–9.
54. Kirschner R, Solot C, Ruotolo R, et al. Speech outcome after surgical management of velopharyngeal dysfunction in 22q11.2 deletion syndrome. Abstract of the annual meeting of the American Cleft Palate Craniofacial Association. Myrtle Beach (SC), April 8, 2005.
55. Zim S, Schelper R, Kellman R, et al. Thickness and histologic and histochemical properties of the superior pharyngeal constrictor muscle in velocardiofacial syndrome. Arch Facial Plast Surg 2003;5:503–10.
56. Sie KC, Tampakopoulou DA, Sorom J, et al. Results with Furlow palatoplasty in management of velopharyngeal insufficiency. Plast Reconstr Surg 2001;108:17–25.
57. Kirschner RE, Solot CB, McDonald-McGinn DM, et al. Speech outcome after cleft palate repair in patients with a chromosome 22q11 deletion. Presented at the 58th Annual Meeting of the American Cleft Palate-Craniofacial Association. Minneapolis (MN), April 27, 2001.
58. Bezuhly M, Fischbach S, Klaiman P, et al. Impact of 22q deletion syndrome on speech outcomes following primary surgery for submucous cleft palate. Plast Reconstr Surg 2012;129:502e–10e.
59. Mehendale FV, Birch MJ, Birkett L, et al. Surgical management of velopharyngeal incompetence in velocardiofacial syndrome. Cleft Palate Craniofac J 2004;41:124–35.
60. Riski JE, Serafin D, Riekfol R, et al. A rationale for modifying the site of insertion of the Orticochea pharyngoplasty. Plast Reconstr Surg 1984;73:882–94.
61. Argamaso RV. Pharyngeal flap surgery for velopharyngeal insufficiency. Oper Tech Plast Surg 1995;2:233–8.
62. Ross DA, Witzel MA, Armstrong DC, et al. Is pharyngoplasty a risk in velocardiofacial syndrome: an assessment of medially displaced carotid arteries. Plast Reconstr Surg 1996;98:1182–90.
63. Ysunza A, Pamplona C, Ramirez E, et al. Velopharyngeal surgery: a prospective randomized study of pharyngeal flaps and sphincter pharyngoplasties. Plast Reconstr Surg 2001;110:1401–7.
64. Spruijt NE, ReijmanHinze J, Hens G, et al. In search of the optimal surgical treatment for velopharyngeal dysfunction in 22q11.2 deletion syndrome: a systematic review. PLoS One 2012;7:e34332.
65. Rouillon I, Leboulanger N, Roger G, et al. Velopharyngoplasty for noncleft velopharyngeal insufficiency. Arch Otolaryngol Head Neck Surg 2009;135:652–6.
66. Widdershoven J, Solot CB, Cohen MA, et al. Surgical management of velopharyngeal dysfunction in 22q11.2 deletion syndrome. Abstract of the 66th Annual Meeting of the American Cleft Palate-Craniofacial Association. Scottsdale (AZ), April 24, 2009.
67. Losken A, Williams JK, Burstein FD, et al. An outcome evaluation of sphincter pharyngoplasty for the management of velopharyngeal insufficiency. Plast Reconstr Surg 2003;112:1755–61.
68. Spruijt NE, Widdershoven JC, Breugem CC, et al. Velopharyngeal dysfunction and 22q11.2 deletion syndrome: a longitudinal study of functional outcome and preoperative prognostic factors. Cleft Palate Craniofac J 2012;49:447–55.

Correction of the Cleft Nasal Deformity: From Infancy to Maturity

Mark D. Fisher, MD[a,b], David M. Fisher, MD, FRCSC[a],
Jeffrey R. Marcus, MD[b],*

KEYWORDS

• Cleft nasal deformity • Dorsal deformity • Cleft lip and nasal repair • Septorhinoplasty

KEY POINTS

• The cleft nasal deformity remains the most likely stigma of the cleft to remain plainly visible despite vigorous and repeated attempts at correction.
• History has witnessed a swinging pendulum in the care of this deformity, starting with ignorance and succeeded by aggressive, numerous, and radical operations.
• Today multiple schools of thought exist, but most recognize that an aggressive early operation does not necessarily negate the need for future operations.
• The cleft nasal deformity is present at birth, but evolves over time. Certain aspects can be treated early, but some, such as the dorsal and septal deformity continue to develop as facial growth proceeds through adolescence.
• This article presents the authors' concept of the mechanism and philosophy of conservative reliable gains starting at the primary operation, with the long-term view of achieving a definitive correction at maturity.
• The diligent student of the cleft nasal deformity who cogently plans the longitudinal care of the deformity from infancy will be rewarded with solid, predictable results.

OVERVIEW

Those who routinely perform cleft rhinoplasty, in addition to cosmetic or functional rhinoplasty in the noncleft patient, readily acknowledge that cleft septorhinoplasty is the single most challenging rhinoplasty to perform. The reasons for this are emphasized in this article, but derive from the complexity of the structural deformity with attendant misconceptions, multiple sites of potential functional obstruction, and the effects of prior surgery. For this reason, those who perform cleft rhinoplasty must not only be highly skilled rhinoplasty surgeons but must also have a strong background of understanding cleft pathoanatomy.

HISTORICAL PERSPECTIVE

Desmond Kernahan's observation in 1980 that "a repaired cleft is revealed more by the associated nasal deformity than by the lip repair" continues to be true today, underscoring the historical difficulty with this complex and dynamic problem.[1] Peter Randall put it this way: "I am reluctant to say correct the cleft lip nose deformity, because, in my experience, it is impossible to really correct the severe deformity."[2]

The early twentieth century saw numerous approaches often characterized by radical external incisions. A review of the myriad of approaches cataloged in Millard's *Cleft Craft*[3] demonstrates

[a] Division of Plastic and Reconstructive Surgery, Cleft Palate and Lip Program, Hospital for Sick Children, Suite 5425, 555 University Avenue, Toronto, ON M5G1X8, Canada; [b] Duke Cleft and Craniofacial Center, Duke Children's Hospital, DUMC 3974, Durham, NC 27710, USA
* Corresponding author.
E-mail address: jeffrey.marcus@duke.edu

Clin Plastic Surg 41 (2014) 283–299
http://dx.doi.org/10.1016/j.cps.2014.01.002
0094-1298/14/$ – see front matter © 2014 Elsevier Inc. All rights reserved.

designs in many ways at odds with the standard of care in aesthetic rhinoplasty at the time. These conflicting approaches were a direct result of similarly conflicting ideas about the underlying mechanism of the deformity.

Then in 1955, counter to patterns prevalent at the time, Gustave Aufricht wrote a treatise on cleft rhinoplasty, urging surgeons to avoid nonanatomic or overly aggressive techniques, in response to the clinical observation that patients treated with these radical techniques were being left with iatrogenic deformities that were nearly impossible to correct. He emphasized the importance of treating all rhinoplasty patients with consistent standards regardless of the presence of a cleft.

However, a more positive sentiment voiced by Gillies and Kilner[4] has become increasingly apt since that time:

optimism… is justified, for the structural defects underlying the deformity are gradually being made more clear and accurate diagnosis is becoming possible. Cure seldom anticipates diagnosis, but it is usually quick to follow it.

In 1984, Harold McComb[5] from New Zealand addressed the question as to whether the nasal deformity was due to intrinsic abnormalities including hypoplasia or malformation versus extrinsic abnormalities including deformation or malpositioning of otherwise normal structures. By performing cadaveric dissections of unoperated clefts in infants, he demonstrated that the cleft-side lower lateral cartilages were actually of normal size and shape, though displaced and tethered posterolaterally, and that symmetric nares could be achieved with release and repositioning.

The tilted tripod model of Hogan[6] was an influential contribution that emphasized the importance of the skeletal base in determining the changes in the cartilages and septum. It is noteworthy that significant inaccuracies were present in both of these models, demonstrating common misconceptions in the field. Contributions since that time, including those of Fisher and Mann,[7] have substantially added to the present-day concept of the deformity and its underlying mechanism. Nowadays a wide philosophic spectrum remains regarding the timing and design of operations.[8–13]

Salyer and colleagues[11] aim at primary correction of the unilateral primary deformity. Their technique involves dissection of the lower lateral cartilage extending onto the normal side through the medial aspect of the incision below the inferior turbinate. The cartilage remains attached to the skin at the dome near the genu, but is otherwise completely freed for repositioning.

Cutting also performs a primary operation designed to allow correction of deformity.[14] The lower lateral cartilages are dissected free at the footplates and ascending medial crura to allow differential positioning of the cartilages. Dissection proceeds to the tip, cleft-side ala, and noncleft upper lateral cartilage to facilitate a Tajima suspension suture. Complete mobilization of the lower lateral cartilages relative to one another and to the piriform enables repositioning in a corrected position. In the bilateral cleft, a retrograde dissection preserving blood supply allows access to cartilages for dissection in the cases of patients treated with nasoalveolar molding.

Guyuron's approach to the secondary unilateral cleft nasal deformity emphasizes the use of standard aesthetic rhinoplasty techniques.[10] Additional techniques designed to deal with specific cleft-related findings are also commonly used. Wedge osteotomy of the bony dorsum may be required to facilitate medial repositioning of the wide and flattened bones. The septoplasty includes resection of vomer and perpendicular plate of ethmoid in addition to quadrangular cartilage resulting from the cleft septal deformity. Direct excision of soft triangle is also noted to be a necessary means of achieving a more elongated, vertically oriented nostril.

The approach of Burget[15] is similar, and he describes significant limitations to primary cleft rhinoplasty attributable to the insubstantial quality of the nascent cartilages of infancy.

THE CLEFT LIP NASAL DEFORMITY

An understanding of the underlying mechanisms responsible for the cleft lip nasal deformity (CLND) is critical if the surgeon wishes to ever reverse the deformity. Although it is often stated that every cleft is different, any individual cleft nasal deformity occurs along a spectrum of potential deformities. It is helpful to look at a series of photographs of patients, from mild through severe. Imagine making a flip-card movie of these photographs. The alterations in the morphology can then be visualized. It is a reversal of this deformation of morphology that must be borne in mind at every step of care.

In 1998, Fisher and Mann[7] presented a model to describe the mechanisms responsible for the cleft lip nasal deformities, mild through severe, unilateral and bilateral. More recently, Fisher and Sommerlad[16] developed a computer-generated animated video of this model. The model is anatomically based. The lobule of the nose is reduced to 2 pairs of arches (**Fig. 1**).[7] The paired

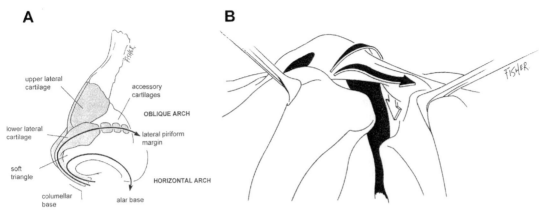

Fig. 1. (*A, B*) The lobule of the nose can be conceived of as 2 pairs of arches. The horizontal arches are formed by the nostril margins. The cartilaginous arches are formed by the lower lateral cartilages, the accessory cartilages, and their investing perichondrium. All arches are based on the skeleton. Predictable alterations in the positions of the skeletal bases result in predictable alterations in the morphology of the arches, which react interdependently because of intervening soft-tissue connections. With progressive degrees of clefting, anterolateral rotation of the premaxilla and hypoplasia of the piriform rim and skeletal alar base are observed. Posterior traction of the cutaneous arch by the cartilaginous arch produces the characteristic recurvatum deformity of the nostril margin. Release of the cartilaginous arch from the lateral piriform rim is required before any rounding of the nostril margin may be achieved.

cutaneous arches are formed by the nostril margins, each being based medially at the columellar base and laterally at the alar base. The paired cartilaginous arches are formed by the lower lateral cartilages, the accessory cartilages, and their investing perichondrium. Each cartilaginous arch is based anteriorly at the premaxilla and posteriorly at the piriform margin at the axial level of the inferior turbinate. The four arches are coincident in the columella. The cartilaginous arches diverge from each other as the medial crura form the middle crura and then the domes. On each side the cutaneous arch diverges from the cartilaginous arch at the soft triangle. Soft-tissue attachments between arches ensure that no single arch is able to move independently of the other arches.

Within the spectrum of the cleft deformity, typical skeletal alterations are observed to varying degrees. Even in the most minor form of cleft there is hypoplasia of the cleft-side piriform margin (**Fig. 2**). Muscular diastasis produces separation of the cleft-side columellar base and alar base.

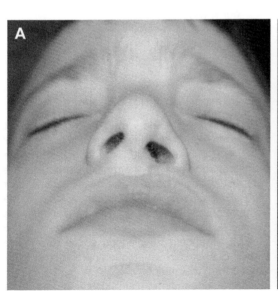
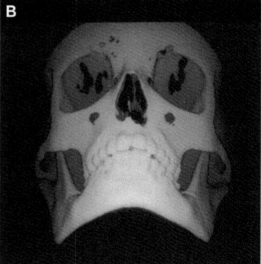

Fig. 2. (*A, B*) Within the spectrum of the cleft deformity, typical skeletal alterations are observed to varying degrees. Even in the most minor form cleft there is hypoplasia of the cleft-side piriform margin.

With greater degrees of clefting, anterolateral rotation of the greater segment accompanies progressive hypoplasia of the piriform rim and skeletal alar base. In the symmetric bilateral case, the premaxilla rotates anteriorly.

As these skeletal asymmetries progress, one observes progressive and predictable changes of arch position and, thus, nasal morphology.

In the unilateral case, separation of the columellar base and alar base is observed. As the greater segment rotates anterolaterally to the noncleft side, the columellar base and caudal septum deviate away from the cleft side. With progressive anterolateral rotation of the greater segment and hypoplasia of the piriform rim, there is increasing deformity of the cleft-side cartilaginous arch that spans these separating bony parts. The footplate deviates away from the midline to the noncleft side, and the lateral crus is pulled posterolaterally. The true dome point migrates posterolaterally as a new genu forms progressively more medially. As a result, one observes shortening of the medial crus and, therefore, of the columella on the cleft side. Posterolateral traction of the lateral cartilaginous arch is transmitted through soft-tissue attachments to the cutaneous arch, and the recurvatum deformity and lateral alar flare can now be observed. The normal overlap of the caudal margin of the upper lateral cartilage by the cranial margin of the lower lateral cartilage is lost. The tension of the cartilaginous arch raises a bowstring elevation of the vestibular lining, the so-called vestibular web.

In a symmetric bilateral cleft, the premaxilla rotates anteriorly and the septum remains midline. Piriform margin hypoplasia and the effects on the lower lateral cartilages occur bilaterally. Bilaterally, the columella is short. The retrodisplaced domes are separated. The vestibular web, recurvatum deformity, and alar flare occur bilaterally.

Because the cleft nasal deformity is the result of an underlying skeletal deformity, this skeletal deformity needs to be corrected before any correction can be fully realized in the nose. Because presurgical orthopedics can only partially improve the deformity (maxillary segment malalignment but not hypoplasia) and because most surgeons do not perform primary bone grafting, it is unrealistic to completely correct the nasal deformity at the primary operation. A plea must be made for patience. There will be future opportunities to augment the skeletal base deficiencies at the time of alveolar bone grafting and orthognathic surgery if indicated; this will set the stage for definitive septorhinoplasty. At this time deformities such as a broad deviated nasal dorsum, which are only obvious after maturity, may be addressed. Definitive secondary septorhinoplasty will be successful only if the cartilages are intact and robust, and if the skin envelope is complete and free of scar.

SURGICAL TECHNIQUE
Primary Cleft Lip and Nasal Repair

Primary cheiloplasty and rhinoplasty can be performed whether or not presurgical orthopedics has occurred. If presurgical orthopedics has corrected the anterolateral rotation of the greater maxillary segment, the required movements will be less, and in all likelihood the degree of recurrence of the deformity will be reduced.

Each surgeon will have his or her own methods and timing for correction of the deformation of the components of the nose already described. Whatever the plan, all interventions should be performed with a reversal of the deformity in mind while avoiding uncorrectable iatrogenic deformities. The author's (D.M. Fisher) plan involves a series of interventions, each improving the deformity to some extent while setting the stage for a definitive septorhinoplasty in the later teens. Presurgical infant orthopedics should narrow the cleft and bring the premaxilla to the midline (**Fig. 3**). Primary rhinoplasty is performed with the following goals in mind:

1. Balanced alar bases (from the anterior view)
2. Columellar base mobilization to the midline
3. Caudal septal release and repositioning
4. Alar base release and repositioning
5. Lateral piriform release and repositioning
6. Anteromedial advancement of the cleft-side dome and lateral crus
7. Creation of the scroll
8. Lateralization of the cleft-side lateral vestibular lining
9. Support
10. No external skin incisions
11. No excision(s) of skin envelope

The authors prefer the anatomic subunit approximation technique for primary lip repair (**Fig. 4**).[17] This technique, like the inferior triangle repair and the straight-line repairs, introduces the least scar at the base of the nose. Balancing of the alar bases should be a primary goal at the time of presurgical marking. The relative positions of the lateral and medial points of closure in the nostril sill should be planned so as to achieve nares of equal circumference and alar base symmetry from the anterior view.

Lip repair begins with incisions in the medial lip element. The cephalic insertion of the orbicularis oris muscle is divided. Dissection to the muscle

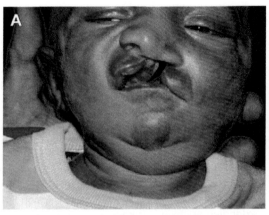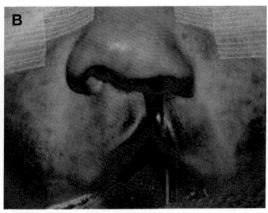

Fig. 3. (*A, B*) Presurgical infant orthopedics should narrow the cleft and bring the premaxilla to the midline.

deep to the columellar base will allow for mobilization of the columella to the midline and access to the anterior nasal spine. The septospinal ligament is divided, allowing for access to the caudal septum. The caudal septum is freed from the premaxilla, and a dissection plane is made between the septum and the noncleft-side mucoperichondrium. The caudal septum can now be easily mobilized to the vertical plane. Maintaining attachments of the cleft-side mucoperichondrium will allow the septum to be drawn toward the cleft side with the closure of the nostril sill.

Attention is then directed to the lateral lip element. The lip incisions are made. The cephalic insertion of the orbicularis oris muscle is divided, and continuation of dissection deep to the muscle will allow for mobilization of the alar base (**Fig. 5**). The alar base can now be mobilized anteromedially; however, this will accentuate the recurvatum deformity and the lateral alar flare because the cartilaginous arch remains attached to the piriform margin. Release of the lower lateral cartilage–accessory cartilage complex from the piriform rim

relieves the tension of the cartilaginous arch on the nostril margin, and will allow the cleft-side nostril margin to become round when the alar base is advanced anteriorly and medially (**Fig. 6**). This lateral piriform release needs to extend to an axial level above the inferior turbinate. It can be performed submucosally in incomplete cases, but with near complete and complete clefts there is also some element of deficiency of vestibular lining, and it is helpful in these cases to divide the mucosa along the piriform rim.

Following the lateral piriform release, the cleft-side dome and lateral crus is advanced anteromedially. Simultaneously, the overlap of the caudal margin of the upper lateral cartilage by the cranial margin of the lower lateral cartilage is created. Both of these movements of the cleft-side dome and lateral crus are maintained with internal nasal

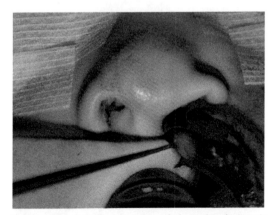

Fig. 5. The cephalic insertion of the orbicularis oris muscle is divided, and dissection continuing deep to the muscle will allow for mobilization of the alar base. The alar base can now be mobilized anteromedially; however, this will accentuate the recurvatum deformity and the lateral alar flare because the cartilaginous arch remains attached to the piriform margin.

Fig. 4. Operative markings for the anatomic subunit approximation technique.

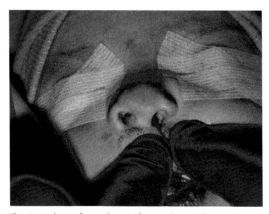

Fig. 6. Release from the piriform relieves the tension of the cartilaginous arch on the nostril margin, and will allow the cleft-side nostril margin to become round when the alar base is advanced anteriorly and medially.

valve plication sutures (**Fig. 7**). These horizontal mattress sutures are placed within the depth of the mucosal scroll and through the caudal margin of the upper lateral cartilage.

Following the release of the lateral lip element and nose from the maxilla, there is a tendency for the cleft-side lateral vestibular lining to adopt an unsupported medial position. The lateral vestibular lining can be lateralized with alar transfixion sutures.

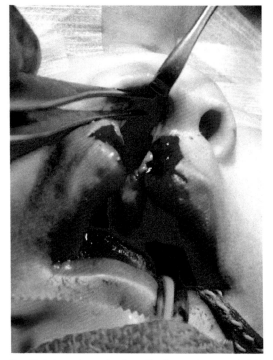

Fig. 7. Internal nasal valve plication sutures maintain the anteromedial movement of the cleft-side dome and lateral crus, and create the mucosal scroll.

Finally, an alar base–columellar base cinch stitch is placed at the height of the lip elements. Care should be made to position this stitch to level the alar bases and to tighten it with the appropriate tension to achieve nostrils of equal circumference.

Support of the movements is maintained during the initial healing period by the absorbable sutures. There will be loss of this support with time. The tendency for relapse may be reduced if the raw area produced by the anteromedial advancement of the lateral lip element is resurfaced with a turbinate flap (**Fig. 8**). Alternatively, an extended nostril-sill closure can be performed. When this is done, the lateral vestibular flap is sutured to an incision line extending posteriorly from the nostril sill along the caudal border of the septum. Nasal stents do not support the tip, and therefore tend to help conform the nostril only when they are used. To be effective, they must be used long term. Some inevitable flattening of the nostril will follow disuse of the stent.

With this primary rhinoplasty, there will be some residual uncorrected primary deformities. Some asymmetry of the alar bases from the inferior view, though perhaps corrected to satisfaction at the primary repair, will likely relapse to some extent because of the uncorrected skeletal base deficiency (**Fig. 9**). This deficiency should be corrected at the time of alveolar bone grafting. Now the stage is set for a successful secondary septorhinoplasty. If the cleft-side lower lateral cartilage and dome remain posterolaterally displaced, they can be mobilized, as described by Potter,[18] as a V-Y chondromucosal flap. Otherwise, standard rhinoplasty techniques can be performed to:

1. Straighten the septum
2. Straighten the nasal pyramid
3. Narrow and augment the nasal dorsum
4. Define, project, and make symmetric the nasal tip

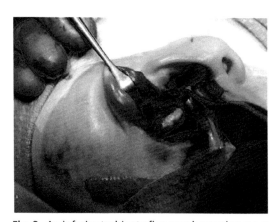

Fig. 8. An inferior turbinate flap may be used to resurface the raw area produced by repositioning of the lateral lip element. This action may prevent relapse.

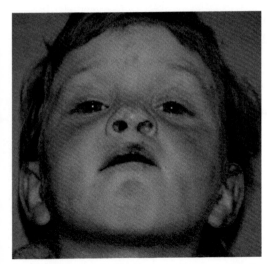

Fig. 9. The patient in **Fig. 5** seen at 3-year postoperative review.

Secondary Cleft Rhinoplasty

Planning
Preoperative planning for a secondary or definitive cleft rhinoplasty should begin even before the primary cleft repair, because the sequence of care adopted profoundly influences the residual cleft deformity seen at maturity. The multiple factors contributing to the secondary CLND can be summarized as:

Residual Primary Deformity
+ Iatrogenic Deformity
+ Growth-related Changes

————————————————

Secondary Cleft Nasal Deformity

The factors of iatrogenic deformity and scar are of particular interest because they are avoidable yet potentially insurmountable obstacles to the outcome desired for patients. The approach detailed in the foregoing sections is designed to reliably achieve conservative gains at every possibly opportunity while minimizing the burden of scar. Hence the long-term plan, beginning from infancy, is aimed at achieving a nose at skeletal maturity ready for a definitive rhinoplasty, with the following characteristics:

1. An untreated upper two-thirds
2. A solid skeletal base with columellar and alar bases in the correct positions
3. An ameliorated septal deformity that has evolved with growth
4. Nares of equal size and reasonable symmetry in the anteroposterior (AP) view
5. A cleft-side dome that has been elevated/advanced, though with some likely relapse

6. No iatrogenic injury to cartilaginous structures
7. Minimal scar; specifically, avoidance of scar within the columella or at its base

Patient assessment at skeletal maturity
Regardless of the plan of care adopted, patient evaluation at the time of skeletal maturity should be comprehensive, including functional and aesthetic concerns. In the authors' practice, the Nasal Obstruction Symptoms Evaluation (NOSE) questionnaire (**Fig. 10**), a validated instrument, aids in stratifying patients according to their subjective obstructive symptoms.[19]

As other investigators have noted, however, patient-reported symptoms can be difficult to interpret in cleft patients who may never have experienced normal airway function. Hence, severe airway obstruction may be underreported. Likewise, the patient may not appreciate dramatic improvements in airflow. Risk factors for adverse outcomes should also be sought through a complete history, physical examination, and review of systems. Goals and expectations should be discussed in detail.

Nasofacial analysis
The physical assessment of the cleft patient should proceed systematically and objectively. Standard approaches to nasofacial analysis provide a solid framework for analysis of any nose, and is well applied to the cleft nasal deformity (**Figs. 11** and **12**).[20] Doing so has the added benefit of lifting clinicians out of "cleft surgeon mode" and reminding us that we really ought to be treating our cleft patients with the same standards, thought processes, and techniques as we would a patient scheduled for aesthetic rhinoplasty. Standard AP, oblique, lateral, and basal views should also be photographed to aid in planning.

Facial symmetry and proportion
Beginning with the AP view, evaluate the overall symmetry and proportionality of the face. The ideal face is divided into thirds divided at the glabella and subnasale. The cleft patient is likely to have restricted midfacial growth, making the middle third of the face and the upper lip disproportionately small relative to the rest of the face.

On profile, this may manifest as a concave appearance with a unilateral cleft with associated malar deficiency. In a bilateral cleft, the protrusive prolabium may result in a convex profile. However, midfacial insufficiency is still present in the malar, piriform, and upper lip areas.

Overall, the facial disproportion and its underlying skeletal causes should be appreciated and properly addressed before definitive rhinoplasty, including orthognathic surgery and alveolar bone

→ To the Patient: Please help us to better understand the impact of nasal obstruction on your quality of life by **completing the following survey.** Thank You!

Over the past _ONE month_, how much of a **problem** were the following conditions for you?

Please (circle) the most correct response

	Not a Problem	Very Mild Problem	Moderate Problem	Fairly Bad Problem	Severe Problem
1. Nasal congestion or stuffiness	0	1	2	3	4
2. Nasal blockage or obstruction	0	1	2	3	4
3. Trouble breathing through my nose	0	1	2	3	4
4. Trouble sleeping	0	1	2	3	4
5. Unable to get enough air through my nose during exercise or exertion	0	1	2	3	4

Fig. 10. The Nasal Obstruction Symptoms Evaluation (NOSE) is a validated questionnaire used to assess patient-reported symptoms before and after functional nasal surgery, specifically septoplasty.

grafting as necessary. In general, it is preferable to complete this work before rhinoplasty, as it sets the foundation for the nose. When cleft rhinoplasty is performed before orthognathic surgery, there is a risk that the nose will shift postoperatively. Significant anterior movement of the maxilla can affect the nasolabial angle as well as the alar base width. Impaction vertically can also cause buckling of the septum, further complicating septal repair.

The nasal dorsum

The degree of dorsal deviation is evaluated by drawing a plumb line from the glabella to the menton. The greater segment draws the nasal dorsum away from the cleft.

The dorsal aesthetic lines should proceed on a gentle curve from the brow toward the tip-defining points. These contours in the cleft patient will be asymmetric and wide, owing to a broad flat and asymmetric dorsum. The upper third is often wide, with asymmetric flaring of the nasal bones. In addition the cleft-side dorsal aesthetic line may become undefined distally, as there may be no clear tip-defining point because of the displacement of the cleft-side dome.

On profile view, the dorsum should be evaluated for its position relative to a cord extending from the radix to the tip-defining points. Contour should also be assessed, including presence of a supra-tip break or dorsal hump that would be addressed according to standard rhinoplasty principles.

A
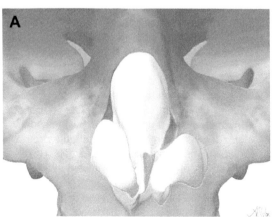

B
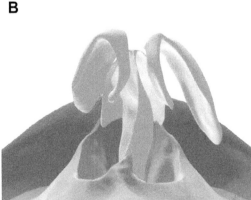

Fig. 11. (_A, B_) The mature cleft nasal deformity. A detailed description of each region is found in the text. These diagrams may be useful in education patients and for use in surgical planning.

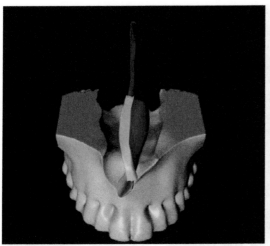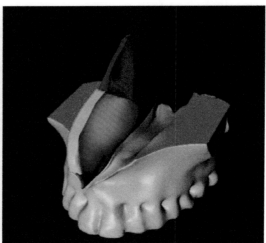

Fig. 12. The complex septal deformity. The caudal septum is associated with the anterior nasal spine, which is deviated off the facial midline to the noncleft side. The cartilaginous midseptum and posterior septum (perpendicular plate) deviate significantly toward the cleft side.

The lower third

The lower third should be assessed in terms of contour, symmetry, and size of the alae and base. On lateral view, projection and rotation should be assessed. The basal view should be evaluated for nostril to infratip lobule ratio and shape.

On the frontal view, typical findings include a wide alar base with a cleft-side dome that is posteriorly and laterally displaced. The angle between the domes (interdomal angle) is obtuse owing to displacement of the cleft-side dome, which produces an asymmetric and wide tip, with tip-defining points similarly affected. The cleft-side alar rim may display recurvatum medially with lateral kinking and flaring, and an overall lower position secondary to tension in the cartilaginous and cutaneous arches of Fisher and Mann.[7] On the lateral view, projection and cephalic rotation will differ from side to side. The cleft side will have diminished cephalic rotation and projection. On the basal view, the ideal nose has a unified equilateral triangle appearance with a nostril to infratip lobule ratio in the range of 2:1. The cleft patient will have widening of the alar base with loss of the triangular shape. Deformation of the paired arches results in deficiency of the infratip lobule and the columella. Deficiency in the infratip lobule is often underappreciated relative to columellar length, and is important to recognize. In addition, the soft tissue of the vestibule is often deficient.

Functional nasal examination

The functional examination should begin with routine use of a symptom assessment, such as the NOSE questionnaire, external observation for internal or external valve collapse, and assessment of the Cottle maneuver.[19] Ameliorative testing using adhesive breathing strips can assist in identifying patients with internal valve collapse.[21] Anterior rhinoscopy assisted with either a headlight or a mirror should evaluate septal deviation and turbinate hypertrophy.[22] The cleft septal deformity is highly complex, and involves not only the quadrangular cartilage itself but also the contiguous perpendicular plate of the ethmoid and the maxillary crest. The latter are markedly abnormal, often incorporate irregular complex spurs, and provide a significant technical challenge. **Fig. 12** presents a diagram of the septal structures in an effort to aid in the understanding of this relatively underreported aspect of the unilateral cleft nasal deformity. The internal examination demonstrates consistent deformation of the septum. The caudal septum is associated with the anterior nasal spine, which is deviated off facial midline to the noncleft side. The cartilaginous midseptum and the osseous posterior septum (perpendicular plate) deviate significantly toward the cleft side, resulting in a complex C-shaped deformity both craniocaudally and anteroposteriorly. The deviation of the cartilaginous septum toward the cleft side narrows the cleft-side airway while enlarging the noncleft cross-sectional area. The noncleft-side turbinate, over many years, hypertrophies to occupy this space on the noncleft side. The cleft-side turbinate is often relatively normal or small in size. **Fig. 13** shows a computed tomography (CT) scan of the complex septal deformity. Nasal endoscopy or CT provide

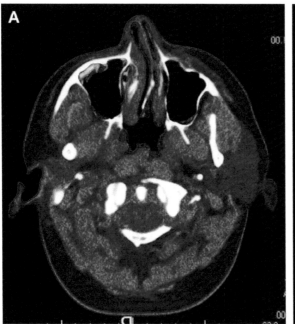
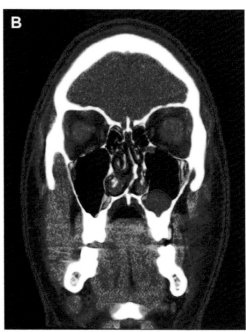

Fig. 13. (*A, B*) Axial computed tomography imaging (cleft side is to the left) demonstrates the C-shaped osseocartilaginous septal deformity in the anteroposterior plane toward the cleft side. Coronal imaging demonstrates the C-shaped deformity in the craniocaudal dimension. Note the osseous spurs of the posterior septum and the maxillary crest. Note also the significant hypertrophy of the noncleft-side inferior turbinate.

visualization beyond that which is visible on anterior rhinoscopy and are useful in surgical planning, particularly if prior nasal surgery has been performed. Rhinomanometry is an accessible objective measure with good attestation in the literature, which can also be used to assess nasal physiology before and following functional maneuvers.[22]

In summary, an understanding of the underlying mechanism of the cleft nasal deformity as well as a methodical history and physical examination, including nasofacial analysis, should yield a comprehensive assessment of the needs of the patient. A typical inventory of issues encountered for the average patient is provided in **Box 1**.

Secondary cleft rhinoplasty

The bad news about cleft rhinoplasty is that it is very difficult, and requires a far greater number and complexity of maneuvers to correct aesthetic and functional issues in comparison with any other rhinoplasty. The good news is that the deformity has remarkable consistency among patients, such that an arsenal of well-orchestrated maneuvers can be used with slight variations from patient

to patient. As variations of the mature deformity based on ethnicity also exist, technique must be adapted as well. Specifics relative to non-Caucasians are relevant, but beyond the scope of this article.

Inferior turbinate reduction

Owing to bowing of the midportion of the septum into the cleft side, a compensatory inferior turbinate hypertrophy prevails on the noncleft side. Inferior turbinate reduction and outfracture is performed on one or both sides depending on the degree of obstruction. Performing this first will avoid problems with bleeding in the ongoing operation. The current method used by the authors is a submucous microdebrider, although this is not the only option. If performing partial turbinectomy, care must be taken to avoid excessive reduction because of the possibility of atrophic rhinitis.

Opening and exposure

An aesthetic inverted V-shaped incision as advocated by Toriumi and colleagues[23] is used by the authors. The nasal tip and nasal dorsum are degloved in a subperichondrial plane, keeping the overlying flap as thick as possible to maintain

Box 1
Typical list of issues regarding secondary cleft nasal deformity

Dorsum

- Dorsal aesthetic lines are wide and asymmetric
- Dorsum deviates away from cleft
- Possible dorsal hump (unrelated to cleft)

Lower Third

- Lower Lateral Cartilage
  - Interdomal angle is obtuse
  - Dome position on the cleft side is posterolateral
  - Domal angles are obtuse
  - Contour on the cleft-side ala has recurvatum, kink, and flare
- Infratip lobule to nostril ratio is less than 2:1 with deficient lobule and columella
- Tip projection is reduced
- Tip rotation is reduced
- Piriform margin is deficient
- Alar base position and contour lack symmetry

Functional

- Septum is deviated and deformed
- Caudal septum is dislocated to the noncleft airway
- Noncleft-side inferior turbinate hypertrophy
- Internal and external valvular collapse

viability. Aggressive prior surgery performed at the time of lip repair, or subsequently, may make this dissection tedious. By staying in the subperichondrial plane, bleeding is reduced and a nonoperated surgical plane can often be elevated.

Next, the septum is approached by dividing the interdomal ligament of the lower lateral cartilages. The upper lateral cartilages are likewise released from the dorsal aspect of the septum. The septum is then degloved bilaterally, completing the wide exposure of the internal nasal deformity. Having already reduced the turbinates at this point, a full view of the complexity of the septal deformity is obtained.

Component reduction of the dorsum

Should a dorsal hump reduction or caudal septal resection be indicated as part of the comprehensive assessment, this should be performed before submucous resection to ensure preservation of an adequate L-strut. One therefore proceeds with a component reduction technique as described by Rohrich and colleagues.[24] The cartilaginous dorsum is reduced under direct vision, sharply followed by a series of graded fomon rasps for the osseous hump.

Treatment of the septum

Having achieved a smooth dorsum, comprehensive treatment of the septum is undertaken, including contour abnormalities and typical dislocation of the caudal septum from the anterior nasal spine into the noncleft-side airway.

The submucous resection of the septum not only provides graft material but treats the septal deformity. The bowing midportion of the cartilaginous septum is resected, leaving behind a 12- to 15-mm L-strut. The L-strut is then scored high on the noncleft side to encourage neutralization of the dorsal deviation. In cases where there is a pronounced S-shaped dorsal deformity, scoring may have to occur on both sides of the septal L-strut. Deviated portions of the perpendicular plate are carefully resected, avoiding transmission of forces cephalad that can injure the cribriform plate. A typically lengthy spur along the maxillary crest is resected using a combination of a 2-mm osteotome and pituitary rongeurs.

Next, the caudal septum is released from its position in the noncleft-side airway and is anchored at the midline into the periosteum of the anterior nasal spine. A drill hole can also be used to facilitate this. Mattressing sutures are placed to quilt the septal mucosa and to nullify the dead space and associated risk for hematoma development. At this point, most of the functional aspects of the rhinoplasty have been completed except for treatment of the internal valve. From another standpoint the nose has been dismantled, and one turns to putting things back together.

Spreader grafts

Spreader grafts fashioned from the harvested septal cartilage will accomplish several goals.[25] Fixing spreader grafts between the septum and the upper lateral cartilages reconstructs the midvault while improving the internal valve and straightening the dorsal angle. The grafts can also be placed asymmetrically with a thicker graft on the cleft side to address concavity, which is often present. Spreader grafts will close the open-roof deformity of the midvault.

Nasal bone osteotomies

At this point the treatment of dorsal angulation is completed, paying attention to the nasal bones. Abnormalities in the bony vault typically include a deviation to the noncleft side, but also a broad and flattened dorsum. Osteotomy and infracture through a nasal, upper buccal sulcus, or percutaneous approach can address both issues. If a dorsal hump has been reduced, lateral low-to-low osteotomies suffice to address the open roof and angulation. If a hump has not required reduction,

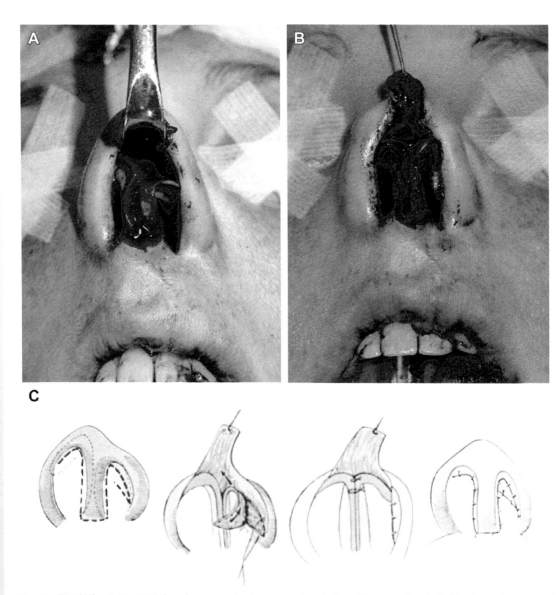

Fig. 14. (A–C) The Potter V-Y chondromucosal advancement is designed to raise the cleft-side dome to an equal position with the noncleft side by fully releasing tethering attachments of mucosa as well as the lateralmost aspect of the lateral crus at the piriform. The authors' modification of the technique (not depicted) incorporates modern rhinoplasty techniques of dome-defining and transdomal sutures, imbrication of the scroll region for vertical elevation, and lateral support using a lateral crural strut. ([C] *Data from* Potter J. Some nasal tip deformities due to alar cartilage abnormalities. Plast Reconstr Surg 1954;13:358. Stockton on Tees, England.)

medial osteotomy(ies) with or without wedge resection may also be needed.

The lower third
Finally, the lower third is addressed. From the perspective of Fisher's paired-arch concept of the lower third, the cleft-side oblique cartilaginous arch is likely to be tethered to the piriform to some extent, even if it has been previously released. Tension on the oblique cartilaginous arch results in deformation of the horizontal cutaneous arch owing to linkage of the 2 arches at the columella and soft triangle; this results in recurvatum medially, and kinking and flaring laterally. Based on these dynamics, tethering of the oblique arch must be addressed to facilitate manipulation of the lower lateral cartilages if one is to avoid actually worsening the kinking and flaring in the horizontal arch.

Potter V-Y advancement
The authors begin with a Potter V-Y advancement on the cleft side, which releases the lateral crus fully and allows repositioning (**Fig. 14**).[18] A mucocartilaginous incision is taken along the caudal margin of the lower lateral cartilage/accessory cartilage complex to the piriform, followed by a intercartilaginous back-cut. Tethering to the piriform is widely released, and the lateral crus and dome are advanced anteriorly and medially while closing the defect in V-Y fashion.

Shape and support of the lower lateral cartilages
With the cleft-side oblique arch now released and advanced, deforming lines of tension will have been diminished if not completely released. One can then move on to standard aesthetic rhinoplasty techniques for supporting and shaping the lower lateral cartilages. The lower lateral cartilages must be unified with aesthetic contour, projection, and rotation. Common maneuvers used to achieve these goals include a cephalic trim leaving at least 6 mm behind, dome-defining sutures to set the angle of the genu, and a transdomal or interdomal suture to set the tip-defining points. Experience with the Potter technique has also led to the observation that additional support is needed to retain the advancement of the lateral crus. An underlay lateral crural strut, anchored securely at the piriform, is placed to prevent relapse and correct lateral crus concavity. When combined with a strong, columellar strut, the tripod concept of

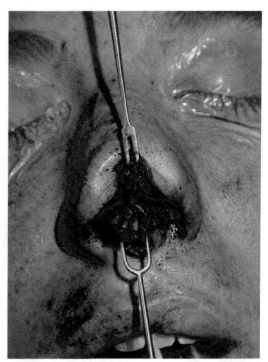

Fig. 15. The shape and support of the tip are finalized with a cephalic trip of the lower lateral cartilages, placement of dome-defining (intradome) sutures, placement of a lateral crural strut on the cleft side, placement of a strong columellar strut, and a transdomal or interdomal suture.

lower lateral cartilages is stabilized with desired tip rotation (**Fig. 15**). Finally, imbrication of the cleft-side scroll area is performed by placing mattress sutures internally to raise the lateral crus cephalad. A case example is provided in **Fig. 16**.

In the authors' experience tip grafts have rarely been necessary, although this may be more of a consideration in the multiply operated nose in which projection is inadequate. In this scenario, standard grafts such as the Sheen[26] and Peck[27] grafts are preferable.

Other issues that may have to be addressed, depending on the history of the patient, include residual asymmetries in the alar bases and piriform. Readvancement and rerotation of the alar base, as well as alar base or Weir excisions, can be used without introducing new scar. Several excellent examples are demonstrated in Millard's *Cleft Craft*.[3] Deficiency in the sill can also be addressed with dermal fat grafts or Alloderm.

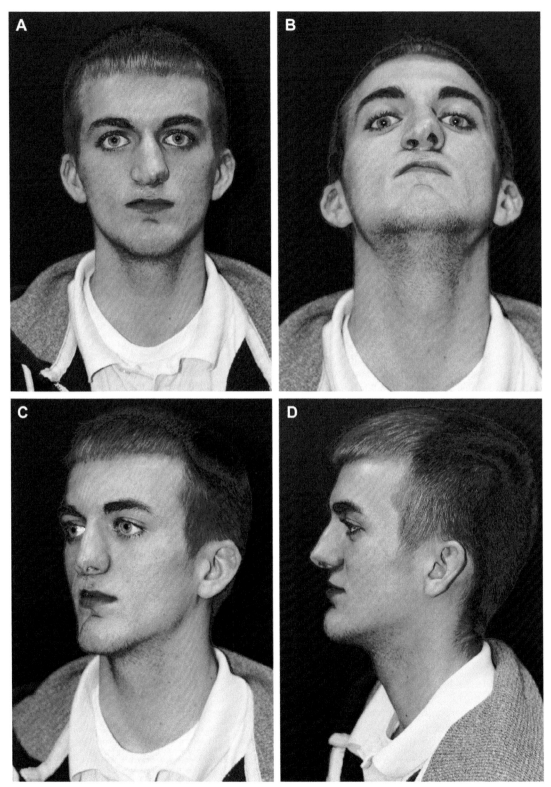

Fig. 16. (*A–H*) This young man presented with a classic nasal deformity including the upper, middle, and lower third. He was treated according to the sequence provided herein. He has achieved significant improvement in dorsal height and angulation, upper-third width, balance to the lower third, correction of alar base discrepancy, and dramatic improvement in his nasal airway as demonstrated in postoperative NOSE scores.

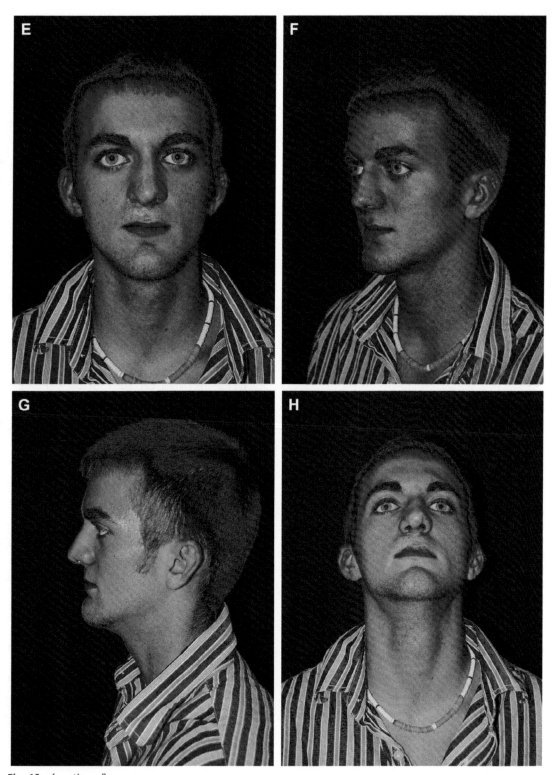

Fig. 16. (*continued*)

SUMMARY

Cleft care continues to improve in quality and efficiency as developing concepts are implemented in team-care and meaningful outcomes research. The cleft nasal deformity remains a challenging area, and may be one of the last domains of cleft care to truly be solved across the discipline, for reasons of the multiple important considerations discussed in this article.

Misconception regarding the underlying mechanism of the deformity persists; as is often said, the eye cannot see what the mind does not know. Hence, operations that approach the nasal deformity without addressing the underlying mechanism may be prone to relapse in the long term. The 2-arches model of the lobule proposed by Fisher and Mann is helpful in conceiving the architecture in question, particularly when considering how clefting deforms the arches, leading to the externally visible changes in the skin.[7]

Even with an understanding of the forces at play, the familiar issues of growth and development add another layer to the problem. How aggressive should one be with the nose at the primary operation? Which maneuvers will achieve a lasting benefit? In the authors' opinion, the cleft nasal deformity is heavily influenced by several key factors not amenable to correction at the index operation, including the ungrafted alveolar arch and long-term growth and development of the septum and nose. Patience must therefore be emphasized if one is to achieve the best possible correction in the most efficient manner. Measured and conservative gains can me made throughout childhood, leading to a nose set up for success with a definitive rhinoplasty at maturity. With the advantage of a minimally scarred field, the surgeon may then proceed with a definitive rhinoplasty characterized by standard aesthetic techniques.

REFERENCES

1. Kernahan DA, Bauer BS, Harris GD. Experience with the Tajima procedure in primary and secondary repair in unilateral cleft-lip nasal deformity. Plast Reconstr Surg 1980;66(1):46–53.
2. Randall P. History of cleft-lip nasal repair. Cleft Palate Craniofac J 1992;29(6):527–30.
3. Millard R. Cleft craft. Evolution of its surgery. Boston: Little Brown and Company; 1977.
4. Gillies H, Kilner T. Hare-lip operations for the correction of secondary deformities. Lancet 1932; 2:1369–75.
5. McComb H. Primary correction of unilateral cleft-lip nasal deformity—a 10-year review. Plast Reconstr Surg 1985;75(6):791–7.
6. Hogan VM. Secondary deformities of unilateral cleft lip and nose. Boston: Little, Brown, and Company; 1971.
7. Fisher D, Mann R. A model for the cleft lip nasal deformity. Plast Reconstr Surg 1998;101(6):1448–56.
8. Cutting CB. Secondary cleft lip nasal reconstruction: state of the art. Cleft Palate Craniofac J 2000;37(6): 538–41.
9. Mulliken J. Repair of bilateral complete cleft lip and nasal deformity—state of the art. Cleft Palate Craniofac J 2000;37(4):342–7.
10. Guyuron B. MOC-PS(SM) CME article: late cleft lip nasal deformity. Plast Reconstr Surg 2008; 121(Suppl 4):1–11.
11. Salyer KE, Genecov ER, Genecov DG. Unilateral cleft lip-nose repair: a 33-year experience. J Craniofac Surg 2003;14(4):549–58.
12. Mulliken J. Primary repair of bilateral cleft lip and nasal deformity. Plast Reconstr Surg 2001;108(1):181–94.
13. Khosla RK, McGregor J, Kelley PK, et al. Contemporary concepts for the bilateral cleft lip and nasal repair. Semin Plast Surg 2012;26(4):156–63.
14. Hopper R, Cutting C, Grayson B. Cleft lip and palate. In: Thorne CH, editor. Grabb and Smith's plastic surgery. Lippincott Williams & Wilkins; 2007. p. 208–12.
15. Burget G. Definitive rhinoplasty for adult cleft lip nasal deformity. In: Losee J, Kirschner R, editors. Comprehensive cleft care. McGraw Hill Medical; 2009. p. 499–507.
16. Fisher DM, Sommerlad BC. Cleft lip, cleft palate, and velopharyngeal insufficiency. Plast Reconstr Surg 2011;128(4):342E–60E.
17. Fisher DM. Unilateral cleft lip repair: an anatomical subunit approximation technique. Plast Reconstr Surg 2005;116(1):61–71.
18. Potter J. Some nasal tip deformities due to alar cartilage abnormalities. Plast Reconstr Surg 1954;13(5): 358–66.
19. Stewart MG, Witsell DL, Smith TL, et al. Development and validation of the Nasal Obstruction Symptom Evaluation (NOSE) Scale. Otolaryngol Head Neck Surg 2004;130(2):157–63.
20. Woodard C, Park S. Nasal and facial analysis. Clin Plast Surg 2010;37(2):181–9.
21. Gruber RP, Lin AY, Richards T. Nasal strips for evaluating and classifying valvular nasal obstruction. Aesthetic Plast Surg 2011;35(2):211–5.
22. Murrell GL. Components of the nasal examination. Aesthet Surg J 2013;33(1):38–42.
23. Toriumi DM, Mueller RA, Grosch T, et al. Vascular anatomy of the nose and the external rhinoplasty approach. Arch Otolaryngol Head Neck Surg 1996;122(1):24–34.

24. Rohrich RJ, Muzaffar AR, Janis JE. Component dorsal hump reduction: the importance of maintaining dorsal aesthetic lines in rhinoplasty. Plast Reconstr Surg 2004;114(5):1298–308.
25. Sheen JH. Spreader graft—a method of reconstructing the roof of the middle nasal vault following rhinoplasty. Plast Reconstr Surg 1984; 73(2):230–7.
26. Sheen JH. Tip graft—a 20-year retrospective. Plast Reconstr Surg 1993;91(1):48–63.
27. Peck GC. The onlay graft for nasal tip projection. Plast Reconstr Surg 1983;71(1):27–37.

Secondary Lip and Palate Surgery

Laura A. Monson, MD*, David Y. Khechoyan, MD,
Edward P. Buchanan, MD, Larry H. Hollier Jr, MD

KEYWORDS

- Bilateral cleft lip revision • Unilateral cleft lip revision • Buccal fat pad flap • Palatal fistulas

KEY POINTS

- Secondary deformities of unilateral cleft lip repair present a unique set of challenges to the cleft surgeon.
- Some deformities are amenable to correction, whereas some may be difficult to address and reverse completely.
- In general, if more than one conspicuous deformity is present, it is best to consider performing a full lip revision by complete takedown of the previous repair and rerepair.
- A cleft surgeon who performs a large number of lip revisions learns first-hand the critical value of a well-executed, meticulous primary cleft lip repair.
- Historically, there has always been some level of acceptance for revisionary surgery of the lip and nose. In the current era, the need for major revision is generally avoidable and should be viewed with greater scrutiny.

INTRODUCTION

Secondary cleft deformities are common and require thorough workup and evaluation by the treating cleft surgeon. Timing and sequence of surgical correction of secondary deformities are contingent on the type and severity of the problem. Cleft lip revision is typically performed before a child enters a social setting where stigmatization and/or isolation from peers may take place. By contrast, closure of oronasal fistulae is undertaken whenever the fistula is deemed "symptomatic," manifested as speech dysfunction or oronasal reflux. This article reviews surgical strategies to address secondary deformities following unilateral and bilateral cleft lip repair, as well as management of oronasal fistulae following cleft palate repair.

Secondary Cleft Lip Deformities Following a Unilateral Cleft Lip Repair

On initial evaluation of a patient who presents with persistent or iatrogenic stigmata of cleft following repair of a unilateral cleft lip deformity, it is necessary to deduce the type of repair that was initially performed. Each different repair type can be associated with specific, consistent, potential problems, the patterns of which can be addressed with a reliable corrective action. Close inspection of the patient's lip repair will provide a good sense of the type of previous repair. It is helpful to review previous operative reports and to discuss the circumstances of initial cleft lip repair. Questions regarding any complications following the initial repair (infection, dehiscence, suture reaction); what type of suture material was used; whether

Meeting Presentations: None.
Financial Disclosures/Commercial Associations: None.
Devices/Products: None.
Division of Plastic Surgery, Michael E. Debakey Department of Surgery, Baylor College of Medicine, 6701 Fannin Street, Houston, TX 77030, USA
* Corresponding author. Division of Plastic Surgery, Michael E. Debakey Department of Surgery, Baylor College of Medicine, 6701 Fannin Street, Suite 610, Houston, TX 77030.
E-mail address: Laura.monson@bcm.edu

Clin Plastic Surg 41 (2014) 301–309
http://dx.doi.org/10.1016/j.cps.2013.12.008
0094-1298/14/$ – see front matter © 2014 Elsevier Inc. All rights reserved.

post-operative nasal stents were used; and whether primary rhinoplasty was performed may all help to identify contributing factors that can then help guide subsequent decisions.

Patients can present at any age for evaluation of a prior cleft lip repair. In some cases, the parents may seek additional opinion to correct residual deformity; in other cases, families may be establishing team care following a move or adoption. In the former setting, the surgeon's opinion is specifically sought to answer the question as to whether additional surgery has a likelihood of improving on the result. In the latter, the family may not specifically be dissatisfied with the result; therefore, the surgeon must carefully bring the matter to discussion if he/she feels that revision would provide significant benefit now or in the future. Cleft lip revision is most typically entertained before a child enters school or earlier if persistent deformity is highly disfiguring. Although the goal of primary surgery is to avoid the need for revision, parents should be counseled early that lip revision may be beneficial before starting first grade.

Common deformities that are seen following a unilateral cleft lip repair include: [1,2]

- Vermilion discontinuity with medial notching
- Poor cutaneous roll continuity or obliteration of cutaneous roll by prominent scar
- Vertically short (more common) or a vertically long cleft-side (lateral) lip element
- Wide and prominent cutaneous scar
- Conspicuous transverse hatch marks from sutures that were tied too tightly or left in place too long (**Fig. 1**)

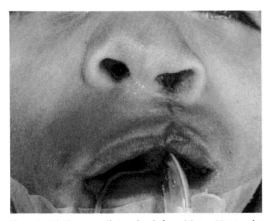

Fig. 1. Distinct unilateral deformities. Note the asymmetric vertically short lateral lip, cutaneous roll discontinuity, vermilion asymmetry, and prominent suture hatch-marks. In addition, the cleft-side alar base position is inferiorly displaced and the nostrils asymmetric.

Associated nasal deformity, resulting from either incomplete correction at time of primary cleft lip repair or from overzealous primary rhinoplasty, may also include: [3–5]

- Alar base malposition
- Nostril asymmetry
- Effacement of nostril sill
- Micronostril deformity
- Persistent, uncorrected deviation of caudal septum to the noncleft side
- Excessive scarring (see **Fig. 1**)

In rare instances, especially with an improperly executed primary rotation-advancement lip repair, one can observe a complete shift of the Cupid's bow to the cleft side with a high point of noncleft Cupid's bow peak found in the midline. This finding may also be observed in patients who have had multiple previous revisions with vertical scar excision and rerepair in whom normal Cupid's bow and philtrum landmarks have been virtually obliterated.

Failure to completely release and approximate orbicularis oris can also result in common deformities. Abnormal upper lip animation may be evident if continuity of the orbicularis oris muscle was not achieved. Asymmetric fullness (muscle bulge) on the superior aspect of the cleft-side upper lip subjacent to subalare may reflect inadequate initial dissection between the muscle and the overlying skin envelope. Problems related to muscle discontinuity most often require takedown, rerelease, and rerepair of skin and muscle, even when the skin repair itself is nonproblematic. This underscores the need for proper muscle alignment and repair at the initial surgery because it reintroduces the risk of cutaneous scarring, which is greater among older children than it was during infancy.

SURGICAL CORRECTION OF SECONDARY CLEFT LIP DEFORMITIES FOLLOWING UNILATERAL CLEFT LIP REPAIR

The approach to surgical correction depends on the degree and severity of the presenting deformity. In general, if sufficient residual lip tissue is present and more than one deformity (problem) is present, the authors recommend complete takedown of previous repair and rerepair via either a rotation-advancement (Millard) cleft lip repair (LM) or a conversion to a Fisher repair[2] (DK, EB). More minor or isolated problems may be amenable to simpler approaches: fat graft augmentation of medial (central) vermilion deficiency (**Fig. 2**); an asymmetric Z-plasty at vermilion-mucosal junction (**Fig. 3**); transverse wedge excision at the

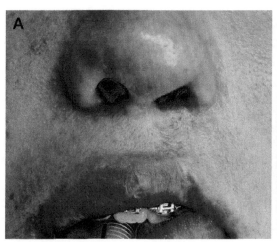

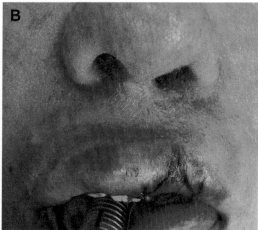

Fig. 2. Treatment of vermilion deficiency with fat grafting. (*A*) Minor soft tissue deficiency of vermilion following unilateral cleft lip repair. (*B*) Immediate post-operative result following autologous fat grafting. The authors routinely overgraft the deficient tissue to account for anticipated atrophy of the graft.

vermilion-cutaneous junction for lateral lip element vermilion fullness; deepening of the upper sulcus; or simple linear scar excision and closure. Secondary nasal deformities should also be addressed; these are covered in detail in the article "Correction of the Cleft Nasal Deformity: From Infancy to Maturity" by Mark D. Fisher, David M. Fisher, and Jeffrey R. Marcus elsewhere in this issue of the Clinics.

Challenging Deformities

Some deformities are extremely difficult, if not impossible, to correct. One example is an excessively wide cutaneous scar, particularly in the setting of a deficiency in transverse lip length. In this setting, complete excision of the scar would further tighten the upper lip and negatively affect animation.

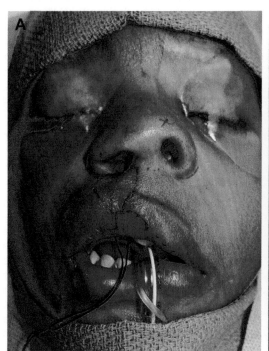

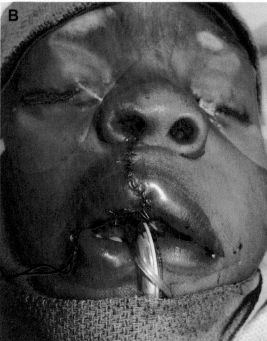

Fig. 3. Asymmetric Z-plasty at vermilion-cutaneous junction. (*A*) Preoperative markings for the asymmetric Z-plasty to correct asymmetric medial and lateral vermilion heights. (*B*) Immediate post-operative result following repair.

Another example is a concentration of scar tissue at the lip-columella junction following an improperly inset C-flap in a rotation-advancement repair. In such cases, the extent of scarring present may preclude complete excision, as it would yield a significant soft tissue deficiency vertically. Revisionary surgery is elective, and as such, one must judge the likelihood and potential extent of improvement to help the family build appropriate expectations as they make a decision whether to have their child undergo another surgical procedure (and anesthetic). The discussion should include timing of the procedure and consideration of future or concurrent needs.

When revising a wide or prominent vertical cutaneous scar from previous repair, it is key to recognize that subsequent straight-line closure may asymmetrically lengthen the upper lip on the cleft side. A concomitant single or double wedge excision either just above the cutaneous roll and/or immediately medial to subalare may be required to balance out the lip height. These wedge excisions have a transverse orientation with their base medially. Alternatively, the vertical scar excision may be extended bidirectionally into the nasal sill or caudally past the vermilion-mucosal junction as a "dog-ear" where the excess length may be camouflaged intranasally or corrected via a transverse wedge excision, respectively. A vertically short lip may benefit from length augmentation with an appropriately sized lateral cutaneous triangle immediately above the white roll that is inset into a back-cut on the medial lip element, as a form of an asymmetric Z-plasty. Reducing scar burden and proper reorientation and realignment of key landmarks may make the residual, now narrowed scar, appear more camouflaged.

Secondary Cleft Lip Deformities Following a Bilateral Cleft Lip Repair

Some inherent characteristics in the secondary bilateral cleft lip and nose deformity must be taken into consideration. These include paucity of tissue of the central lip, an inadequate or diminutive columella, and a limited blood supply to the prolabium. Each of these affects treatment management and outcomes.

"Whistle" Deformity

The most common secondary deformity seen in the vermilion of the bilateral cleft lip is a relative deficiency. The deformity can be caused by both the lack of normal musculature and mucosa in all dimensions, as well as an inappropriate primary repair.[6] Some state that this "whistle deformity" can be adequately corrected by reapproximation

of the orbicularis oris muscle.[7] In mild cases, various local tissue rearrangements may compensate or camouflage the central vermilion deficiency.[8-10] Fat augmentation can also be used for correction of mild to moderate central vermilion deficiency. These grafts can be injected micrografts or full-thickness dermal fat grafts. For more substantial defects, the main issue is usually an inadequate primary repair, and the vermilion deficiency will be accompanied by a widened philtrum, deficient columella, and widened nasal base (**Fig. 4**). The proper correction will involve a complete takedown and rerepair. The approach to correcting central vermilion deficiency is thus predicated on the extent of the deformity. For the severe whistle deformity or transversely deficient (tight) lip an Abbe flap may be required.[11] This approach is particularly helpful when local measures of tissue rearrangement have been exhausted. It is the only available procedure that can reconstruct a natural-looking philtrum, Cupid's bow, and central tubercle while augmenting the transverse dimension, thereby alleviating tightness.[12] When designing the flap dimensions, emphasis should be placed on reconstructing the entire philtral unit, which will release the abnormal tightness and provide a balanced profile. It is also advisable to harvest the flap from the center of the lower lip and place it in the aesthetic center of the upper lip.[12,13] This facilitates the appearance of a central vermilion tubercle and cupid's bow.[13] It should be designed slightly smaller than the intended neophiltrum; this facilitates closure of the lower lip donor site and allows for stretching of the flap once in position. Finally, the authors recommend dividing the flap on postoperative day 10 to day 14. To assure viability, one can compress the native labial artery pedicle and check capillary refill of the inset flap.

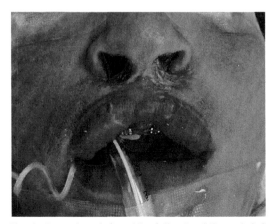

Fig. 4. Secondary deformities following bilateral cleft lip repair. Note the wide philtrum; vermillion deficiency; and short, scarred columella base.

The Manchester repair, which is now used by far fewer surgeons, merits specific mention. In the Manchester repair, central vermilion is retained from the prolabial segment with the prolabial shield, rather than being derived from the lateral lip elements and meeting in the midline. The vermilion height of the prolabial segment is significantly different than that of the lateral elements and therefore is consistently conspicuous as a mismatch with unsightly, dry and flaky vermilion from the original prolabium. When the patient has had this type of initial repair, there will likely also be orbicularis oris discontinuity, an absence of white roll within Cupid's bow, and a shallow sulcus. The only option in this setting is to perform a total lip revision according to more contemporary methods (refer to article on "Modern Tenets for Repair of Bilateral Cleft Lip" elsewhere in this issue by Alexander C. Allori and Jeffrey R. Marcus). Total revision involves removal of the abnormal vermilion from the prolabium, replacement with the fuller, muscle-containing vermilion of the lateral lip elements, and deepening of the sulcus by bringing lateral mucosa to the midline.

Excessive Scarring

Often, the most noticeable and striking stigmata of a repaired bilateral cleft lip is an unsightly scar. A poor scar is one that even after 18 months remains hyperpigmented, raised, or foreshortened. Contributing factors at the time of cleft repair include inadequate orbicularis oris muscle release and repair, a protruding premaxilla, and excessive cleft width. All these conditions result in a tight lip closure. This leads to tension and subsequent widening of the lip scar over time. Permanent sutures used at the time of primary repair, taken with excessively wide bites and left in for more than a few days, will result in a scar with cross-hatching as well. Although some feel that the cutaneous lip should never be reopened for revision,[14,15] the authors advocate full-thickness scar excision, from the prolabial side of the repair, and muscle reapproximation if continuity is lacking.[13] An adequate muscle repair is the basis for successful, permanent correction of widened and prominent scars.[16]

Goals of Reconstruction

The goal of primarily reconstructing the orbicularis oris sphincter and obtaining lip muscle continuity cannot be overemphasized. The literature is replete with examples documenting its importance.[8,9,13,16–22] With regard to the soft tissues, a discontinuous orbicularis oris has been implicated in widened lip scars, wide and convex philtra, and whistle deformities. Furthermore, failure to fully dissect, release, reorient, and unite the muscle fibers from the alar bases will contribute to persistent bulging of the discontinuous lateral lip musculature with attempted animation.[8,9,13,18,19] If evaluation reveals functional abnormality of the orbicularis oris and a telltale "muscle bulge" on animation, it should be released from all of its abnormal attachments and repaired.

The philtrum truly is the keystone of the upper lip. In the bilateral cleft lip, the philtrum has a tendency to become progressively wide and convex in shape over time. The action of the orbicularis oris, combined with the persistent presence of tension from the primary repair, leads to a horizontal widening of the prolabial soft tissue and further loss of convexity of an already abnormal philtrum.[13,17,23] Excision of the excess philtral tissue, with reapproximation of the orbicularis to the newly redesigned philtrum, is the surgical optimum.[18] When considering the subtleties of the philtral subunit, one must include Cupid's bow. Although there is a tremendous anatomic variety in individuals, the presence of a Cupid's bow is an essential feature of a "normal-appearing" upper lip. The bilateral cleft lip often has a shallow or absent buccal sulcus and a tethering of the upper lip to the anterior aspect of the alveolus.[17,24] An adequate sulcus, although often underemphasized, is essential for cleft lip reconstruction, and it can be created by adequate elevation of the prolabium from the premaxilla during primary repair and coverage of the resultant raw premaxilla with an inferiorly based mucosal flap.[7] The creation of an adequate sulcus and normal anatomy enhances proper lip function and facilitates appropriate fitting of orthodontic appliances.[7,25] Several surgical techniques have been described for the treatment of the shallow buccal sulcus and fall primarily into 2 categories: mucosal grafts[7,13,23,25,26] and local flaps.[7,25] Although mucosal grafts are not ideal and have been associated with contraction, readhesion, and sulcus obliteration,[25,26] these complications can be minimized with the use of a dental amalgam stents.[13]

Palatal Fistulas

For all cleft surgeons, palatal fistulas remain a considerable challenge whether they are encountered in the authors' own patients, as referrals from other surgeons, or on mission trips. Many small, early post-operative fistulas can be managed conservatively. They may eventually close without intervention. Fistulas may be clinically significant when they lead to nasal air escape, speech distortion, or regurgitation of liquids and solids. Larger fistulas may also lead to velopharyngeal insufficiency, thereby complicating speech management.

The published rate of post-operative fistulas varies widely, from 0% to 70%.[27–29] This in part is because of the lack of a standard classification scheme, which hinders both communication and research efforts. At the authors' institution, the authors use the Pittsburgh Fistula Classification System, described by Losee and colleagues,[30] due to its ease of use. The Pittsburgh Fistula Classification System includes 7 fistula types: those at the uvula or bifid uvulae (type I); in the soft palate (type II); at the junction of the soft and hard palates (type III); within the hard palate (type IV); at the incisive foramen or junction of the primary and secondary palates (type V; this designation is reserved for use with Veau type IV clefts); lingual-alveolar (type VI); and labial-alveolar (type VII). Fistulas are then further classified into functional or nonfunctional depending on their impact on speech and the presence of nasal regurgitation.

Fistulas are difficult to repair definitively; the recurrence rate after repair reportedly approaches 65%.[31] Many strategies to repair and decrease the incidence of post-operative palatal fistulas have been reported over the years that have ascended the reconstructive ladder.[31–50] From direct cauterization by Obermeyer in 1967, to an appliance/obturator by Berkman, to the myriad of local flap designs by von Langenbeck to Gabka in 1964, and to free conchal grafts by Ohsumi and colleagues,[35,46,48,51] the options put forth for closure of palatal fistulas have been numerous. Guerrero-Santos and Altamirano popularized the tongue flap in the 1960s and 1970s, which has remained a mainstay at some centers for closure of larger anterior fistulas.[42,52] Multiple pedicle flaps, including the facial artery myomucosal flap, have been described to treat those most difficult large anterior fistulas as well.[33,38,42,52,53] Even free tissue transfer[34,37,41,45,47,48] has been described for when all other modalities have been exhausted. As with many situations in plastic surgery, when there are numerous procedures described, it is often because no one option works reliably in all cases. The most recent innovations in fistula treatment have been the use of acellular dermal matrix as described by Kirschner and colleagues[43,44] and the use of the buccal fat pad flap.[54]

In general, the larger the fistula, the larger the surgery required to address it. Small local flaps have the inherent problem of using already scarred, stiff tissue that is often friable and difficult to work with due to the constant exposure of regurgitating nasal and oral contents. The well-described procedures such as the FAMM flap and tongue flap have the benefit of bringing in vascularized, unscarred tissue, but at the expense of considerable donor site morbidity, technical difficulty, considerable postoperative care, and need for a second surgery.

The preferred method at the authors' institution for fistulas of the soft palate only is a direct excision and repair, often in conjunction with a conversion Furlow palatoplasty if the fistula occurs in the presence of velopharyngeal insufficiency.

Fistulas of the hard palate, including those at the junction of the hard and soft palate, require considerably more than direct excision and closure due to their nature and paucity of malleable local tissue. The local transposition flaps described in various textbooks are often inadequate for complete closure, as the arc of rotation often falls short. In the authors' experience, it is the rare hard palate fistula that does not require complete re-elevation of either unipedicled or bipedicled flaps for adequate oral mucosal closure.

Nasal lining closure is often the more difficult of the 2 layers to achieve watertight repair for. This is because of the inherent friability of the tissues that have been exposed to constant reflux of fluids through the fistula. If local nasal tissue proves to be inadequate, palatally based hinge flaps or nasal septal flaps may be used. Another option, based on the work of Kirschner and colleagues,[43,44,55–58] is the use of acellular dermal matrix as an adjunct when local soft tissue options prove inadequate for a watertight closure. They advocate for use of a thin piece of acellular dermal matrix for augmentation of nasal closure and have data to support its use in all fistula types, except those of the soft palate only, with a recurrent fistulas rate of 3.6%.[43,44,55]

Another option, when local tissue is insufficient for closure of either the nasal or the oral lining, is use of the buccal fat pad flap. This flap has been widely described for closure of palatal defects both in the head and neck literature and in the cleft palate literature.[59–61] It has several advantages over other options and has become the preferred method for closure of larger fistulas of the hard palate at the authors' institution. It is a simple flap to raise, is reliable, and has minimal donor morbidity. The flap does not require tunneling, a second operation, or use of a bite block. The flap can easily reach the midline or the lingual central incisors. Additionally, it is well-vascularized, autologous tissue that epithelializes readily and can be used for either nasal or oral closure.

In the care of fistulas, as in most secondary cleft surgery, prevention of complications is key. A well-executed primary palatoplasty is the best defense against later fistula formation. A tension-free closure and careful post-operative care are crucial in prevention. To achieve tension-free closure, the surgeon should use relaxing incisions as necessary, perform a complete intravelar veloplasty, completely release the neurovascular bundle with optional osteotomy of the bony foramen, and use meticulous surgical precision to avoid unnecessary handling or crushing of the mucosal edges. The cleft palate surgeon will be rewarded more from preventing palatal fistulas than from correcting them.

SUMMARY

The care of children with cleft lip and palate is often challenging, but perhaps even more so when confronted with difficult secondary deformities. The most important first step when evaluating one of these patients is to properly diagnose the underlying problem. This often necessitates a good working understanding of the original repair technique that was performed. Recognizing the common pitfalls of certain repairs will help facilitate the surgical planning process and assist the surgeon during future procedures. Although there is no doubt that the execution and results of these procedures can be less than satisfactory for the surgeon, the patient truly benefits from a revision if the original repair did not adhere to modern standards of cleft surgery. Not only will that patient gain from a repair that brings them closer to a "normal" functional and aesthetic state, but in caring for these patients, the authors' understanding of the cleft condition is advanced and their primary patients surely benefit as well.

REFERENCES

1. Fisher DM, Sommerlad BC. Cleft lip, cleft palate, and velopharyngeal insufficiency. Plast Reconstr Surg 2011;128(4):342e–60e.
2. Fisher DM. Unilateral cleft lip repair: an anatomical subunit approximation technique. Plast Reconstr Surg 2005;116(1):61–71.
3. Fisher DM, Mann RJ. A model for the cleft lip nasal deformity. Plast Reconstr Surg 1998;101(6): 1448–56.
4. Cutting CB. Secondary cleft lip nasal reconstruction: state of the art. Cleft Palate Craniofac J 2000;37(6):538–41.
5. Losee JF, Kirschner RE. Comprehensive cleft care. New York: McGraw-Hill Companies, Inc; 2008.
6. Viale-Gonzalez M, Barreto F, Ortiz-Monasterio F. Surgical management of the bilateral cleft lip. Plast Reconstr Surg 1973;51(5):530–5.
7. Jackson IT, Fasching MC. Secondary deformities of cleft lip, nose, and cleft palate. In: McCarthy JG, editor. Plastic and reconstructive surgery, vol. 4. Philadelphia: WB Saunders; 1990. p. 2771.
8. Stal S, Hollier LH. Correction of secondary cleft lip deformities. Plast Reconstr Surg 2002;109(5): 1672–81.
9. Cohen M. Residual deformities after repair of clefts of the lip and palate. Clin Plast Surg 2004;31:331–45.
10. Jackson IT. Cleft lip and palate. In: Mustarde JC, Jackson IT, editors. Plastic surgery in infancy and childhood. 3rd edition. London: Churchill Livingstone; 1988. p. 1–40.
11. Abbe R. A new plastic operation for the relief of deformity due to double harelip. Plast Reconstr Surg 1968;42(5):481–3.
12. Lewis MB. Secondary soft tissue procedures for cleft lip and palate. In: Cohen M, editor. Mastery of plastic and reconstructive surgery. Boston (MA): Little, Brown, and Company; 1994. p. 605–18.
13. Stal S, Hollier LH. Secondary deformities of the cleft lip, nose, and palate. In: Mathes SJ, editor. Plastic Surgery, vol. 4, 2nd edition. Philadelphia (PA): Elsevier and Saunders; 2005. p. 339–63.
14. Mulliken JB, Wu JK, Padwa BL. Repair of bilateral cleft lip: review, revisions, and reflections. J Craniofac Surg 2003;14(5):609–20.
15. Mulliken JB. Bilateral cleft lip. Clin Plast Surg 2004; 31(2):209–20.
16. Meijer R. Secondary repair of the bilateral cleft lip deformity. Cleft Palate J 1984;21(2):86–90.
17. Garza JR, Pessa JE, Futrell JW. Secondary deformities of the cleft lip and nose. In: Bentz ML, editor. Pediatric plastic surgery. Valley Stream (NY): Appleton and Lange; 1998. p. 81–92.
18. McCarthy JG, Cutting CB. Secondary deformities of cleft lip and palate. In: Georgiade GS, Riefkohl R, Levin LS, editors. Georgiade: plastic, maxillofacial, and reconstructive surgery. 3rd edition. Philadelphia (PA): Williams and Wilkins; 1997. p. 247–57.
19. Oneal RM, Greer DM, Nobel GL. Secondary correction of bilateral cleft lip deformities with Millard's midline muscular closure. Plast Reconstr Surg 1974;54(1):45–51.
20. Black PW, Scheflan M. Bilateral cleft lip repair: "putting it all together". Ann Plast Surg 1984; 12(2):118–27.
21. Tessier P, Tulasne JF. Secondary repair of cleft lip deformities. Clin Plast Surg 1984;11(4):747–60.
22. Rees TD, Swinyard CA, Converse JM. The prolabium in the bilateral cleft lip. Plast Reconstr Surg 1962;30(6):651–62.
23. Gillies H, Kilner TP. Hare-lip: operations for the correction of secondary deformities. Lancet 1932; 2:1369–75.

24. Stal S, Hollier LH. Correction of secondary deformities of the cleft lip nose. Plast Reconstr Surg 2002;109(4):1386–92.
25. Erol OO, Agaoglu G. Reconstruction of the superior labial sulcus in secondary bilateral cleft lip deformities: an inverted U-shaped flap. Plast Reconstr Surg 2001;108(7):1871–3.
26. Brown JB, McDowell F. Secondary repair of cleft lips and their nasal deformities. Ann Surg 1941; 114:101–17.
27. Bardach J, Morris H, Olin W, et al. Late results of multidisciplinary management of unilateral cleft lip and palate. Ann Plast Surg 1984;12:235–42.
28. Maeda K, Ojimi H, Utsugi R, et al. A T-shaped musculomucosal buccal flap method for cleft palate surgery. Plast Reconstr Surg 1987;79:888–96.
29. Senders CW, Sykes JM. Modifications of the Furlow palatoplasty (six- and seven-flap palatoplasties). Arch Otolaryngol Head Neck Surg 1995;121: 1101–4.
30. Smith D, Vecchione L, Jiang S, et al. The Pittsburgh Fistula Classification System: a standardized scheme for the description of palatal fistulas. Cleft Palate Craniofac J 2007;44:590–4.
31. Schultz RC. Management and timing of cleft palate fistula repair. Plast Reconstr Surg 1986;78: 739–47.
32. Thaller SR. Staged repair of secondary cleft palate deformities. J Craniofac Surg 1995;6:375–81.
33. Assuncao AG. The design of tongue flaps for the closure of palatal fistulas. Plast Reconstr Surg 1993;91:806–10.
34. Batchelor AG, Palmer JH. A novel method of closing a palatal fistula: the free fascial flap. Br J Plast Surg 1990;43:359–61.
35. Berkman MD. Early non-surgical closure of postoperative palatal fistulae. Plast Reconstr Surg 1978; 62:537–41.
36. Brusati R, Mannucci N. Repair of the cleft palate without lateral release incisions: results concerning 124 cases. J Craniomaxillofac Surg 1994;22: 138–43.
37. Chen HC, Ganos DL, Coessens BC, et al. Free forearm flap for closure of difficult oronasal fistulas in cleft palate patients. Plast Reconstr Surg 1992; 90:757–62.
38. Coghlan K, O'Regan B, Carter J. Tongue flap repair of oro-nasal fistulae in cleft palate patients: a review of 20 patients. J Craniomaxillofac Surg 1989; 17:255–9.
39. Cohen SR, Kalinowski J, LaRossa D. Cleft palate fistulas: a multivariate statistical analysis of prevalence, etiology, and surgical management. Plast Reconstr Surg 1991;87:1041–7.
40. Denny AD, Amm CA. Surgical technique for the correction of postpalatoplasty fistulae of the hard palate. Plast Reconstr Surg 2005;115:383–7.
41. Eufinger H, Machtens E. Microsurgical tissue transfer for rehabilitation of the patient with cleft lip and palate. Cleft Palate Craniofac J 2002;39: 560–7.
42. Guerrero-Santos J, Altamirano JT. The use of lingual flaps in repair of fistulas of the hard palate. Plast Reconstr Surg 1966;38:123–8.
43. Kirschner RE, Cabiling DS, Slemp AE, et al. Repair of oronasal fistulae with acellular dermal matrices. Plast Reconstr Surg 2006;118: 1431–40.
44. Kirschner RE, LaRossa DD, Losee JE, et al. Repair of oronasal fistulae using acellular dermal matrices: preclinical study and clinical case series. Presented at the 60th Annual Meeting of the American Cleft Palate-Craniofacial Association, Asheville (NC), April 10–13, 2003.
45. Krimmel M, Hoffmann J, Reinert S. Cleft palate fistula closure with a mucosal prelaminated lateral upper arm flap. Plast Reconstr Surg 2005;116: 1870–2.
46. Millard DR. Cleft craft: the evolution of its surgery. 1st edition. Boston: Little, Brown; 1976.
47. Ninkovic M, Hubli EH, Schwabegger A, et al. Free flap closure of recurrent palatal fistula in the cleft lip and palate patient. J Craniofac Surg 1997;8: 491–5.
48. Ohsumi N, Onizuka T, Ito Y. Use of a free conchal cartilage graft for closure of a palatal fistula: an experimental study and clinical application. Plast Reconstr Surg 1993;91:433–40.
49. Rintala AE. Surgical closure of palatal fistulae: follow-up of 84 personally treated cases. Scand J Plast Reconstr Surg 1980;14:235–8.
50. Wilhelmi BJ, Appelt EA, Hill L, et al. Palatal fistulas: rare with the two-flap palatoplasty repair. Plast Reconstr Surg 2001;107:315–8.
51. Obermeyer P. Early closure of suture dehiscence after uranoplasty by means of a conservative method. Dtsch Stomatol 1967;17:168–73 [in German].
52. Guerrero-Santos J, Fernandez JM. Further experience with tongue flap in cleft palate repair. Cleft Palate J 1973;10:192–202.
53. Ashtiani AK, Emami SA, Rasti M. Closure of complicated palatal fistula with facial artery musculomucosal flap. Plast Reconstr Surg 2005;116: 381–8.
54. Levi B, Kasten SJ, Buchman SR. Utilization of the buccal fat pad flap for congential cleft palate repair. Plast Reconstr Surg 2009;123: 1018–21.
55. Smith DM, Vecchione L, Jiang S, et al. Progress in palatoplasty: strategies to eliminate fistulae. Presented at the 64th Annual Meeting of the American Cleft Palate-Craniofacial Association, Broomfield (CO), April 23–28, 2007.

56. Clark JM, Saffold SH, Israel JM. Decellularized dermal grafting in cleft palate repair. Arch Facial Plast Surg 2003;5:40–5.

57. Cole P, Horn TW, Thaller S. The use of decellular-ized dermal grafting (AlloDerm) in persistent oro-nasal fistulas after tertiary cleft palate repair. J Craniofac Surg 2006;17:636–41.

58. Steele MH, Seagle MB. Palatal fistula repair using acellular dermal matrix: the University of Florida experience. Ann Plast Surg 2006;56:50–3.

59. Hanazawa Y, Itoh K, Mabashi T, et al. Closure of or-oantral communications using a pedicled buccal fat pad graft. J Oral Maxillofac Surg 1995;53: 771–6.

60. Baumann A, Ewers R. Application of the buccal fat pad in oral reconstruction. J Oral Maxillofac Surg 2000;58:389–93.

61. Samman N, Cheung LK, Tideman H. The buccal fat pad in oral reconstruction. Int J Oral Maxillofac Surg 1993;22:2–6.

Measuring Outcomes in Cleft Lip and Palate Treatment

Thomas J. Sitzman, MD[a],*, Alexander C. Allori, MD, MPH[b],
Guy Thorburn, FRCS (Plastic Surgery), MA[c]

KEYWORDS

- Cleft lip • Cleft palate • Cleft surgery • Evidence base • Outcomes measurement • Outcome data

KEY POINTS

- Outcome measurement is essential to document quality and to facilitate improvement.
- Cleft surgeons should choose outcome measures that are valid, reliable, practical to implement, and broadly adopted.
- New measures are under development, and existing measures will continue to evolve in all aspects of cleft care. Measures should focus on outcomes most relevant to patients and include input from providers and health care purchasers.

> If you can not measure it, you can not
> improve it.
>
> —Lord Kelvin

WHY MEASURE OUTCOMES?

Once the sole purview of clinical and health-services research, *outcome assessment* has become a core component of clinical practice. Generally speaking, outcome measurement may be used for accountability, quality improvement, and health-system design (eg, resource allocation, purchasing decisions, and policy development) (**Box 1**). *Accountability* refers to the demonstration that a particular surgeon's or team's results are within accepted standards. *Quality improvement* is a process of combining domain expertise with knowledge of systems, variation, and psychology to effect meaningful improvement. Originally developed in the manufacturing and service industries, quality improvement is now widely applied to health care delivery systems.[1]

It is intuitive that regularly reviewing one's outcomes is useful and instructive for improving patient care. For some time, the American Board of Medical Specialties' Maintenance of Certification process has required demonstration of quality-improvement practices in an individual's clinical practice.[2] However, it is important to underscore that routine collection and reporting of clinical outcomes are increasingly emphasized in the public sphere. There is a growing movement to tie reimbursement to outcomes, and organizations such as the Leapfrog group and the Agency for Healthcare Research and Quality have advocated public reporting of these data. The American College of Surgeons' National Surgical Quality Improvement Program was conceived as a volunteer program to help hospitals monitor specific clinical outcomes (particularly the so-called never events) that are already being tied to reimbursement. Recently, the Centers for Medicare and Medicaid Services announced its intention to require a proven level of performance to be eligible for payment.[3] In the future, payers will be increasingly

[a] Division of Plastic Surgery, Cincinnati Children's Hospital Medical Center, 3333 Burnet Avenue, MLC 2020, Cincinnati, OH 45229, USA; [b] Division of Plastic, Maxillofacial, and Oral Surgery, Children's Health Center, Duke University Hospital, Durham, NC, USA; [c] Department of Plastic Surgery, North Thames Cleft Centre, Great Ormond Street Hospital for Children NHS Foundation Trust, London, UK
* Corresponding author.
E-mail address: Thomas.Sitzman@cchmc.org

Clin Plastic Surg 41 (2014) 311–319
http://dx.doi.org/10.1016/j.cps.2013.12.001
0094-1298/14/$ – see front matter © 2014 Elsevier Inc. All rights reserved.

Box 1
Applications of outcome measurement in
health care

Accountability
  Accreditation
  Quality assurance
  Public reporting
Quality improvement
  Improve clinical care
  Research
  Board certification
Health-system design
  Resource allocation
  Value-based purchasing
  Policy development

sensitive to objective data on outcomes when deciding where care should be directed and when negotiating fees.

OUTCOMES ASSESSMENT AND QUALITY IMPROVEMENT REQUIREMENTS IN CLEFT CARE

Specific to cleft care, the American Cleft Palate Association (ACPA) established minimum requirements for accreditation.[4] These requirements include that "the Team has mechanisms to monitor its short-term and long-term treatment outcomes" by documenting "its treatment outcomes, including base-line performance and changes over time" and conducting "periodic retrospective or prospective studies to evaluate treatment outcomes."[4] Similar requirements exist in the United Kingdom.[5] To date, the ACPA offers no specific recommendations regarding *which* outcomes should be assessed, nor *how* these data are to be collected, analyzed, and interpreted. Consequently, the onus is on each cleft team to conceive and develop its own system of outcomes assessment, monitoring, and quality assurance.

OUTCOMES ASSESSMENT IN THE LITERATURE

Cleft lip and palate treatment has been the subject of innumerable studies in the surgical, medical, and allied health literature. Most of the evidence base is level IV and level V evidence—that is, most data derive from case series, experiential reports, and expert opinion. Few papers have been

subjected to the rigors of contemporary clinical trial design or systematic review and metanalysis.

Some outcome data do exist. Perhaps the most complete early report was a 1984 study by Bardach and colleagues[6] describing the long-term esthetic, dental, facial growth, and speech outcomes of 45 patients with unilateral cleft lip and palate. In 1987, the Third International Symposium on Early Treatment of Cleft Lip and Palate initiated a collaborative investigation, in which cephalograms and treatment records from 15 international centers were reviewed to evaluate the effects of individual treatment protocols on facial growth.[7] Attendees from the symposium later developed novel measures for objective comparison of treatment outcomes, such as the Great Ormond Street, London, and Oslo (GOSLON) yardstick for assessing dental arch alignment[8] and a validated instrument for rating nasolabial esthetic results.[9]

In the late 1980s and early 1990s, Eurocleft was founded to study treatment outcomes from 6 European cleft centers.[10–14] The Eurocleft study included Caucasian children with nonsyndromic, complete unilateral cleft lip and palate. Initial outcomes of interest were dental arch alignment, midfacial growth and facial profile, and nasolabial esthetics. Follow-up studies also considered orthognathic outcomes at skeletal maturity, speech, burden of care, and patient satisfaction.[15–20] Results are summarized in **Table 1** but highlighted much disparity in protocols and outcomes between centers. Results of the Eurocleft studies kindled a desire for quality improvement in the cleft-care community at large. With funding from the European Union, a registry of European cleft teams was created. It issued a policy statement that delineated practice guidelines for the treatment of children with clefts and that recommended minimum recordkeeping standards for teams. EUROCRAN was conceived to help organize clinical and genetic research and to foster collaboration.[21,22] Many of the Eurocleft researchers also participated in the World Health Organization's (WHO) development of an international strategy to craniofacial research, bringing Eurocleft's quality-improvement aims to a worldwide audience.[23]

In response to poor outcomes obtained by British centers participating in the Eurocleft studies, the Clinical Standards Advisory Group (CSAG) performed an audit of all 5- and 12-year-old children in the United Kingdom with unilateral cleft lip and palate. Results were poor across all measures (see **Table 1**).[24–27] CSAG proposed specific methods for restructuring the cleft-care-delivery process and created specific service specifications for providers. Based on

Table 1
Selected outcomes from intercenter outcomes studies (see text for relevant citations)

Patient Characteristics					
Cleft Type	Age at Evaluation	No. Enrolled	No. of Centers	Location(s)	Measures Reported
Eurocleft					
cUCLP	8–10	151	6	UK, Sweden, Denmark, Netherlands, Norway	Craniofacial form (cephalometry)
	11–14	131	6		Dental arch relationships (GOSLON)
	12, 17	124	5		Nasolabial appearance (Asher-McDade scale)
					Speech (structured, multilingual)
					Burden of care
					Craniofacial form (cephalometry)
					Dental arch relationships (GOSLON)
					Nasolabial appearance (Asher-McDade scale)
					Patient/parent satisfaction questionnaire
CSAG					
cUCLP	5, 12	457	50	UK	Craniofacial form (cephalometry)
					Dental arch relationships (5-year-old index, GOSLON)
					Success of alveolar bone grafting (modified Bergland)
					Nasolabial appearance (Asher-McDade scale)
					Patient/parent satisfaction questionnaire
					Speech (modifed CAPS)
Americleft					
cUCLP	6–12	172	5	US, Canada	Craniofacial form (cephalometry)
					Dental arch relationships (GOSLON)
					Nasolabial appearance (Asher-McDade scale)
					Speech (pending)
Scandcleft					
cUCLP	5	445	10	Denmark, Sweden, Finland, Norway, UK	Craniofacial form (cephalometry)
					Dental arch relationships (5-year-old index)
					Nasolabial appearance (Asher-McDade scale)
					Speech (structured, multilingual, nasometry)

Abbreviation: cUCLP, complete unilateral cleft lip and palate.

these findings and recommendations, the National Health Service made reorganization of cleft-care services a national priority in 1999, a process that was completed in 2005.[28] A key principle established when cleft services were centralized in the United Kingdom was that results should be routinely collected and assessed. A national database, CRANE, was set up (https://www.crane-database.org.uk/); use of electronic databases in individual units was made the norm, and the Craniofacial Society of Great Britain and Ireland (CFSGBI) set out an agreed minimum dataset for audit. Recently, a follow-up cross-sectional study, Cleft Care UK, was begun to monitor improvement in outcomes of 5-year-old children treated following the reorganization of services.

Inspired by the success of the Eurocleft project, the ACPA convened a taskforce in 2006 to establish a similar multicenter collaborative effort in North America. Named Americleft, the 5 participating centers compared outcomes using existing clinical records and the methodology described in the Eurocleft studies.[29–33] Results are summarized in **Table 1**.

The rich history of collaborative research in cleft care underscores the complexity and considerable difficulty inherent in retrospective comparisons of outcomes from diverse institutions. These studies also demonstrate the great potential of multicenter collaborations. Presently, new collaborations are underway in Scandinavia, Japan, India, Brazil, and Australia. In particular, the 10-center Scandcleft collaborative has progressed beyond retrospective observational studies to use randomized controlled trials for the evaluation of surgical technique, timing of individual interventions, and sequence of interventions (see **Table 1**).[34] The planning and execution of prospective research methods mark a significant advance in cleft research.

CONCEPTUALIZING OUTCOMES IN CLEFT CARE
What to Measure in Cleft Outcomes?

From a *holistic* perspective, the patient should be conceptualized as the center of the health care delivery process (**Fig. 1**). Three principal domains for outcomes are clinical, psychosocial, and systems-based parameters. The *clinical* domain includes aspects common to traditional clinical outcomes studies and includes many subdomains such as general pediatrics (eg, physical and cognitive development), surgery, dental/orthodontic, speech, and audiology. The *psychosocial* domain is arguably equally important and includes aspects related to psychological well-being and social functioning. Some psychosocial elements may be intricately related to traditional clinical outcomes; for example, self-perception of appearance may be related to nasolabial appearance, and academic performance may be related to cognitive development. However, these qualitative elements carry the additional semantic value of "how does this matter to the patient?" missing from traditional

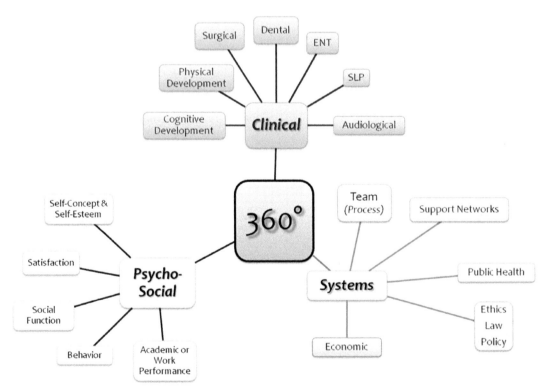

Fig. 1. "Outcomes" viewed from a holistic perspective would conceptualize the patient with cleft lip and palate at the center and at least 3 main domains that directly affect the patient. *Clinical* outcomes include traditional subdomains such as surgery, dental/orthodontics, speech, and audiology. Arguably equally important are *psychosocial* outcomes, which pertain to concepts such as self-esteem, behavior, and social functioning. *Systems*-based outcomes consider economic concepts such as value, team performance, public health, and policy.

quantitative clinical outcomes. A third domain in the conceptualization of outcomes in cleft care is *systems-based parameters*. These elements may pertain to cost, resource allocation, process of care (eg, efficiency), supplemental/ancillary services, and so on and are typically used in value assessments and continuous quality improvement endeavors.

When to Measure Cleft Outcomes?

Compared with many clinical problems, outcomes assessment in cleft care is particularly challenging. First, the child can be considered a "moving target" (**Fig. 2**); that is, treatment of the condition typically requires several sequential steps that include operative and nonoperative interventions delivered over time, all while the child is growing physically, cognitively, and developmentally. The questions then arise: When is the best time to measure an outcome? Is it better to measure outcomes (particularly surgical outcomes) before and after a particular intervention, in the short or long term? Or is it better to look at outcomes at a particular age or developmental stage? Or perhaps at the very end of a treatment protocol?

There is perhaps no single right answer, and arguments can be made for each strategy. Typically, single institutions in their case series tend to look at short- and long-term outcomes surrounding a particular intervention of interest. These types of data tend to generate evidence of efficacy. However, this approach is problematic when attempting to compare results from multiple institutions to generate evidence of effectiveness under different conditions. The Eurocleft collaboration,

for example, highlighted that because of diversity of protocols, it was impossible to look at short- and long-term results of a specific intervention. Therefore, it adopted the approach of looking at the long-term results following an entire treatment protocol, which included numerous interventions. Although a practical and reasonable decision, it was impossible to derive conclusions regarding the effectiveness or relative worth of a treatment, the appropriateness of its timing within the protocol, or of the experiences that the child has during this time frame.

How to Measure Cleft Outcomes?

Every domain and each outcome of interest can be viewed from a different vantage point (**Fig. 3**). Consequently, each outcome of interest may be measured in a different way. For example, nasolabial appearance might be measured quantitatively via direct or indirect anthropometry, semi-quantitatively through expert panel assessment of photographs, or qualitatively by way of a patient-reported outcome measure. It is therefore critical to choose an appropriate and practical method of outcome measurement.

At a minimum, measures should be valid and reliable. Measurement validity ensures accurate conclusions are made regarding superior or

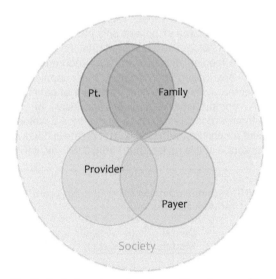

Fig. 3. Each domain and each specific outcome of interest can be viewed from a different vantage point, specifically, from that of the patient, family, clinical care providers, payers, or society as a whole. The perspective(s) chosen will affect which specific outcomes are chosen for assessment and the methods that are used for their assessment (for example, direct quantitative measurement vs qualitative or semi-quantitative patient-reported outcome measures).

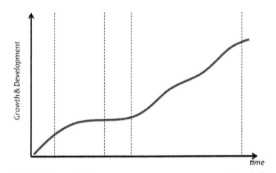

Fig. 2. One challenge to outcomes assessment in cleft care is that the child with cleft lip and palate undergoes several operations and nonsurgical interventions at different stages, all while he is growing and developing physically, cognitively, and psychologically. The question arises: Is it better to measure "outcomes" at a specific biologic age, developmental stage, surrounding an intervention (in the short- or long-term), or at the very end of a treatment protocol?

inferior treatment methods. Reliability allows comparison between different patients, surgeons, or teams and improves the ability to detect differences in outcome. Ideally measures should also be practical to implement, able to discriminate between different outcomes, and consistently adopted.[35]

Nearly all cleft surgery outcome measures contain a subjective component and can be a limiting factor even for well-validated measures. In the research setting, study methodologies are able to minimize potential bias from this subjective component. However, in clinical practice (audits and public reporting), controlling for bias (particularly selection bias, measurement bias, and unblinded assessment) is more difficult.

When deciding which measures to use in your individual practice, the importance of considering complexity for record collection and analysis cannot be underestimated. Measures that are under development or lack validation, or which require patient involvement beyond routine care, should be approached with caution.

Specific Measures

Several national and international groups have published recommendations for a minimum set of treatment records. The Eurocleft investigators and WHO international collaborative made identical recommendations in 2001 (**Table 2**).[21,23] The CFSGBI adapted these recommendations to include measures of patient and parent satisfaction, psychology evaluation, dental health, and general feeding and growth.[36] All recommendations are based on records that should be collected during the routine treatment of patients.

A comprehensive critical appraisal of all outcome measures existing and under development for children with cleft lip and palate is beyond the scope of this review, but **Table 3** lists available validated measures. Other articles in this issue of *Clinics in Plastic Surgery* expound on specific measures useful to a particular purpose.

PERFORMING OUTCOME MEASUREMENT

After considering which outcomes should be included and when they should be measured, a framework should be built to facilitate the systematic collection of records during routine clinical practice. This is challenging, but fortunately, models exist for the routine assessment of treatment outcomes within the framework of team-based cleft care. The North Thames Regional Cleft Centre uses a specially structured "audit clinic" to collect its outcomes. This clinic is distinct from a clinical care appointment, and its sole purpose is to obtain standardized data for subsequent review. Depending on age and cleft type, a patient may require any or all of the following: Great Ormund Street Speech Assessment (GOS.SP.ASS) speech profile with audiovisual recording for subsequent assessment using the Cleft Audit Protocol for Speech-Augmented (CAPS-S)[37]; clinical photographs and dental impressions for esthetics and 5-year index of facial growth[38]; dental health assessment with the Decayed, Missing, Filled, and Treated (DMFT) index; audiology; psychology; height and weight. The audit review is conducted by the team at a later date, which allows each clinician time to analyze any outcomes between the audit clinic and the review. An important guiding principle is that a surgeon *other than the original operating surgeon* leads the review for a particular child. The team can then highlight any technical issues of the repair, discuss any outstanding issues or learning points, and make a management plan. If specific concerns arise, a normal clinic appointment is booked soon after the review.

Table 2
WHO recommendations for minimum record collection and timing, complete cleft lip, and palate (see text for relevant citation)

Timing	Dental Models	Lateral Skull Radiograph	Photographs	Speech/ Tympanometry	Audiometry	Patient/Parent Satisfaction
Primary surgery	X		X			
3 y				X	X	
5/6 y	X		X	X	X	
10 y	X	X	X	X	X	
18+ y	X	X	X	X		X

From World Health Organization. Global strategies to reduce the health-care burden of craniofacial anomalies: report of WHO meetings on International Collaborative Research on Craniofacial Anomalies, Geneva, Switzerland, 5–8 November 2000 ; Park City, Utah, USA 24–26 May 2001. Geneva: World Health Organization, 2002; with permission.

Table 3
Selected measures for evaluating treatment outcomes (see text for relevant citations)

Type	Measure
Aesthetic	
Passive	Asher-McDade
Active	
Craniofacial form	Cephalometrics
Dental arch relations	GOSLON
	5-year-old index
	Eurocran index
	Bilateral index
Speech	CAPS-A
	Universal parameters (Speech Parameters Group)
	Nasometry
Dental	DMFS/Dmfs
Oral health	Child Oral Health Impact Profile (COHIP) (under development)
Audiometry	
Psychosocial	Peds-QL
	Child Health Questionnaire (CHQ)
	Child Oral Health Quality of Life (COHQOL)
	Youth Quality of Life-Facial Differences (YQOLFD)
	CLEFT-Q (under development)
Comprehensive	CLP-360° (under development)

Collated patient data are then presented at an annual meeting with 2 other Cleft Centers. All of the UK Cleft centers are a part of a tricenter or quad-center group. The focus of these meetings is on presenting, discussing, and improving patient outcomes. Finally, certain aspects of the data are submitted for national comparison at the annual meeting of the CFSGBI.

SUMMARY AND FUTURE DIRECTIONS ON OUTCOMES MEASUREMENT

Outcome measurement is an essential component of cleft care that is critical to improving quality and value. Surgeons should lead the way in developing systems for comprehensive appraisal of cleft care—for accountability, quality improvement, and health system design. The system should include systematic methodology built on a sound conceptual framework. Future research should include both development of novel validated measures and effective systems for application of outcome measurement in routine practice, standardization of monitoring methods, and development of automated systems that permit realtime data analysis ("learning health care").

REFERENCES

1. IOM (Institute of Medicine). Best care at lower cost: the path to continuously learning health care in America. Washington, DC: The National Academies Press; 2012.
2. American Board of Medical Specialties. MOC competencies and criteria. 2012. Available at: http://www.abms.org/Maintenance_of_Certification/MOC_competencies.aspx. Accessed June 21, 2013.
3. Phurrough S, Salive ME, Brechner RJ, et al. In: Centers for Medicare & Medicaid Services (CMS), editor. Coverage decision memorandum for bariatric surgery for treatment of co-morbidities associated with morbid obesity. Centers for Medicare & Medicaid Services (CMS); 2006. Available at: http://www.cms.gov/medicare-coverage-database/details/nca-decision-memo.aspx?NCAId=160&ver=32&NcaName=Bariatric+Surgery+for+the+Treatment+of+Morbid+Obesity+(1st+Recon)&bc=BEAAAAAAEAgA&%5D.
4. American Cleft Palate - Craniofacial Association. Standards for Approval of Cleft Palate and Craniofacial Teams. American Cleft Palate - Craniofacial Association. 2010. Available at: http://www.acpa-cpf.org/team_care/standards. Accessed March 31, 2010; June 21, 2013.
5. National Health Service. Cleft lip and palate services: clinical service specification. 2010. Available at: http://www.specialisedservices.nhs.uk/library/37/Cleft_Lip__Palate___Appendix_6.pdf. Accessed June 21, 2013.
6. Bardach J, Morris H, Olin W, et al. Late results of multidisciplinary management of unilateral cleft lip and palate. Ann Plast Surg 1984;12(3):235–42.
7. Ross RB. Treatment variables affecting facial growth in complete unilateral cleft lip and palate. Cleft Palate J 1987;24(1):5–77.
8. Mars M, Plint DA, Houston WJ, et al. The Goslon Yardstick: a new system of assessing dental arch relationships in children with unilateral clefts of the lip and palate. Cleft Palate J 1987;24(4):314–22.
9. Asher-McDade C, Roberts C, Shaw WC, et al. Development of a method for rating nasolabial appearance in patients with clefts of the lip and palate. Cleft Palate Craniofac J 1991;28(4):385–90 [discussion: 390–1].
10. Asher-McDade C, Brattstrom V, Dahl E, et al. A six-center international study of treatment outcome in patients with clefts of the lip and palate: part 4. Assessment of nasolabial appearance. Cleft Palate Craniofac J 1992;29(5):409–12.

11. Mars M, Asher-McDade C, Brattstrom V, et al. A six-center international study of treatment outcome in patients with clefts of the lip and palate: part 3. Dental arch relationships. Cleft Palate Craniofac J 1992;29(5):405–8.

12. Molsted K, Asher-McDade C, Brattstrom V, et al. A six-center international study of treatment outcome in patients with clefts of the lip and palate: part 2. Craniofacial form and soft tissue profile. Cleft Palate Craniofac J 1992;29:398–404.

13. Shaw WC, Asher-McDade C, Brattstrom V, et al. A six-center international study of treatment outcome in patients with clefts of the lip and palate: part 1. Principles and study design. Cleft Palate Craniofac J 1992;29(5):393–7.

14. Shaw WC, Dahl E, Asher-McDade C, et al. A six-center international study of treatment outcome in patients with clefts of the lip and palate: part 5. General discussion and conclusions. Cleft Palate Craniofac J 1992;29(5):413–8.

15. Semb G, Brattstrom V, Molsted K, et al. The Eurocleft study: intercenter study of treatment outcome in patients with complete cleft lip and palate. Part 1: introduction and treatment experience. Cleft Palate Craniofac J 2005;42(1):64–8.

16. Brattstrom V, Molsted K, Prahl-Andersen B, et al. The Eurocleft study: intercenter study of treatment outcome in patients with complete cleft lip and palate. Part 2: craniofacial form and nasolabial appearance. Cleft Palate Craniofac J 2005;42(1):69–77.

17. Molsted K, Brattstrom V, Prahl-Andersen B, et al. The Eurocleft study: intercenter study of treatment outcome in patients with complete cleft lip and palate. Part 3: dental arch relationships. Cleft Palate Craniofac J 2005;42(1):78–82.

18. Semb G, Brattstrom V, Molsted K, et al. The Eurocleft study: intercenter study of treatment outcome in patients with complete cleft lip and palate. Part 4: relationship among treatment outcome, patient/parent satisfaction, and the burden of care. Cleft Palate Craniofac J 2005;42(1):83–92.

19. Shaw WC, Brattstrom V, Molsted K, et al. The Eurocleft study: intercenter study of treatment outcome in patients with complete cleft lip and palate. Part 5: discussion and conclusions. Cleft Palate Craniofac J 2005;42(1):93–8.

20. Grunwell P, Brondsted K, Henningsson G, et al. A six-centre international study of the outcome of treatment in patients with clefts of the lip and palate: the results of a cross-linguistic investigation of cleft palate speech. Scand J Plast Reconstr Surg Hand Surg 2000;34(3):219–29.

21. Shaw WC, Semb G, Nelson P, et al. The Eurocleft project 1996-2000: overview. J Craniomaxillofac Surg 2001;29(3):131–40 [discussion 141–2].

22. The EUROCRAN Project. 2013. Available at: http://www.eurocran.org/content.asp?contentID=1&sid=132836. Accessed June 21, 2013.

23. Global strategies to reduce the health care burden of craniofacial anomalies: report of WHO meetings on international collaborative research on craniofacial anomalies. Cleft Palate Craniofac J 2004;41(3):238–43.

24. Bearn D, Mildinhall S, Murphy T, et al. Cleft lip and palate care in the United Kingdom–the Clinical Standards Advisory Group (CSAG) Study. Part 4: outcome comparisons, training, and conclusions. Cleft Palate Craniofac J 2001;38(1):38–43.

25. Sandy JR, Williams AC, Bearn D, et al. Cleft lip and palate care in the United Kingdom–the Clinical Standards Advisory Group (CSAG) Study. Part 1: background and methodology. Cleft Palate Craniofac J 2001;38(1):20–3.

26. Sell D, Grunwell P, Mildinhall S, et al. Cleft lip and palate care in the United Kingdom–the Clinical Standards Advisory Group (CSAG) Study. Part 3: speech outcomes. Cleft Palate Craniofac J 2001;38(1):30–7.

27. Williams AC, Bearn D, Mildinhall S, et al. Cleft lip and palate care in the United Kingdom–the Clinical Standards Advisory Group (CSAG) Study. Part 2: dentofacial outcomes and patient satisfaction. Cleft Palate Craniofac J 2001;38(1):24–9.

28. Currie G, Starr T, White L, et al. In: N.I.f.H.R.S.D.a.O. Programme, editor. Comparative evaluation of children's services networks: analysing professional, organisational and sector boundaries in Paediatric Nephrology, Children's Safeguarding and Cleft Lip and Palate Networks. London: Queen's Printer and Controller of HMSO; 2010. Available at: http://www.nets.nihr.ac.uk/__data/assets/pdf_file/0016/64321/FR-08-1718-149.pdf.

29. Daskalogiannakis J, Mercado A, Russell K, et al. The Americleft study: an inter-center study of treatment outcomes for patients with unilateral cleft lip and palate part 3. Analysis of craniofacial form. Cleft Palate Craniofac J 2011;48:252–8.

30. Hathaway R, Daskalogiannakis J, Mercado A, et al. The Americleft study: an inter-center study of treatment outcomes for patients with unilateral cleft lip and palate part 2. Dental arch relationships. Cleft Palate Craniofac J 2011;48(3):244–51.

31. Long RE Jr, Hathaway R, Daskalogiannakis J, et al. The Americleft study: an inter-center study of treatment outcomes for patients with unilateral cleft lip and palate part 1. Principles and study design. Cleft Palate Craniofac J 2011;48:239–43.

32. Mercado A, Russell K, Hathaway R, et al. The Americleft study: an inter-center study of treatment outcomes for patients with unilateral cleft lip and palate part 4. Nasolabial aesthetics. Cleft Palate Craniofac J 2011;48(3):259–64.

33. Russell K, Long RE Jr, Hathaway R, et al. The Americleft study: an inter-center study of treatment outcomes for patients with unilateral cleft lip and palate part 5. General discussion and conclusions. Cleft Palate Craniofac J 2011;48:265–70.

34. Semb G, Enemark H, Friede H, et al. Scandcleft randomized trials: overview of the project, in 12th International Congress on Cleft Lip/Palate and Related Craniofacial Anomalies. Lake Buena Vista, May 8, 2013.

35. Love R, Walters M, Southall P, et al. Dental arch relationship outcomes in children with complete unilateral cleft lip and palate treated at Princess Margaret Hospital for Children, Perth, Western Australia. Cleft Palate Craniofac J 2012;49(4):456–62.

36. Craniofacial Society of Great Britain and Ireland. Recommendations for minimum records for cleft audit. 2005. Available at: http://www.craniofacialsociety.org.uk/info/audit.html. Accessed April 14, 2005; June 21, 2013.

37. John A, Sell D, Sweeney T, et al. The cleft audit protocol for speech-augmented: a validated and reliable measure for auditing cleft speech. Cleft Palate Craniofac J 2006;43(3):272–88.

38. Atack NE, Hathorn IS, Semb G, et al. A new index for assessing surgical outcome in unilateral cleft lip and palate subjects aged five: reproducibility and validity. Cleft Palate Craniofac J 1997;34(3):242–6.

Index

Note: Page numbers of article titles are in **boldface** type.

Clin Plastic Surg 41 (2014) 321–323
http://dx.doi.org/10.1016/S0094-1298(14)00013-3
0094-1298/14/$ – see front matter © 2014 Elsevier Inc. All rights reserved.

plasticsurgery.theclinics.com

Moving?

Make sure your subscription moves with you!

To notify us of your new address, find your **Clinics Account Number** (located on your mailing label above your name), and contact customer service at:

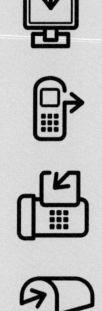

Email: journalscustomerservice-usa@elsevier.com

800-654-2452 (subscribers in the U.S. & Canada)
314-447-8871 (subscribers outside of the U.S. & Canada)

Fax number: 314-447-8029

Elsevier Health Sciences Division
Subscription Customer Service
3251 Riverport Lane
Maryland Heights, MO 63043

*To ensure uninterrupted delivery of your subscription, please notify us at least 4 weeks in advance of move.

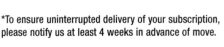

Printed and bound by CPI Group (UK) Ltd, Croydon, CR0 4YY

03/10/2024

01040382-0016